CMOS

Nanoelectronics

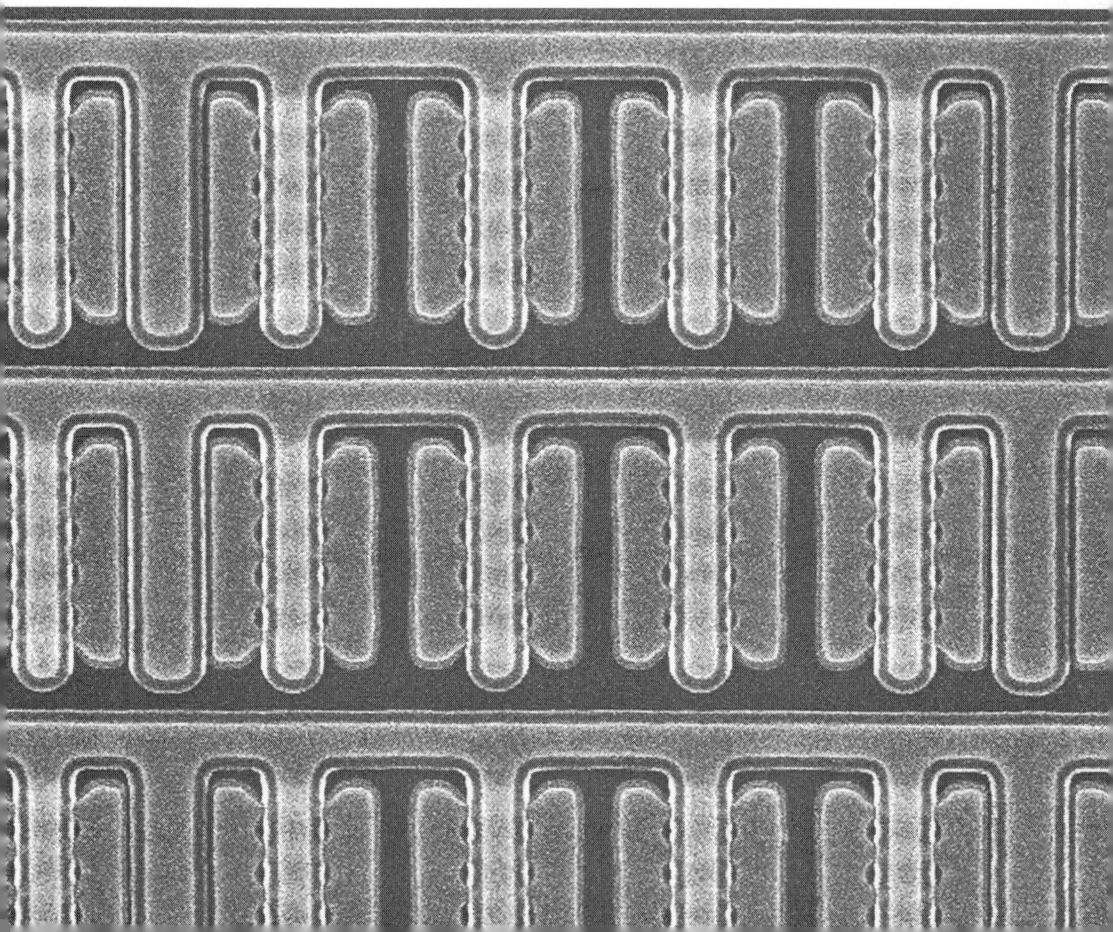

CMOS Nanoelectronics

INNOVATIVE DEVICES, ARCHITECTURES, AND APPLICATIONS

edited by
Nadine Collaert

PAN STANFORD PUBLISHING

Published by

Pan Stanford Publishing Pte. Ltd.
Penthouse Level, Suntec Tower 3
8 Temasek Boulevard
Singapore 038988

Email: editorial@panstanford.com
Web: www.panstanford.com

British Library Cataloguing-in-Publication Data
A catalogue record for this book is available from the British Library.

CMOS Nanoelectronics: Innovative Devices, Architectures, and Applications

ISBN 978-981-4364-02-7 (Hardcover)
ISBN 978-981-4364-03-4 (eBook)

Printed in the USA

Contents

Preface

In 1965, Gordon Moore published his legendary paper "Cramming more components onto integrated circuits." In this paper, he described that the number of components in integrated circuits had doubled every year since the invention of the integrated circuit in 1958 until 1965 and that this trend would continue for at least 10 more years. Now, almost five decades later, industry is still following Moore's law, even though its end has been predicted on many occasions and even by Moore himself.

Indeed, one needs to point out that since the development of the 130 nm technology node, it has become more and more difficult to scale down the traditional MOSFET structure in order to keep up with the pace of Moore's law. Especially in the last decade, many innovations such as high-k/metal gate and strain engineering have been introduced to ensure the required performance improvement with every new technology node. However, these material innovations are not enough to control the ever-increasing off-state leakage problem in these advanced devices. New device architectures such as multi-gate devices have emerged as a means to solve this issue by increasing the gate control through geometry. Although proposed already in the beginning of the 1980s, multi-gate devices (Delta FET, FinFET, tri-gate, etc.) and more generally fully depleted transistors have long been considered the exotic devices that somehow were no real contenders to replace the planar bulk MOSFET. With Intel's announcement to introduce the tri-gate architecture on bulk substrates at the 22 nm technology node, a new era of MOSFET scaling arrived. It is expected that more companies will follow and introduce multi-gate devices at future technology nodes.

This book tries to give the reader an insight into the theory, technology, and circuit aspects of FinFET-based multi-gate transistors. It also goes one step further and extends the scope to nanowires and derived device architectures such as the junctionless nanowire FET. Further, some of the chapters discuss the new characterization and mathematical tools to predict the behavior of nanoscale structures.

As such, the book is divided into three main parts with a total of 11 chapters, each written by experts in the field:

Part I: Integration of Multi-Gate Devices (FinFET)

Chapter 1, "Introduction to Multi-Gate Devices and Integration Challenges," by Nadine Collaert, gives an overall introduction to multi-gate devices. It briefly reviews the history of multi-gate devices and discusses their specific advantages over standard bulk devices. Although the integration of these devices is very similar to their planar counterparts, a number of integration challenges are highlighted in this chapter.

Chapter 2, "Dry Etching Patterning Requirements for Multi-Gate Devices," by Efraín Altamirano-Sánchez, Tom Vandeweyer, Marc Demand, and Werner Boullart, describes the challenges of patterning high-density FinFET devices for the 22 nm technology node and beyond. Apart from the 193 nm lithography-based fin patterning, the use of full-field extreme ultraviolet (EUV) lithography is addressed in this chapter.

Chapter 3, "High-k Dielectrics and Metal Gate Electrodes on SOI MuGFETs," by Isabelle Ferain, covers the processing of high-k dielectrics/metal gate electrodes on fully depleted SOI MuGFETs or finFETs. In the second section of this chapter, several methods used for controlling and tuning the work function in MuGFETs with metal gates are described.

Chapter 4, "Doping, Contact and Strain Architectures for Highly Scaled finFETs" by Rob Lander, tackles one of the most important integration challenges of FinFET-based devices and thin Si film devices: reduction of the parasitic source/drain resistance. Next to that, more insight is given into strain engineering techniques in multi-gate devices.

Part II: Circuit-Related Aspects

Chapter 5, "Variability and Its Implications for FinFET SRAM," by Emanuele Baravelli, Luca De Marchi, and Nicolò Speciale, discusses physical-level models for fin and gate line-edge roughness (LER) that can be applied to estimate their impact on the FinFET electrical performance. Six-transistor (6T) SRAM is used as a benchmark to evaluate the impact of line-edge roughness at the circuit level.

Chapter 6, "Specific Features of MuGFETs at High Temperatures over a Wide Frequency Range," by Valeriya Kilchytska, Jean-Pierre Raskin, and Denis Flandre, focuses on the high-temperature behavior of SOI-based FinFET devices with a specific focus on analog and RF applications. Although FinFETs show excellent short-channel behavior, it is not clear if they maintain their performance advantages at high temperatures. Some particular features of the high-temperature behavior of advanced FinFETs are highlighted in this chapter.

Chapter 7, "ESD Protection in FinFET Technology," by Steven Thijs, deals with the Electro-Static Discharge (ESD) robustness of multi-gate architectures. Especially, the early FinFET devices showed very low ESD robustness, which demonstrated the need of considering ESD already in a very early technology development phase. The impact of the different geometrical parameters and technology options is the focus of this chapter.

Part III: Exploratory Devices and Characterization Tools

Chapter 8, "The Junctionless Nanowire Transistor" by Bart Sorée, Ahn-Tuan Pham, Dries Sels, and Wim Magnus, introduces the junctionless nanowire transistor as an alternative device concept to the inversion mode nanowire MOSFET. An analytical model is used to describe the basic working principle. Furthermore, the impact of scaling down both the wire radius and the gate length is addressed in this chapter. Finally, an advanced transport model is used to investigate the impact of strain on the short-channel junctionless nanowire FET.

Chapter 9, "The Variational Principle: A Valuable Ally Assisting the Self-Consistent Solution of Poisson's Equation and Semi-Classical Transport Equations," by Wim Magnus, Hamilton Carrillo-Nuñez, and Bart Sorée, attempts to give the reader some insight into the increasing mathematical complexity that is encountered when nanoscale devices are to be modeled with acceptable accuracy. Specifically, the variational principle is explored as a numerical tool to self-consistently solve Poisson's equation and a set of semi-classical transport equations to describe transport in nanoscale structures.

Chapter 10, "New Tools for the Direct Characterisation of FinFETs," by G. C. Tettamanzi, A. Paul, S. Lee, G. Klimeck, and S. Rogge, discusses how classical transport theories such as the thermionic emission in combination with state-of-the-art tight binding simulations can be used as a powerful tool for the study of the complex transport mechanisms in FinFETs.

Chapter 11: "Dopant Metrology in Advanced FinFETs," by G. Lansbergen, R. Rahman, G. C. Tettamanzi, J. Verduijn, L. C. L. Hollenberg, G. Klimeck, and S. Rogge, describes a new approach to atomistic impurity metrology. The method offers opportunities for non-invasive characterization down to the level of a single donor and could be a future tool in the guidance of device processing.

Finally, I would like to thank all the authors for making this book a diverse yet comprehensive text in which different aspects of nanoscale devices are addressed. Many thanks as well to everyone who indirectly contributed to this work. In particular, I would like to thank my husband, Gunther, and my children, Michiel and Karen, for their continuous support.

Nadine Collaert
July 2012

Part I

Integration of Multi-Gate Devices (FinFET)

Chapter 1

Introduction to Multi-Gate Devices and Integration Challenges

Nadine Collaert
IMEC, Kapeldreef 75, 3001 Heverlee, Belgium
collaert@imec.be

1.1 Introduction

In May 2011 Intel announced the introduction of the tri-gate architecture at the 22 nm technology node [1]. As such, Intel was the first big player in the semiconductor industry to use a 3D device, going from a pure 2D structure that had been introduced in 1960 [2] and that had basically not changed much during almost five decades of scaling to a new device architecture that was still a MOSFET but with some new complexities and advantages: in this architecture the gate is wrapped around a thin conducting channel, also called "fin."

Tri-gate or multi-gate devices (MuGFET) in general have been the subject of much research, especially over the last 10 years. Until Intel's announcement there was still a big debate at what technology node and, if ever, they would be introduced.

CMOS Nanoelectronics: Innovative Devices, Architectures, and Applications
Edited by Nadine Collaert

ISBN 978-981-4364-02-7 (Hardcover), 978-981-4364-03-4 (eBook)
www.panstanford.com

The first double-gate device, called XMOS, was proposed by the Electrotechnical Laboratory (ETL) under the Agency for Industrial Science and Technology (former AIST) in 1984 [3]. The paper demonstrated that significant reduction of short-channel effects (SCE) can be achieved by considering a fully depleted channel with more than one gate. By the end of the 1980s more publications had appeared introducing different multi-gate architectures, amongst them the Gate-All-Around (GAA) transistor [4] and the DELTA FET [5]. However, although most structures demonstrated superior electrostatics as compared to the standard bulk devices, it never came to a real breakthrough at that time.

The renewed interest was triggered by a publication at the International Electron Devices Meeting (IEDM) 1998 [6]. Although the device architecture, called FinFET (Fin Field Effect Transistor), was pretty much the same as in [5], it came at a time when CMOS scaling started to become much more challenging. The era of "happy scaling" was over: with the 90 nm technology node, leakage reduction started to become extremely challenging. So the time was right to put this device architecture in the picture again.

Many different flavors of FinFETs have been proposed over the last decade and typically they can be classified in terms of number of gates or channels and fin aspect ratio: pi-gate [7], omega gate [8] and tri-gate [9].

An overview of the most important multi-gate architectures, based on the FinFET concept, is shown and compared in Fig. 1.1. The figure shows device architectures fabricated on silicon-on-insulator (SOI) substrates; however, as we will see later, standard bulk substrates can be used as well to realize these devices. In the remainder of the chapter, we will also refer to the FinFET-based multi-gate devices as MuGFETs.

Next to FinFETs and vertical transistors [10], which can be seen as GAA, planar double-gate structures have been proposed: the silicon-on-nothing (SON) architecture [11] and the use of wafer bonding [12]. A quasi double-gate device that has gained a lot of interest lately is the ultra-thin buried oxide (UTBOX) fully depleted silicon-on-insulator (FDSOI). The BOX, scaled down to 10 nm and

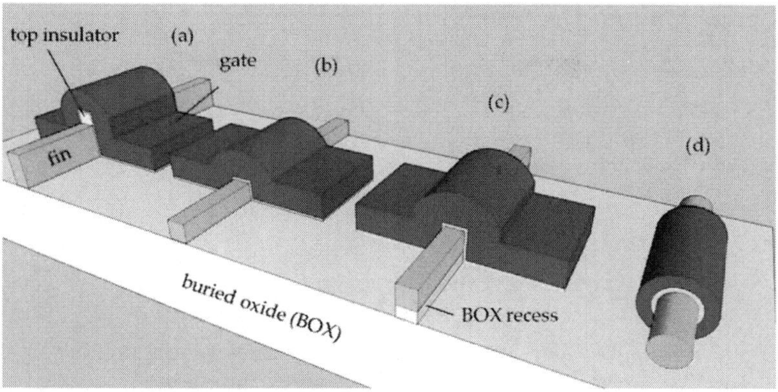

Figure 1.1. Comparison of different device architectures, the devices are schematically presented after gate patterning: (a) the originally proposed FinFET was a double-gate device, having a thick insulator on the top channel, (b) tri-gate device as proposed by Intel with a 1:1 fin aspect ratio, (c) a pi-gate device, where the recess in the buried oxide or STI allows to create a quasi fourth gate; (d) a horizontal gate-all-around nanowire.

even below, allows back gate biasing with low voltages for tuning the device performance [13].

1.2 It Is All in the Lambda...

Why are these multi-gate devices so interesting? As already mentioned in Section 1.1, until the 90 nm technology node, CMOS scaling was pretty straightforward. It was mostly lithography driven, where with every new technology node the dimensions of the MOSFET were scaled down with a factor α and the voltages with a factor k. This is known as the "constant field" scaling and was first proposed by Dennard *et al.* in 1974 [14]. Gate oxide scaling, by far the most important way of boosting the device performance, reached its limit at the 90 nm technology node and material innovations like high-k/metal gates and mobility enhancement techniques were introduced. However, it was clear that it would become more and more difficult to keep the SCE like drain-induced barrier lowering (DIBL) and the degradation of the sub-threshold swing under control in a standard planar bulk device

1.2.1 *Where do These Short-Channel Effects Come From?*

The ideal MOSFET behavior is disturbed by the presence of the source and drain areas. For long channel devices, the impact is small and the threshold voltage V_T, off-state leakage I_{OFF} and the sub-threshold swing S are well defined and independent of the gate length and drain bias. As the channel length is scaled down, the shorter distance between source and drain will lower the potential barrier and make it dependent on the drain bias V_{DS}. A large barrier is mandatory in order to prevent the carriers from flowing to the drain when the transistor is switched off, i.e., when the gate voltage is (in absolute value) lower than $|V_T|$. This is shown in Fig. 1.2.

As a consequence V_T shows a typical roll-off behavior and DIBL increases. The latter is a measure for the V_{DS} dependency of the V_T and is defined as DIBL $= (V_T(V_{D2}) - V_T(V_{D1}))/(V_{D2} - V_{D1})$ with $V_{D1} < V_{D2}$. The latter is the case for an nMOS. Ideally the DIBL should be as low as possible because any reduction in V_T leads to increasing I_{OFF} and S (Fig. 1.3).

Multi-gate devices in general have more than one gate and allow increasing the gate control and thus the vertical electric field, thereby reducing the lateral field and the off-state leakage. In order to explain this, we will use the characteristic length lambda λ as a

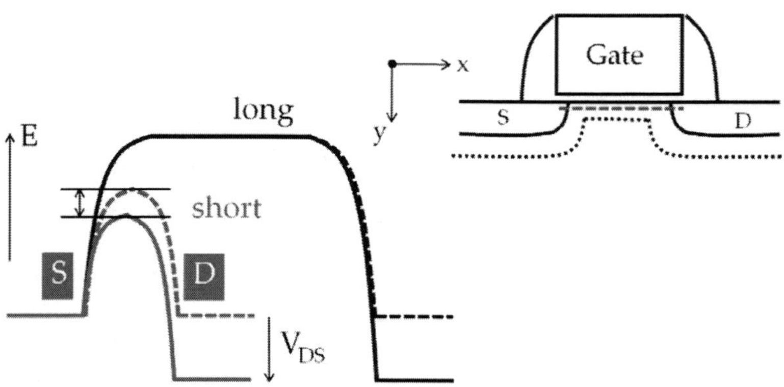

Figure 1.2. Schematic presentation of the impact of the drain bias on the potential barrier of a long channel device and a short-channel device; the potential is taken at the interface between the channel and the gate dielectric, S = source and D = drain.

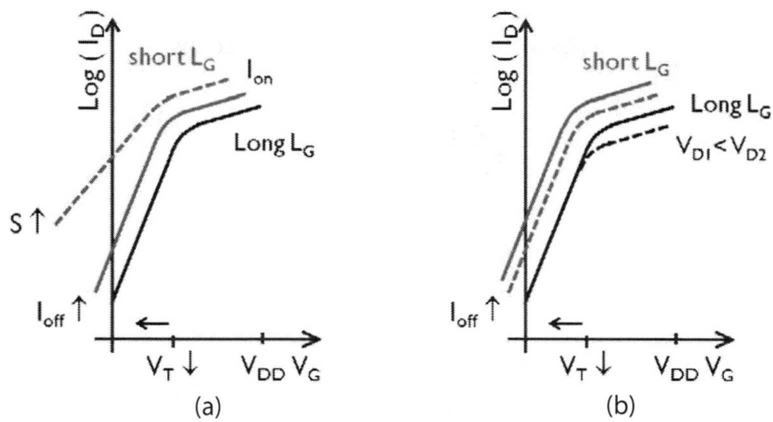

Figure 1.3. $I_{DS}-V_{GS}$ characteristics showing the impact of (a) L_G scaling and (b) the V_{DS} impact on the characteristics of short-channel devices (red curves). See also Color Insert.

figure of merit to compare different device architectures. The 3D Poisson equation is the fundamental electrostatic equation that can be used to derive the channel potential in semiconductor devices. It is usually simplified to its 2D form (Eq. 1.1).

$$\frac{\partial^2 \psi}{\partial x^2} + \frac{\partial^2 \psi}{\partial y^2} = \frac{-\rho}{\varepsilon} \tag{1.1}$$

where Ψ represents the 2D electrical potential in the channel, ρ the total charge and ε the dielectric constant of the semiconductor used in the channel.

Many quasi 2D expressions of Ψ can be found in literature, amongst them the equation that can be found below (Eq. 1.2):

$$\psi(x, y) = \psi_o(y) + (V_{bi} + V_{DS} - \psi_o(y)) \frac{\sinh\left(\frac{x}{\lambda}\right)}{\sinh\left(\frac{L_G}{\lambda}\right)} + (V_{bi} - \psi_o(y)) \frac{\sinh\left(\frac{L_G - x}{\lambda}\right)}{\sinh\left(\frac{L_G}{\lambda}\right)} \tag{1.2}$$

where Ψ_o is the long channel surface potential, V_{bi} the built-in potential, V_{DS} the drain bias, x is the position along the channel and L_G the gate length.

An important parameter in this equation is the characteristic length λ which represents the steepness or fall-off of the potential

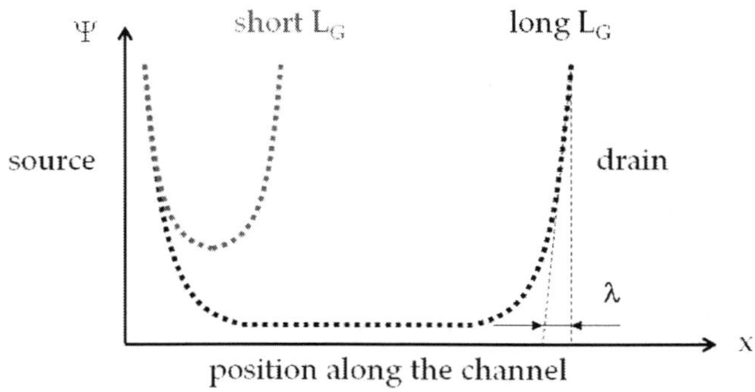

Figure 1.4. Surface potential as a function of a position x along the channel; the characteristic or natural length λ is indicated. See also Color Insert.

as shown in Fig. 1.4. A smaller λ will give rise to a steeper potential and thus lower SCE. As a rule of thumb $L \gg 2\lambda$ is needed to keep SCE under control.

Parameter λ results from the boundary conditions and is different for different device architectures (Table 1.1).

Table 1.1 clearly shows that SCE in planar devices can be reduced by either increasing the channel doping N_{SUB} (through X_{dep}) or reducing the gate dielectric thickness. Introduction of higher k

Table 1.1. Comparison of the characteristic length for various architectures; t_{ox} = gate dielectric thickness, ε_{ox} = permittivity of the gate dielectric, ε_{Si} = permittivity of the semiconductor (in this case Si), X_{dep} = maximum depletion depth and t_{Si} = Si film thickness.

Device architecture	Characteristic length λ
Planar bulk	$\lambda = \sqrt{\frac{\varepsilon_{Si}}{\varepsilon_{ox}} t_{ox} X_{dep}}$
FDSOI	$\lambda = \sqrt{\frac{\varepsilon_{Si}}{\varepsilon_{ox}} t_{ox} t_{Si}}$
Double gate	$\lambda = \sqrt{\frac{\varepsilon_{Si}}{2\varepsilon_{ox}} t_{ox} t_{Si}}$
Tri-gate	$\lambda \approx \sqrt{\frac{\varepsilon_{Si}}{3\varepsilon_{ox}} t_{ox} t_{Si}}$
Gate-all-around of quadruple gate	$\lambda \approx \sqrt{\frac{\varepsilon_{Si}}{4\varepsilon_{ox}} t_{ox} t_{Si}}$
Cylindrical gate-all-around	$\lambda = \sqrt{\frac{2\varepsilon_{Si} t_{Si}^2 \ln\left(1 + \frac{2t_{ox}}{t_{Si}}\right) + \varepsilon_{ox} t_{Si}^2}{16\varepsilon_{ox}}}$

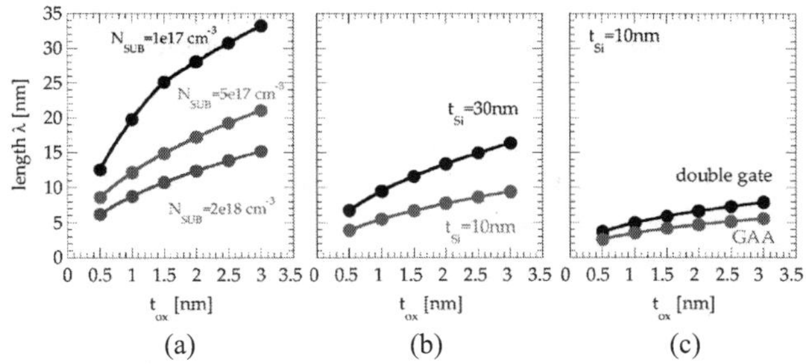

Figure 1.5. The characteristic or natural length λ is shown as function of the gate oxide thickness; in this case SiO_2 ($\varepsilon_r = 3.9$) has been assumed; (a) planar devices with different channel doping N_{SUB}, (b) FDSOI with different Si film thickness t_{Si}, (c) double-gate and GAA devices are compared. See also Color Insert.

materials like HfO_2 as gate dielectric will also be beneficial since by increasing the dielectric permittivity ε_r, λ will be decreased. The depletion depth in fully depleted devices like FDSOI, double-gate, Gate-All-Around (GAA) is defined by the Si film thickness t_{Si} or fin width W_{FIN}, as such, the natural length can be reduced significantly as is shown in Fig. 1.5.

It is clear from Fig. 1.5 that t_{Si} and t_{ox} are interchangeable: going to thin-film devices will relax the scaling requirement for the gate dielectric and vice versa. The additional benefit of going from double gate devices to Tri-gate and GAA might seem small, but one needs to realize that these device architectures will be finally considered for the sub 22 nm technology nodes where every nm counts.

Apart from the natural length other figures of merit like the electrostatic integrity EI [15] have been proposed to compare architectures and provide guidelines for device design. As a rule of thumb, typically the minimum gate length for a FinFET device needs to fulfill $L_{gmin} \geq 1.5\ W_{FIN}$ in order to have a good electrostatic control and reduce the SCE.

1.3 SOI MuGFET Versus Bulk MuGFET

A typical single fin SOI MuGFET is shown in Fig. 1.6. All relevant device dimensions are indicated. Increase of the total transistor width is usually done by patterning several fins in parallel.

FinFET-based multi-gate devices can be fabricated on SOI substrates but also on standard bulk substrates. This architecture was first proposed in 2003 [16]. Bulk FinFET uses a fabrication scheme very close to standard bulk processing. After the Shallow-Trench-Isolation (STI), the STI oxide is recessed in order to define the fin height H_{FIN} as is shown in Fig. 1.7. During active area patterning, hard mask (HM) and resist trimming are typically used

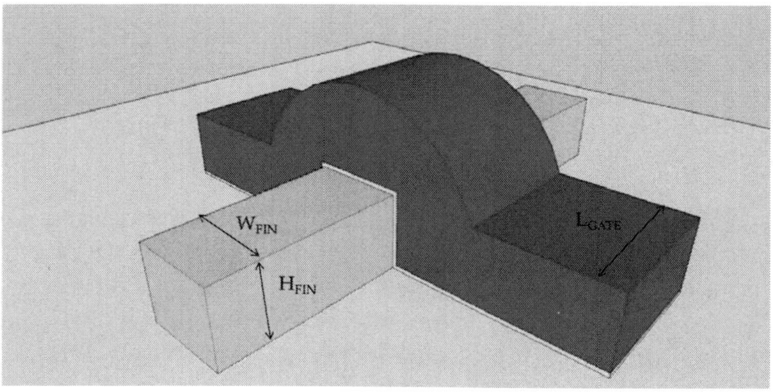

Figure 1.6. Schematic presentation of a single fin SOI MuGFET; the fin width W_{FIN}, fin height H_{FIN}, fin pitch and gate length L_{GATE} have been indicated.

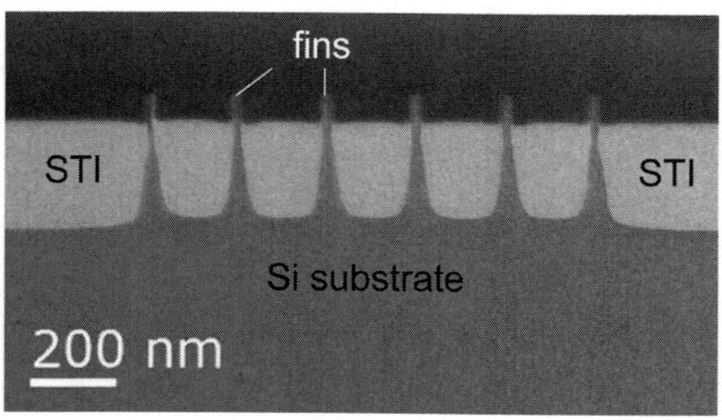

Figure 1.7. Cross section TEM showing a bulk FinFET device with six fins in parallel; the recessed STI in between the fins is visible thereby defining the fin height H_{FIN} [17].

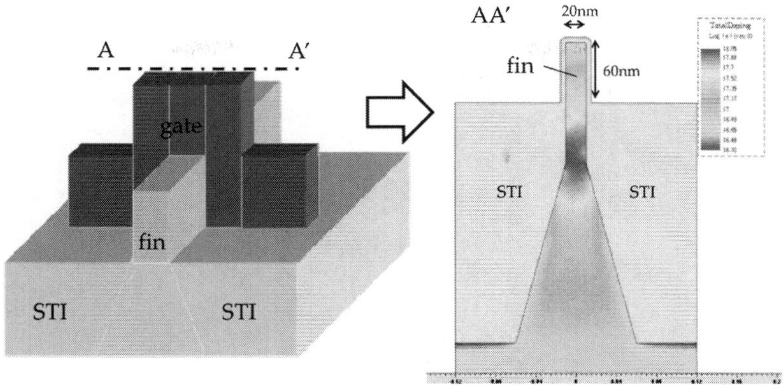

Figure 1.8. Schematic presentation of a bulk FinFET device indicating the fin/channel implantation profile; the implantation profile was obtained by TCAD process simulations [20]; in the cross section, the gate stack has been omitted. See also Color Insert.

to define the narrow fins. Well and ground plane (GP) implantations are used to reduce the leakage between transistors and between fins (Fig. 1.8). After gate stack deposition, the gate is patterned in such a way that it is wrapped around the top part of the active area.

The overall advantage of bulk FinFET is the lower cost of the substrate and the easy co-integration with standard planar bulk CMOS. The multi-gate architecture that will be used in Intel's 22 nm technology node is a bulk tri-gate device. Many other companies [18, 19] are actively looking into bulk FinFET for future technology nodes.

Finally, one needs to point out that Hisamoto's DELTA FET [5] was fabricated on a standard bulk substrate. However, local oxidation was used to finally isolate the channel from the underlying substrate.

1.4 A Typical MuGFET Process Flow

Figure 1.9 shows a schematic presentation of a MuGFET flow. For completeness, both the SOI and bulk MuGFET flows are shown. Apart from the fin patterning and channel implantations, both flows are identical from the gate patterning steps on. The figure

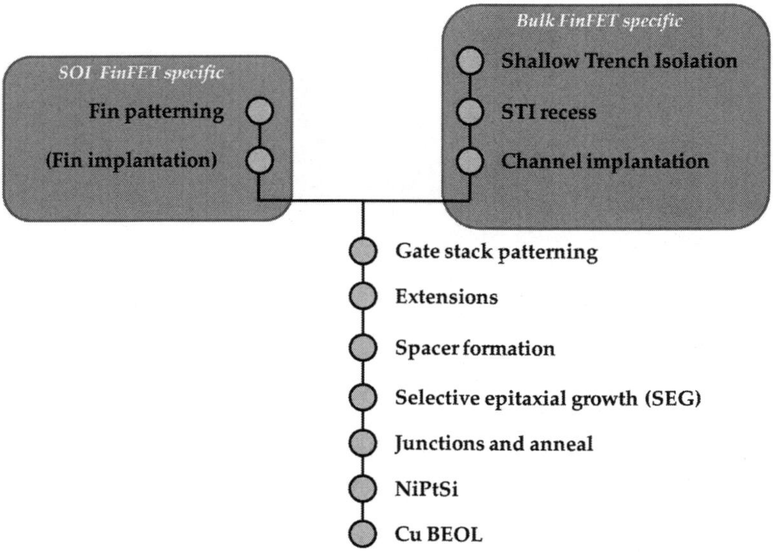

Figure 1.9. Schematic presentation of a MuGFET flow. Comparison between the SOI and bulk MuGFET flow has been made.

shows that the MuGFET fabrication follows a quite conventional Si processing. However, some specific process steps or modules will require additional restrictions and optimization, e.g., fin critical dimension (CD) control and fin height control. Next to that, process modules such as selective epitaxial growth of Si or SiGe (SEG), optional in planar bulk processing (as stressor), will be mandatory in MuGFET fabrication.

In the following sections, some of the technological challenges like fin patterning, workfunction engineering and strain engineering will be briefly addressed. In part I, some selected topics will be discussed in detail.

1.4.1 *Challenges*

1.4.1.1 Fin width patterning

One of the most important challenges in MuGFET integration is the formation of sub-10 nm wide fins. As we have seen in Section 1.2, narrow fins are required to fully benefit from the increased short-channel control in multi-gate devices. A standard way of defining the fins is by optical lithography and dry etch. The MuGFET device layout can be very diverse depending on the application, for example, standalone single fins are used in the case of SRAMs while multiple fin devices with large source and drain pads are more suitable for ring-oscillators etc. Each of these different device layouts requires optimization of the lithography settings in order to control the fin width [21]. As such the development of a model-based Optical Proximity Correction (OPC) is needed.

The requirement at litho level is very stringent: assuming a target fin width of 10 nm and allowing a maximum variation in fin width of 10% in order to keep the maximum V_T shift at $L_{GATE} = 20$ nm smaller than 70 mV, this would mean that at litho level only a litho CD variation of 1.5% can be allowed taking into account a specific and constant etch bias (which is in this case 60 nm). However, this assumes that W_{FIN} variation is the main cause of V_T variability. Other important sources of variability are L_{GATE} and fin height H_{FIN} variations. The latter is especially important for bulk MuGFET. Figure 1.10 shows the V_{T_lin} dependency on fin width and L_{GATE}. In this case, the results are for SOI MuGFETs. For short (< 70 nm) gates, the W_{FIN} dependency on V_{T_lin} is found to be surprisingly weak, while for longer gate lengths, a strong V_{T_lin} increase is observed, especially for narrow fins. This increase can be attributed to fin width fluctuations, as is confirmed by Monte Carlo simulations accounting for the quantum confinement. The largest impact on variability is seen for long gates and narrow fins. In Chapter 2, the trade-offs that need to be considered for fin patterning in high density circuits will be further detailed out.

An alternative fin fabrication technique is the spacer defined patterning technique. This technique can provide double and even quadruple fin density with less stringent lithography requirements [23]. In this case, a dummy pattern (typically SiGe or oxide) is defined and then spacers are formed next to the dummy pattern, which will eventually define the fin spacing. The dummy areas are removed selectively towards the spacers and the spacers are used as a hard mask during the formation of the fins. This can finally also be done in combination with optical lithography if, for example, large source/drain pads need to be patterned. A schematic

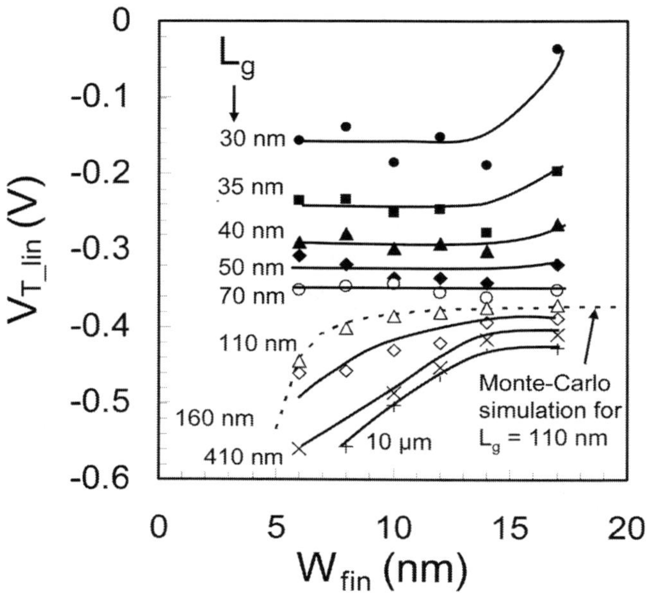

Figure 1.10. pMOS V_{T_lin} *vs.* W_{FIN} for various L_{GATE}. The dashed line corresponds to the simulation of a device with L_{GATE} = 110 nm including W_{FIN} fluctuations [22].

view of the process flow is shown in Fig. 1.11. Although the processing is somewhat more complex and only allows patterning even number of fins, it has quite some advantages: it provides a more uniform pattern size, thereby reducing the fin width variability, and much higher device density than the current optical lithography. Devices and circuits with a fin pitch as small as 50 nm have been demonstrated in [23].

Apart from the ability to fabricate these narrow fins, metrology tools have to guarantee a high enough accuracy to measure features far below 10 nm. For example, a 5 nm accuracy error would correspond to a 30% change in CD when dealing with a 15 nm feature, which is unacceptable. Next to that, Line Width Roughness (LWR) and sidewall roughness have a direct impact on device performance. A robust metrology to characterize these elements in both development and production is required [24].

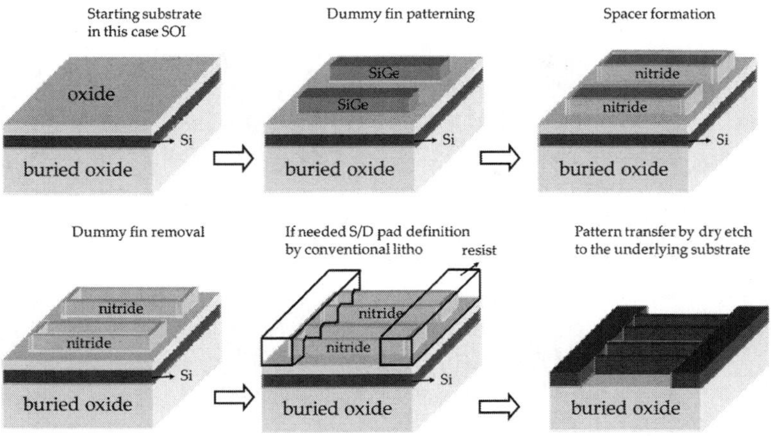

Figure 1.11. A schematic presentation of the spacer defined MuGFET process flow.

1.4.1.2 Work function engineering

Work function engineering relates to the V_T setting and tuning and will be discussed in more details in chapter three. The threshold voltage setting and tuning in planar devices is usually achieved by increasing or decreasing the channel implant, using halo implantations for the short gate lengths, scaling the gate dielectric or using a metal gate to tune the work function (Eqs. 1.3 and 1.4):

$$V_T = 2\varphi_F + V_{FB} + \frac{\sqrt{2q\varepsilon_{Si}N_{sub}\,|2\varphi_F + V_{BS}|}}{C_{ox}} \quad (1.3)$$

$$\varphi_F = \frac{kT}{q}\ln\left(\frac{N_{sub}}{n_i}\right) \quad (1.4)$$

with φ_F the fermi voltage, V_{FB} the flatband voltage, C_{ox} the gate capacitance per unit area, k the Boltzmann constant, T the temperature, q the electron charge, V_{BS} the substrate bias and N_{sub} the channel doping.

In the case of MuGFET devices, the full depletion of the fin makes threshold voltage setting and tuning with implantation very difficult [25]: the depletion width of the transistor is determined by the Si film thickness and cannot be changed by mere channel implantation. One needs to note that this is also the case in narrow bulk FinFET devices. The well and GP implants, in this case, are only used to prevent a large subsurface leakage current from flowing.

Therefore work function tuning with metal gate is the most efficient way of setting the V_T in MuGFET devices. Integration of a single metal gate is the preferred solution when considering process complexity. A single mid-gap metal like TiN or TaN on planar bulk devices typically results in either high threshold voltages or poor short-channel control. In MuGFET, the mid-gap work function leads to almost symmetric threshold voltages for nMOS and pMOS, which are able to fulfill the LSTP requirements [26]. However, different flavors of V_T are needed: low, medium, high V_T. Different from planar bulk devices, MuGFETs need less shifting from the mid-gap work function in order to reach the low V_T targets [27]. Different techniques have been considered for V_T tuning: implantation into the metal gate [28], TiN thickness variation [29] and the use of dielectric capping layers [30]. Recently also the use of buried channel architectures has been considered. Especially Si/SiGe buried channels for pMOS allow reducing the V_T by more than 300 mV (for $Si_{55}Ge_{45}$) [31] while using a metal gate with a work function closer to the n-type band edge.

These are all "gate first" fabrication schemes, where the final gate stack (electrode and gate dielectric) is fabricated quite early in the process flow. Over the last years, there has also been a shift from "gate first" to "gate last" processing [32]. In the latter fabrication scheme, a dummy gate is patterned. The dummy gate is removed after source/drain silicidation and replaced by the final gate stack. Several combinations are possible: either both electrode and gate dielectric are replaced or only the gate electrode is replaced. One of the advantages of the "gate last" process is that the final metal gate is not exposed to the high activation anneal for the junctions. As a result, a better controlled work function for nMOS and pMOS can be achieved.

All these techniques, typically used in planar bulk devices, need to be compatible with the higher topography in MuGFETs. This requires highly conformal deposition techniques for the gate electrode and dielectric, and in the "gate last" process this also requires a careful optimization of the dummy gate processing and subsequent Chemical Mechanical Polishing (CMP) of this dummy gate in order to be able to remove it efficiently after silicidation.

1.4.1.3 Access resistance

For the 22 nm technology node and beyond, fin widths smaller than 10 nm will be needed to maintain good short-channel behavior as was discussed in Section 1.2. Just like in fully depleted SOI (FD SOI) where ultra-thin Si films are needed to obtain good electrostatic control, the access resistance is very high in narrow fin devices [33]. Many publications [34] have addressed the issue and it will be briefly discussed in this section. Chapter 4 will give a more detailed overview of the challenges and solutions to reduce the access resistance.

Overall the parasitic source/drain resistance $R_{S/D}$, which becomes more dominant when the gate length is scaled down, consists of the following contributions [35]:

$$R_{S/D} = R_{CON} + R_{SH} + R_{SP} + R_{ACC} \quad (1.5)$$

where R_{CON} represents the contact resistance, R_{SH} the sheet resistance of the deep source/drain areas with uniform current flow, R_{SP} the spreading resistance and R_{ACC} the accumulation resistance under the gate overlap. Especially the early MuGFET devices suffered from very high R_{CON}. One way to reduce the contact resistance is increasing the contact area. This can be achieved by the implementation of selective epitaxial growth of Si or SiGe (SEG) on the source and drain areas. At the same time, SEG reduces the over-silicidation that occurs in aggressively scaled fins. This problem is more severe for nMOS than for pMOS since p-type dopants like boron typically retard the Ni-silicidation. As a consequence, the NiSi thickness on n-type areas is overall much thicker than on p-type areas. Next to that, the multi-directional consumption of Si during the silicidation and the limited amount of available Si can lead to a full silicidation of the fin. In the worst case, the silicide can overrun the source and drain areas since the Ni is the diffusing species and it will look for available Si to form NiSi. This silicide encroachment will not only lead to an increase in source/drain resistance but also an increase in gate-induced drain leakage (GIDL) [36]. A typical

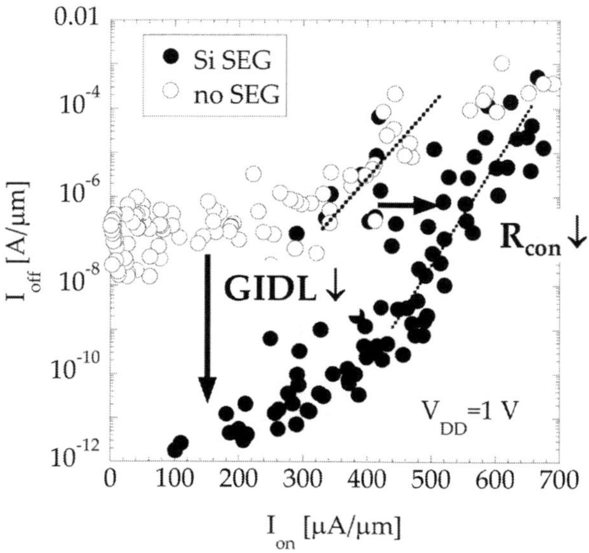

Figure 1.12. $I_{\mathrm{ON}} - I_{\mathrm{OFF}}$ characteristics comparing nMOS devices with and without Si S/D SEG; the fin width of the devices is 25 nm and the SEG thickness is 30 nm [36].

Schottky barrier FET behavior is seen and this leads to an increased off-state leakage. Also here, the use of SEG can reduce the GIDL significantly (Fig. 1.12).

In order to meet the ITRS requirements for the 22 nm technology node and beyond [26], other contributors like the spreading and sheet resistance will need to be addressed. In [38] it was shown that one of the root causes for the high access resistance in aggressively scaled fins is related to the full amorphization of the fins during source/drain implant and its problematic recrystallization during the high temperature anneal. In sub-20 nm wide fins, surface proximity suppresses crystal regrowth and promotes the formation of twin boundary defects in the implanted region. If solid-phase epitaxy (SPE) is significantly retarded, random nucleation and growth (RNG) may take place and part of the fin transforms into polysilicon. Therefore, alternative implantation techniques like plasma doping and vapor phase doping can bring some extra benefits in forming conformal junctions with limited amorphization of the fins. The latter techniques might also solve the problem of implant tilt limitation in high density circuits like SRAMs. The close proximity of the implant masks and the small fin-to-fin spacing do not allow high implantation angles. Consequently, the implantation profile is largely non-conformal (the implantation of the top is different from the sidewalls). Device simulations have shown that this reduces the on-state current of the devices significantly. Some groups have proposed the use of one-sided implants to partially overcome this issue [39].

1.4.1.4 Strain engineering

Since the 90 nm technology node, strain engineering techniques like SiGe S/D stressors and strained contact etch stop layers (sCESL) have been very efficient in boosting the performance of planar bulk devices. MuGFET devices in general do not require channel implants and intrinsically the mobility can be higher than the standard planar devices. However, the different crystal orientation of the sidewalls as compared to the top, can either improve the mobility or decrease it [40]. The former situation is valid for pMOS when the sidewall orientation/current direction is (110)/<110> while this combination of crystal plane and current direction is more detrimental for nMOS devices. Next to that, the fin patterning reactive ion etch (RIE) leads to increased sidewall roughness thereby reducing the channel mobility. Surface smoothening by H_2 anneal [41] has been demonstrated to increase the mobility. However, the impact of the H_2 anneal is quite layout dependent and careful optimization of the process conditions is needed. One of the most straightforward and efficient ways of introducing strain into both planar and multi-gate devices is the use of intrinsically strained SiN layers or sCESL. Publications [43] have shown that the nMOS performance can be improved significantly by the use of tensile sCESL (Fig. 1.13). With the help of TCAD [43] it has been demonstrated that downscaling of the fin width and increase of the fin height will lead to higher top-down and longitudinal stress components. Both are beneficial for nMOS mobility. Furthermore it has been demonstrated that tensile sCESL can also be used on pMOS without degradation of the current. This allows a more simple

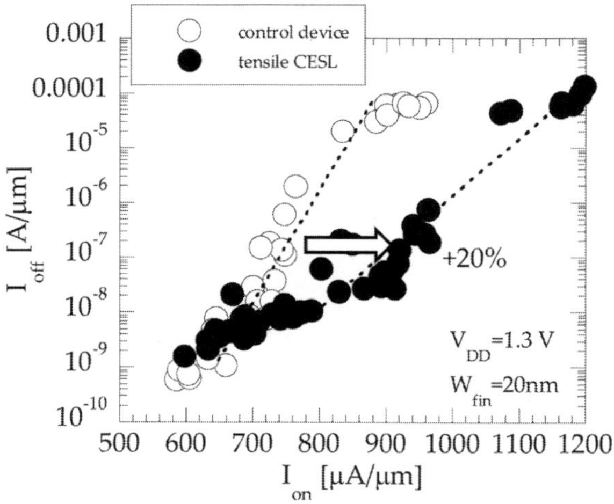

Figure 1.13. I_{ON}–I_{OFF} of nMOS devices with W_{fin} = 20 nm and H_{fin} = 65 nm; the impact of tensile sCESL is shown [46].

process scheme where a single tensile sCESL can be used to improve nMOS without negative impact on the pMOS. sCESL can also be combined with substrate level stressor like strained SOI (SSOI) for nMOS [44] or strained SiGe (SGOI) for pMOS [45].

However, it is important to point out that the efficiency of sCESL is reduced or altered when the fin and poly pitch are scaled down and the device layout is different, e.g., single vs. multiple fins.

The use of embedded SiGe S/D for pMOS [46] and Si:C for nMOS has also been demonstrated in MuGFET devices [48]. In SOI MuGFETs, typically the impact on the mobility is small as the recess depth is limited due to the Si film thickness. This stressor has shown to be more efficient in planar bulk devices [49].

Finally, all strain need to be compatible with "gate last" processing which is considered the most feasible way of introducing metal gates. Only a small amount of publications have appeared on the latter topic but it can be noticed that the overall trends in MuGFET devices are the same as compared to planar bulk. Stressors like sCESL give higher improvement when combined with a "gate last" process [50].

1.5 From MuGFET to Nanowires

Nanowires are devices with a diameter of 10 nm and less, even down to a few nanometers. These devices demonstrate unique properties because, at this scale, quantum mechanical effects cannot be neglected anymore [51]. A wide variety of nanowires have been studied and processed, some are non-Si like carbon nanotubes (CNTs) [52] and they can have a wide variety of applications, but most Si nanowire transistors are FinFET-based. Typically, the fins are scaled down by sacrificial oxidation and HF wet etch [53] or rounded by H_2 anneal [54], and the gate is completely wrapped around the wire. The gate all-around structure allows for the most optimal electrostatic control and these devices have shown excellent scalability [55, 56]. Publications have also demonstrated that the gate length can be reduced to the extent that quasi-ballistic transport occurs [57, 58]. However, the quantum confinement, which is a result of the aggressive scaling of the channel diameter, leads to an unwanted increase in threshold voltage [59]. The carriers in the channel start to occupy discrete energy levels where the lowest energy level is located at a higher level than the bottom of the conduction band. This is different from the traditional continuum of energy levels or bands found in bulk materials. As such, more band bending is required to form the inversion layer in the channel.

Different groups have also described the observation of oscillations in the drain current versus gate voltage at low temperatures, but even at room temperature when the drain bias is low enough [60, 61]. These oscillations can be attributed to the filling of the consecutive 1-D energy sub-bands by electrons as the gate voltage is increased. Next to horizontal devices, vertical nanowire FETs [62] and multi-stacked nanowires, based on the SON technology, have been demonstrated [63].

Apart from their use in standard CMOS applications, there are many possible applications that can benefit from the specific properties of nanowire devices: optics, mechanics, sensors etc. Due to the high surface-to-volume ratio, they can be used as highly sensitive biosensors [64]. Solar cell applications benefit from the reduced reflection, extreme light trapping, improved band gap tuning, easy strain relaxation and increased defect tolerance [65].

1.6 Conclusions

In this introductory chapter, we have briefly reviewed the history of multi-gate devices, starting with the very first demonstrations in the early 1980s up to Intel's announcement to introduce the tri-gate architecture, fabricated on a standard bulk substrate, at the 22 nm technology node.

The advantages of these devices lie in their excellent electrostatic control and SCE robustness. The significant reduction of the off-state leakage as compared to the standard planar bulk MOSFETs make them into excellent candidates for low voltage-low power applications.

For more than a decade, FinFET-based multi-gate devices have been studied by many research groups and although the integration of these devices is very similar to their planar counterparts, the challenges lie in the process control of specific steps like fin and gate patterning. Similar to the thin film in FDSOI, the scaled fin gives rise to an increased external resistance which has typically been seen as one of the possible showstoppers. Introduction of SEG and novel doping techniques has provided a solution to the aforementioned problem. Next to that, strain engineering techniques will be required to enhance the mobility, similar to planar bulk technology.

The ultimate MOSFET architecture will be a gate all-around device where the gate stack is wrapped around a nanowire of only a few nanometers. These devices demonstrate unique features like quantum confinement and possible ballistic transport when the gate length is scaled down. Apart from the standard CMOS applications, there is a growing interest of using nanowires in, for example, bio-applications and solar cells.

Acknowledgments

I would like to thank the former EMERALD (Emerging Alternative Devices IIAP program) team and the many assignees of imec's core partners involved in this program for the inspiring and very successful collaboration over the years.

References

1. www.intel.com
2. Dawon K., "Electric field controlled semiconductor device," U.S. Patent No. 3,102,230 (filed May 31, 1960, issued August 27, 1963).
3. Sekigawa T. and Hayashi Y., "Calculated threshold-voltage characteristics of an XMOS transistor having an additional bottom gate," *Solid State Electron*, **27**, 827–828, 1984.
4. Colinge J. P., Gao M. H., Romano A., Maes H. and Claeys C., "Silicon-on-insulator 'gate-all-around' MOS device," *IEDM Tech Digest*, 595, 1990.
5. Hisamoto D., Kaga T., Kawamoto Y. and Takeda E., "A fully depleted lean-channel transistor (DELTA) — A novel vertical ultra thin SOI MOSFET," *IEDM Tech. Digest*, 833–836, 1989.
6. Hisamoto D., *et al.*, "A folded-channel MOSFET for deep-sub-tenth micron era," *IEDM Tech. Digest*, 1032–1034, 1998.
7. Park J.-T., Colinge J.-P. and Diaz C. H., "Pi-gate SOI MOSFET," *IEEE Electron. Device Lett*, **22(8)**, 405–406, 2001.
8. Fu-Liang Yang *et al.*, "25nm CMOS omega FETs," *IEDM Tech. Digest*, 255–258, 2002.
9. Doyle B. S., Datta S., Doczy M., Hareland S., Jin B., Kavalieros J., Linton T., Murthy A., Rios R. and Chau R., "High performance fullydepleted tri-gate CMOS transistors," *IEEE Electron. Device Lett*, **24(4)**, 263–265, 2003.
10. Schulz T., Rosner W., Risch L., Korbel A. and Langmann U., "Short-channel vertical sidewall MOSFETs," *IEEE Trans. Electron. Devices*, **48(8)**, 1783–1788, 2001.
11. Jurczak M., Skotnicki T., Paoli M., Tormen B., Martins J., Regolini J. L., Dutartre D., Ribot P., Lenoble D., Pantel R. and Monfray S., "Silicon-on-nothing (SON) — An innovative process for advanced CMOS," *IEEE Trans. Electron. Device*, **47(11)**, 2179–2185, 2000.
12. Vinet M., Poiroux T., Licitra C., Widiez J., Bhandari J., Previtali B., Vizioz C., Lafond D., Arvet C., Besson P., Baud L., Morand Y., Rivoire M., Nemouchi F., Carron V. and Deleonibus S., "Self-aligned planar doublegate MOSFETs by bonding for 22-nm node, with metal gates, high κ dielectrics, and metallic source/drain," *IEEE Electron. Device Lett*, **30(7)**, 748–750, 2009.
13. Liu Q., *et al.*, "Impact of back bias on ultrathin body and BOX (UTBB) devices," *VLSI Tech. Symp*, 160–161, 2011.

14. Dennard R., *et al.*, "Design of ion-implanted MOSFETs with very small physical dimensions," *IEEE J. Solid State Circuits*, **SC-9(5)**, 256–268, 1974.
15. Skotnicki T., "Materials and structures for sub-32nm CMOS nodes," *Microelectron Eng*, **84**, (9–10), 1845–1852, 2007.
16. Park T., Choi S., Lee D. H., Yoo J. R., Lee B. C., Kim J. Y., Lee C. G., Chi K. K., Hong S. H., Hyun S. J., Shin Y. G., Han J. N., Park I. S., Chung U. I., Moon J. T., Yoon E. and Lee J. H., "Fabrication of bodytied FinFETs (Omega MOSFETs) using bulk Si wafers," *VLSI Tech. Symp*, 135–136, 2003.
17. Redolfi A., Sleeckx E., Devriendt K., Shamiryan D., Vandeweyer T., Horiguchi N., Togo M., Wouter J. M. D., Jurczak M., Hoffmann T., Cockburn A., Gravey V. and Diehl D. L., "Bulk FinFET fabrication with new approaches for oxide topography control using dry removal techniques," *12th International Conference on Ultimate Integration on Silicon (ULIS)*, 1–3, 2011.
18. Okano K., Izumida T., Kawasaki H., Kaneko A., Yagishita A., Kanemura T., Kondo M., Ito S., Aoki N., Miyano K., Ono T., Yahashi K., Iwade K., Kubota T., Matsushita T., Mizushima I., Inaba S., Ishimaru K., Suguro K., Eguchi K, Tsunashima Y. and Ishiuchi H., "Process integration technology and device characteristics of CMOS FinFET on bulk silicon substrate with sub-10nm fin width and 20nm gate length," *IEDM Tech. Digest*, 725–728, 2005.
19. Yeh C.-C., *et al.*, "A low operating power FinFET transistor module featuring scaled gate stack and strain engineering for 32/28nm SoC technology," *IEDM Tech. Digest*, 772–775, 2010.
20. *Sentaurus Process and Device Reference Manual*, D-2010.03 ed., 2010.
21. Ercken M., Delvaux C., Baerts C., Locorotondo S., Degroote B., Wiaux V., Nackaerts A., Rooyackers R., Verhaegen S. and Pollentier I., "Challenges in patterning 45nm node multiple-gate devices and SRAM cells," *Proceedings of the 41st Interface Symposium*.
22. Collaert N., De Keersgieter A., Dixit A., Ferain I., Lai L., Lenoble D., Mercha A., Nackaerts A., Pawlak B., Rooyackers R., Schulz T., San K., Son N., Van Dal M., Verheyen P., von Arnim K., Witters L., De Meyer K., Biesemans S. and Jurczak M., "Multi-gate devices for the 32 nm technology node and beyond," *Solid State Electron*, **52(9)**, 1291–1296, 2008.
23. Rooyackers R., *et al.*, "Doubling or quadrupling MuGFET fin integration scheme with higher pattern fidelity, lower CD variation and higher layout efficiency," *IEDM Tech. Digest*, 993–996, 2006.

24. Lorusso G. F., *et al.*, "Comprehensive approach to MuGFET metrology" in *Metrology, Inspection, and Process Control for Microlithography XX, Proc. SPIE*, 6152, 615219, 2006.
25. Collaert N., Demand M., Ferain I., Lisoni J., Singanamalla R., Zimmerman P., Yim Y. S., Schram T., Mannaert G., Goodwin M., Hooker J. C., Neuilly F., Kim M. C., De Meyer K., De Gendt S., Boullart W., Jurczak M. and Biesemans S., "Tall triplegate devices with TiN/HfO_2 gate stack," *VLSI Tech. Symp*, 108–109, 2005.
26. *ITRS Roadmap*, Semiconductor Industry Association, San Jose, CA, 2009.
27. Kranti A. and Armstrong G. A., "Device design considerations for nanoscale double and triple gate FinFETs," *IEEE SOI Conf*, 96–98, 2005.
28. Witters L., Son N. J., Ferain I., San T., Singanamalla R., Kerner C., Collaert N., De Meyer K. and Jurczak M., "Threshold voltage modulation in FinFET devices through arsenic ion implantation into TiN/HfSiON gate stack," *IEEE SOI Conf*, 31–32, 2007.
29. Ferain I., Collaert N., O'Sullivan B., Conard T., Popovici M., Van Elshocht S., Swerts J., Jurczak M. and De Meyer K. "Metal gate thickness optimization for MuGFET performance improvement," *Eur Solid-State Device Res. Conf. (ESSDERC)*, 202–205, 2008.
30. Kubicek S., *et al.*, "Low V_T CMOS using doped Hf-based oxides, TaC-based metals and laser-only anneal," *IEDM Tech. Dig*, 49–52, 2007.
31. Witters L., *et al.*, "8Å T_{inv} gate-first dual channel technology achieving low-V_t high performance CMOS," *VLSI Tech. Symp*, 181–182, 2010.
32. Veloso A., *et al.*, "Gate-last vs. gate-first technology for aggressively scaled EOT logic/RF CMOS," *VLSI Tech. Symp*, 34–35, 2011.
33. Kedzierski J., Ieong M., Nowak E., Kanarsky T. S., Zhang Y., Roy R., Boyd D., Fried D. and Wong H.-S. P., "Extension and source/drain design for high-performance FinFET devices," *IEEE Trans. Electron. Device*, **50(4)**, 952–958, 2003.
34. Dixit A., Kottantharayil A., Collaert N., Goodwin M., Jurczak M. and De Meyer K., "Analysis of the parasitic source/drain resistance in multiple gate field effect transistors," *IEEE Trans. Electron. Device*, **52(6)**, 1132–1140, 2005.
35. Ng K. and Lynch W. T., "Analysis of the gate-voltage dependent series resistance of MOSFETs," *IEEE Trans. Electron. Devices*, **33**, 965–972, 1986.
36. Hoffmann T., *et al.*, "S/D engineering in advanced HfO_2/TiN FinFET devices: A view on GIDL (gate-induced drain leakage) and Schottky barriers S/D leakages," *IEDM Tech. Digest*, 743–746, 2005.

37. Collaert N., Rooyackers R., Hikavyy A., Dixit A., Leys F., Verheyen P., Loo R., Jurczak M. and Biesemans S., "Multi-gate devices for the 32 nm technology node and beyond: challenges for selective epitaxial growth," *Thin Solid Films*, **517(1)**, 101–104, 2008.
38. Duffy R., van Dal M. J. H., Pawlak B. J., Kaiser M., Weemaes R. G., Degroote B., Kunnen E., and Altamirano E., "Solid phase epitaxy versus random nucleation and growth in sub-20 nm wide fin field-effect transistors," *Appl. Phys. Lett*, 90, 241912, June 2007.
39. Kawasaki H., *et al.*, "Demonstration of highly scaled FinFET SRAM cells with high κ /metal gate and investigation of characteristic variability for the 32 nm node and beyond," *IEDM Tech. Digest*, 237–240, 2008.
40. Iyengar V. V., Kottantharayil A., Tranjan F. M., Jurczak M. and De Meyer K., "Extraction of the top and sidewall mobility in FinFETs and the impact of finpatterning processes and gate dielectrics on mobility," *IEEE Trans Electron Devices*, **54(5)**, 1177–1184, 2007.
41. Xiong W., Gebara G., Zaman J., Gostkowski M., Nguyen B., Smith G., Lewis D., Cleavelin C. R., Wise R., Yu S., Pas M., King T.-S. and Colinge J. P., "Improvement of FinFET electrical characteristics by hydrogen annealing," *IEEE Electron. Device Lett*, **25(8)**, 541–543, 2004.
42. Suthram S., Hussain M. M., Harris H. R., Smith C., Cheng H.-H., Jammy R. and Thompson S. E., "Comparison of uniaxial wafer bending and contact-etch-stop-liner stress induced performance enhancement on double-gate FinFETs," *IEEE Electron. Device Lett*, **29(5)**, 480–482, 2008.
43. Collaert N., De Keersgieter A., Anil K. G., Rooyackers R., Eneman G., Goodwin M., Eyckens B., Sleeckx E., de Marneffe J.-F., De Meyer K., Absil P., Jurczak M. and Biesemans S., "Performance improvement of tall triple gate devices with strained SiN layers," *IEEE Electron. Device Lett*, **26(11)**, 820–822, 2005.
44. Collaert N., Rooyackers R., Clemente F., Zimmerman P., Cayrefourcq I., Ghyselen B., San K. T., Eyckens B., Jurczak M. and Biesemans S., "Performance enhancement of MUGFET devices using super critical strained–SOI (SC-SSOI) and CESL" *VLSI Tech. Symp*, 52–53, 2006.
45. Irisawa T., Numata T., Tezuka T., Usuda K., Nakaharai S., Hirashita N., Sugiyama N., Toyoda E. and Takagi S., "High performance multi-gate pMOSFET using uniaxially-strained SGOI channels," *IEDM Tech. Digest*, 709–712, 2005.
46. Collaert N., Rooyackers R., De Keersgieter A., Verheyen P., Clemente F., Kottantharayil A., Jurczak M. and Biesemans S., "Strain engineering in multi-gate devices," *SEMI Technology Symposium*, Japan, December 2006.

47. Verheyen P., Collaert N., Rooyackers R., Loo R., Shamiryan D., De Keersgieter A., Eneman G., Leys F., Dixit A., Goodwin M., Yim Y.S., Caymax M., De Meyer K., Absil P., Jurczak M. and Biesemans S., "25% drive current improvement for p-type multiple gate FET (MuGFET) devices by the introduction of recessed $Si_{0.8}Ge_{0.2}$ in the source and drain regions," *VLSI Tech. Symp*, 194–195, 2005.

48. Liow T.-Y., Tan K.-M., Lee R. T. P., Du A., Tung C.-H., Samudra G. S., Yoo W.-.J., Balasubramanian N. and Yeo Y.-C., "Strained N-channel FinFETs with 25 nm gate length and silicon–carbon source/drain regions for performance enhancement," *VLSI Tech. Symp*, 56–57, 2006.

49. Eneman G., Verheyen P., Rooyackers R., Nouri F., Washington L., Schreutelkamp R., Moroz V., Smith L., De Keersgieter A., Jurczak M. and De Meyer K., "Scalability of the $Si_{1-x}Ge_x$ source/drain technology for the 45-nm technology node and beyond," *IEEE Trans. Electron. Devices* **53(7)**, 1647–1656, 2006.

50. Auth C., *et al.*, "45 nm high-k + metal gate strain-enhanced transistors," *VLSI Tech. Symp*, 128–129, 2008.

51. Afzalian A., Chi-Woo Lee, Akhavan N. D., Ran Yan, Ferain, I. and Colinge J., "Quantum confinement effects in capacitance behavior of multigate silicon nanowire MOSFETs," *IEEE Trans. Nanotechnol*, **10(2)**, 300–309, 2011.

52. Chen Z., Farmer D., Xu S., Gordon R., Avouris P. and Appenzeller J., "Externally assembled gate-all-around carbon nanotube field-effect transistor" *IEEE Electron. Device Lett*, **29(2)**, 183–185, 2008.

53. Singh N., Lim F. Y., Fang W. W, Rustagi S. C., Bera L. K., Agarwal A., Tung C. H., Hoe K. M., Omampuliyur S. R., Tripathi D., Adeyeye A. O., Lo G. Q. Balasubramanian N. and Kwong D. L., "Ultra-narrow silicon nanowire gate-all-around CMOS devices: Impact of diameter, channel-orientation and low temperature on device performance," *IEDM Tech. Digest,* 1–4, 2006.

54. Hashemi P., Teherani J. T. and Hoyt, J. L., "Investigation of hole mobility in gate-all-around Si nanowire p-MOSFETs with high κ/metal-gate: Effects of hydrogen thermal annealing and nanowire shape," *IEDM Tech. Digest*, 788–791, 2010.

55. Lee H., Yu L.-E., Ryu S.-W, Han J.-W., Jeon K., Jang D.-Y., Kim K.-H., Lee J., Kim J.-H., Jeon S. C., Lee G. S., Oh J. S., Park Y. C., Bae W. H. and Lee H. M., Yang J. M., Yoo J. J., Kim S. I. and Choi Y.-K. Sub-5 nm allaround gate FinFET for ultimate scaling," *VLSI Tech. Symp*, 58–59, 2006.

56. Singh N., Agarwal A., Bera L. K., Liow T. Y., Yang R., Rustagi S. C., Tung C. H., Kumar R., Lo G. Q., Balasubramanian N. and Kwong D.-L., "High-

performance fully depleted silicon nanowire (diameter $\leq$ 5 nm) gate all around CMOS devices," *IEEE Electron. Device Lett*, **27(5)**, 383–386, 2006.

57. Wang R., Zhuge J., Liu C., Huang R., Kim D.-W., Park D. and Wang Y., "Experimental study on quasi-ballistic transport in silicon nanowire transistors and the impact of self-heating effects," *IEDM Tech. Digest*, 1–4, 2008.
58. Cho K. H., Suk S. D., Yeoh Y. Y., Li M., Yeo K. H., Kim D.-W., Hwang S. W., Park D., and Ryu B.-I., "Observation of single electron tunneling and ballistic transport in twin silicon nanowire MOSFETs (TSNWFETs) fabricated by top-down CMOS process," *IEDM Tech. Digest*, 290–293, 2006.
59. Taur Y. and Ning, T. H. *Fundamentals of Modern VLSI Devices*, Cambridge, U.K., Cambridge University Press, 1998.
60. Kobayashi M. and Hiramoto T., "Experimental study on quantum structure of silicon nano wire and its impact on nano wire MOSFET and single electron transistor," *IEDM Tech. Digest*, 855–857, 2006.
61. Akhavan N. D., Afzalian A., Chi-Woo Lee, Ran Yan, Ferain I., Razavi P., Fagas G. and Colinge, J.-P., "Simulation of quantum current oscillations in trigate SOI MOSFETs," *IEEE Trans. Electron. Devices*, **57(5)**, 1102–1109, 2010.
62. Maheshwaram S., Manhas S. K., Kaushal G., Anand B. and Singh N., "Vertical silicon nanowire gate-all-around field effect transistor based nanoscale CMOS," *IEEE Electron. Device Lett*, **32(8)**, 1011–1013, 2011.
63. Tachi K., Casse M., Barraud S., Dupre C., Hubert A., Vulliet N., Faivre M.E., Vizioz C., Carabasse C., Delaye V., Hartmann J.M., Iwai H., Cristoloveanu S., Faynot O. and Ernst T., "Experimental study on carrier transport limiting phenomena in 10 nm width nanowire CMOS transistors," *IEDM Tech. Digest*, 784–787, 2010.
64. Guo-Jun Zhang, Luo Z. H. H., Min Joon Huang, Tay G. K. I., Lim E.-J. A. and Yu Chen, "Highly sensitive and selective label-free detection of cardiac biomarkers in blood serum with silicon nanowire biosensors," *IEDM Tech. Digest*, 1–4, 2009.
65. Garnett E. C., Brongersma M. L., Cui Yi and McGehee M. D., "Nanowire solar cells," *Ann. Rev. Mater. Res*, **41**, 269–295, 2011.

Chapter 2

Dry Etching Patterning Requirements for Multi-Gate Devices

Efraín Altamirano-Sánchez, Tom Vandeweyer, and Werner Boullart
IMEC, Kapeldreef 75, 3001 Heverlee, Belgium
efrain.altamirano.sanchez@gmail.com

2.1 Introduction

The FinFET architecture leads to a more complex plasma etching processing, especially for active fins with a critical dimension (CD) below 25 nm targeting straight profiles, needed for controlling the short channel effects (SCE) [1]. Patterning such silicon fins becomes more challenging when the structure density increases and the CD is scaled down to less than 15 nm. When a node is scaled down, among many other parameters, the fin pitch changes, provoking drifts between the plasma and exposed surface, i.e., etching rates (ER) and etched profiles shapes. In this chapter we present the evolution of the plasma etching processes from a 130 nm-like node to 16 nm node, in other words, from a "relax" fin pitch of 350 nm to an aggressive 64 nm pitch. In R&D or industrial environment, the etching of fins, gates, spacers, trenches, contact

CMOS Nanoelectronics: Innovative Devices, Architectures, and Applications
Edited by Nadine Collaert

ISBN 978-981-4364-02-7 (Hardcover), 978-981-4364-03-4 (eBook)
www.panstanford.com

holes, etc., is generally carried out in glow discharge reactors, which are commonly referred to as processing plasma's, plasma etching or dry etching. Although, glow discharges are beyond the scope of this chapter, a general overview is needed in order to make the reader familiar with the jargon of plasma etching. A general definition of plasma etching would be: a process that uses a glow discharge of an appropriate gas chemistry as a source of etching species, which in contact with the substrate enables chemical reactions near room temperature[1] producing volatile etching products. For example, in a glow discharge the inert molecule Cl_2 is converted into very reactive species such as Cl atoms that spontaneously react with silicon to form $SiCl_4$ (silicon tetra-chloride) molecules which are very volatile at room temperature. In plasma etching, molecular glow discharges such as CF_4, CH_2F_2, SF_6, HBr, Cl_2, etc., are widely used; these molecules can be used individually or combined depending on the goal of the etching step [2]. A glow discharge is formed whenever a gas is forced to conduct electric current, creating a collection of electrically charged and neutral particles. The density of the negatively charged particles (electrons and negative ions) is equal to the density of positively charge particles (positive ions). This is true for the bulk of the plasma well away from the boundary surfaces. Whenever a plasma is in contact with a surface, a boundary layer known as "sheath" is formed [2, 3]. In a sheath there are more positive charges than electrons because it tends to repel electrons and attracts positive ions, allowing the ion bombardment for etching materials (Figure 2.1). For example the glow discharge of CF_4 can create plasmas that are considered to contain F atoms, CF, CF_2, CF_3 radicals, CF_3^+, CF_2^+, CF^+ ions and smaller quantities of CF_x ions and C_2F_x radicals [4]. Glow discharges entities which consist of electron–atom/molecule collisions are very difficult to understand, even if the discharge consists of chemically unreactive species. This picture is more complex when all the experimental variables associated to the glow discharge reactors are taken into account such as pressure, gas flow, electric field frequency, chamber walls, substrate temperature, etc. Consequently most of the progress and knowledge in plasma

[1]Without the assistance of the plasma much higher temperatures would be required for etching materials.

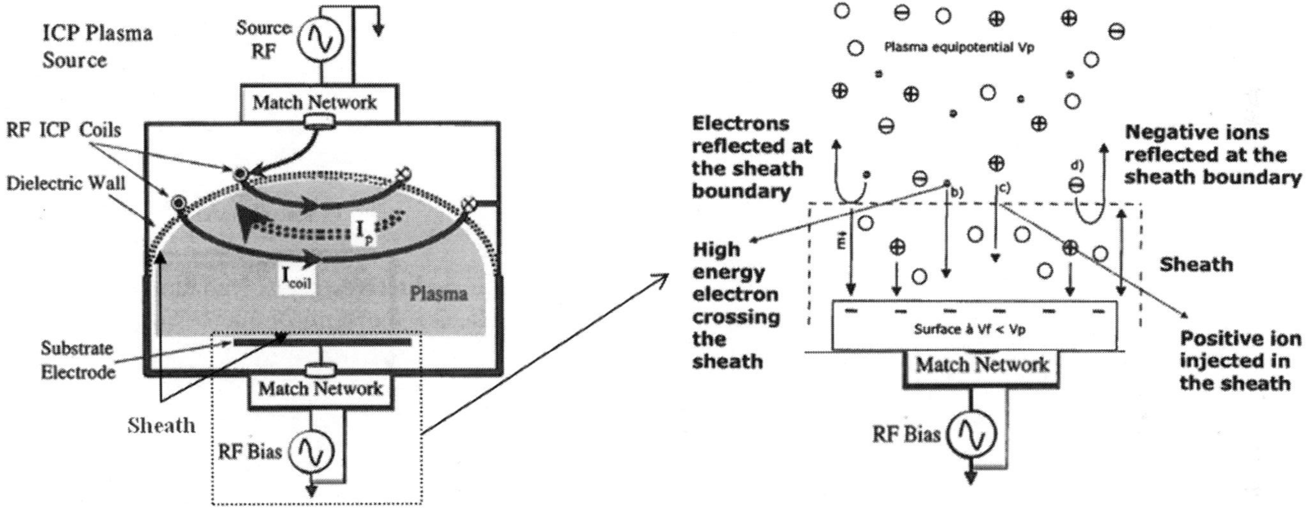

Figure 2.1. Schematic representation of the electric field generated through the sheath: the electric field repels electrons and negative ions and attracts positive ions [modified from ref. [2]].

etching has been accomplished empirically, guided by experience and intuition as suggested by John W. Coburn [2].

Plasma patterning of fins, as well as gates, is carried out in inductively coupled plasma (ICP) reactors. This type of reactor generates high density plasmas in which the source (RF) power is inductively coupled to the plasma providing high ion density and low ion energy ($\sim$100 eV) [2, 3]. In this system, independent control of the ion energy and ion flux can be obtained. Typically the power used in the high density source (source power) is much larger than the power applied to the electrode or electrostatic chuck (ESC) (bias power). In this way, the bias power does not contribute significantly to the plasma density and the ion flux is independent of the bias power.

In general terms the knobs typically used for developing an etching process in an ICP reactor are:

- Pressure: 5 to 100 mTorr.
- Flows: 5 to 500 sccm (standard cubic centimeter per minute).
- Radio frequency power (RF power): 200 W to 1200 W.
- Bias voltage: 50 to 500 V.
- ESC temperature: best practice conditions between 40 and 60 degrees Celsius, but temperatures between 10 and 100 degrees can be used.
- Gases: H_2, He, Ar, HBr, Cl_2, O_2, CF_4, CH_2F_2, CH_3F, SF_6, NF_3, $SiCl_4$, etc.

2.2 Fin Patterning Strategy

Since the patterning of nano-structures is after all a strategy, there are many ways to obtain the same result. Here the strategy that has allowed the scaling of FinFET devices from a 130 nm to a 16 nm node is presented. From 130 to 22 nm technology nodes, the fin mask or template is transferred into the photo resist (PR) using 193 lithography or 193 immersion (193i) lithography. The fin pitch for each node is shown in Table 2.1. The patterning stack consisted of Bottom Anti-Reflective Coating (BARC), Dielectric Anti-Reflective Coating (DARC), and Hard Mask (HM) is shown in Figure 2.2. The PR pattern is transferred into the HM using multiple dry etching

Table 2.1. Fin pitch and CD evolution as function of the technology node

Lithography	Technology node	Fin pitch (nm)	Lithography Fin CD (nm)	Etching fin CD (nm)
193	130	350	78	35
	65	200	78	25
193i	32	125	45	23
	22	90	40	17
EUV	s22	80	40	15
	16	64	35	13

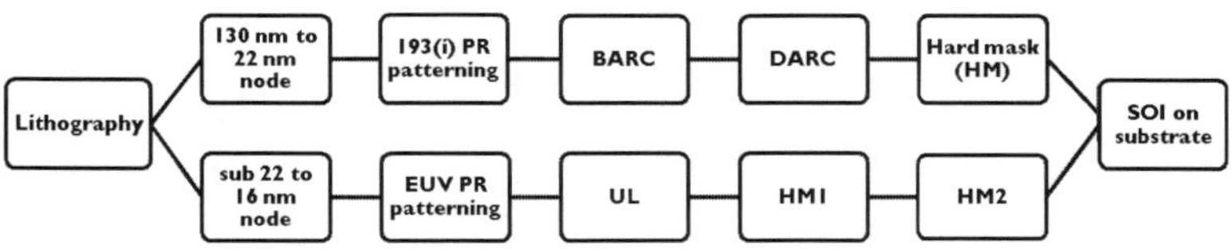

Figure 2.2. Patterning stack for patterning fins on insulator using 193i or EUV lithography.

steps, in order to reach the target critical dimension (CD) for the fin; once the HM has the correct CD, its pattern is transferred into the crystalline silicon (c-Si). The carbon polymer residues are stripped in a microwave chamber followed by a diluted HF clean.

For the sub 22 nm and 16 nm nodes the lithography exposure was carried out using extreme ultraviolet (EUV) lithography. The patterning stack is slightly different from the one used for larger pitches (Figure 2.3). For example, in EUV the lithography community does not talk anymore about BARC because its anti-reflective properties are not needed anymore, consequently now the organic layer below the PR is called "under-layer" mainly used for PR sticking purposes. Using multiple dry etching steps, the PR pattern is transferred into the dual hard mask (HM1 and HM2) where the target CD of the fins is defined and transferred into the c-Si.

2.2.1 *Patterning Stack*

For the 193 dry lithography an ASMLXT:1250 is used in combination with an interfaced TEL ACT12-track, the 193i lithography was performed on an ASML XT: 1900Gi immersion scanner in line

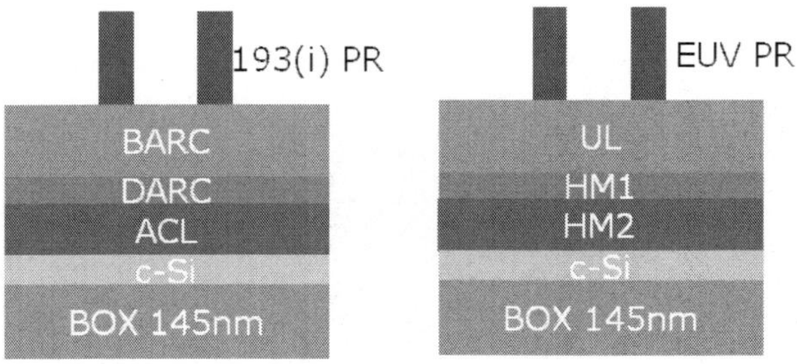

Figure 2.3. Full patterning stack for 193(i) lithography (left) and EUV lithography (right).

with a Sokudo RF3S track. The 193(i) lithography stack for the different nodes is exemplified in Table 2.2 (193(i) lithography stack is referred to as the PR plus the BARC thickness).

EUV Lithography (13.4 nm) was performed on the Alfa Demo Tool (ADT) from ASML, hooked up to an ACT12 (TEL). The litho stack consisted of 24 nm or 10 nm of UL and 80 nm or 60 nm PR (see Table 2.3).

All the process development was carried out on 300 mm Silicon on Insulator (SOI) wafers with 145 nm buried silicon dioxide (BOX) and 65, 40 or 30 nm thick (100) crystalline Silicon (c-Si). The fin structures were patterned in the (110) direction using the stack

Table 2.2. 193i lithography stack and patterning stack thicknesses

Node	Pitch	PR	BARC	DARC (SiOC)	HM (ACL)	c-Si
130	350	165	77	35	70	65
65	200	165	77	35	70	65
32	124	120	85	35	70	40
22	90	105	38	25	70	40

Table 2.3. EUV lithography stack and patterning stack thicknesses

Node	Pitch	PR	UL	HM1 (SiOC)	HM2 (ACL)	c-Si
22	80	80	24	25	70	40
16	64	60	10	15	40	30

described below. On top of the SOI wafers, two chemical vapor deposition (CVD) layers were applied as follows from bottom to top: 70 or 40 nm of amorphous carbon layer (ACL) was used as bottom hard mask; 35, 25 or 15 nm of silicon oxycarbide (SiOC) which was used as top hardmask and supporting the reflection control for lithography (Figure 2.3).

2.3 Fin Patterning: Dry Etching Process Development

In this section, we first describe the fin dry etching process used for the fabrication of an electrically functional device at 130 nm node using 193 nm lithography.

2.3.1 *Process for Fin Patterning on a Multi-Gate Architecture (193 nm Lithography)*

A schematic representation of the dry etching fin patterning process for a 130 nm device is detailed in Figures 2.4 and 2.5. Lithography prints 78 nm CD lines with a final PR height of ~165 nm. The dry etching process starts with BARC opening using a $Cl_2/O_2/He$ plasma chemistry that reduced the PR CD by 3 nm. Then a PR trim step based on $Cl_2/O_2/He$ plasma chemistry with no bias reduced the CD by 25 nm (trim rate, 0.93 nm/s). An additional CD loss of 2 nm was induced during the DARC opening using a CF_4/CH_2F_2 plasma chemistry (Figure 2.4). The DARC trim step with a trim rate of 0.5 nm/s reduced the CD by 15 nm using a CF_4 plasma chemistry (no bias). The HM was etched in two steps. The first step was the partial patterning of the ACL HM (ACL1) using a $Cl_2/O_2/He$ plasma chemistry, during this step ~80% of the ACL was patterned and the CD slightly increased by ~2 nm. The second step patterned the remaining HM (ACL2) using plasma based on CF_4/CH_2F_2 chemistry (Figure 2.5). This ACL2 step has two main purposes: one is to pattern the remaining ACL and the other is to remove the remaining SiOC (DARC).

During the c-Si main etch (ME) step the SiOC could not be completely removed, because the selectivity towards SiOC (1:1.5) and the short etching time. This means that when 65 nm of c-Si

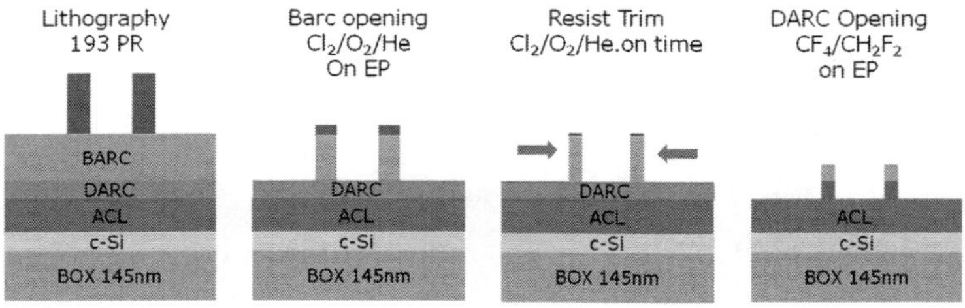

Figure 2.4. Schematic representation of the patterning stack after lithography, BARC opening, PR trim and DARC opening (350 nm fin pitch or 130 nm node).

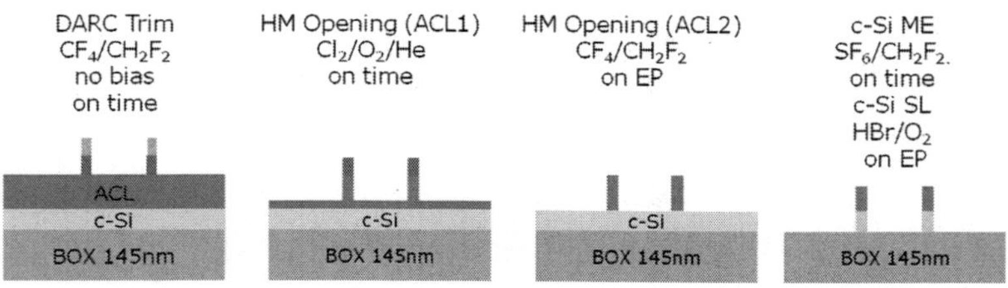

Figure 2.5. Schematic representation of the DARC trim, HM and c-Si patterning (130 nm node).

are etched only ~25 nm of SiOC would be removed. Hence, when the fin etching is completed, a dedicated SiOC removal has to be added. This additional step would induce an undesired Buried Oxide (BOX) recess. Therefore, a CF_4/CH_2F_2 process was developed for consuming SiOC during the ACL2 step. This step slightly increased the CD by 2 nm due to its polymerizing nature [9, 10].

The c-Si etching was done in three steps: in the first step, the ME, is based on a CH_2F_2/SF_6 plasma chemistry, which etches ~80% of the silicon. In the second step is the so-called soft-landing step using a HBr/O_2 plasma chemistry (at low pressure) for etching the remaining Si and tuning the fin profile. The soft-landing is controlled by using a well defined optical emission spectroscopy (OES) end-point algorithm. We defined the end-point as the complete clearance of exposed Si, which is monitored by the optical emission of SiH (414 nm) and Br (827 nm) (Figure 2.6). The last step, the overetch (OE) is based on a HBr/O_2 plasma chemistry (at high pressure), which cleans the remnants of c-Si selectively towards the BOX (>50:1).

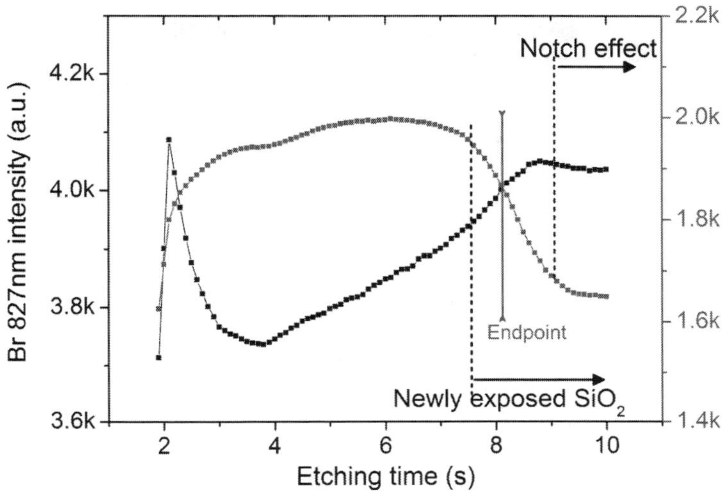

Figure 2.6. Optical emission traces during the soft-landing step. The drop of the 414 nm wave length intensity indicates that the exposed c-Si has been etched, which happens around ~8 s (endpoint). The flat zone of the 827 nm wavelength indicates that the Br species have stopped being consumed by the c-Si etching. See also Color Insert.

After this dry etching was completed, the organic residues on the wafer were stripped on a microwave chamber and cleaned on a diluted HF solution giving a final result fins with a CD of 35 nm (Figure 2.7).

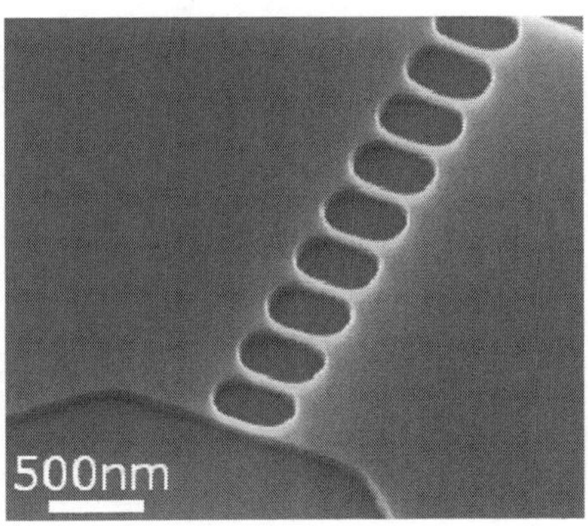

Figure 2.7. Top SEM inspection of fin after dry etching.

Critical dimensions below 25 nm can be achieved at "relax" pitches such as 350 nm and 200 nm. For example, on a multi-gated architecture, the dry etching process for patterning fins with 25 nm CD and 65 nm height on a relaxed 350 nm fin pitch was relatively easily transferred to a 200 nm fin pitch [1]. However, this process could not be transferred to a 124 nm fin pitch (32 nm). In order to obtain fins with 23 nm CD we had to tune the PR trim, the DARC opening and the HM patterning [6]. Moreover, it was observed that this process could not be straightforwardly applied to a 90 nm fin pitch (22 nm node). This time, besides the drifts on the PR trim rate, DARC and HM patterning steps, we also encountered CD increments during the HM patterning, c-Si sidewall roughness (SWR) and tapered fin profiles. In the next section the main changes made for patterning fins on a 90 nm fin pitch are presented.

2.3.2 *Process for Fin Patterning with a 90 nm Fin Pitch for a 22 nm Node 6T-SRAM Cell (193i)*

FinFET architectures lead to a more complex processing, especially for fins with a critical dimension below 25 nm. Patterning such silicon fins becomes more challenging when the structure density increases and the CD is scaled down to 17 nm. We have observed that some of the standard c-Si etching principles are not valid anymore [5].

The dry etching back bone process, developed for a 350 nm pitch (Figures 2.4 and 2.5), was tuned to pattern fins on a 124 nm pitch (32 nm node 0.186 μm^2 6T-SRAM cell) (Figures 2.8 and 2.9); however, this process was not longer functional for a 22 nm node with a 90 nm fin pitch and 17 nm fin CD target. Three main changes were observed when the dry etching process developed for a 32 nm node was directly applied on a 22 nm node cell: 1) the CD was considerably increased, 11 nm larger than the target CD (17 nm); 2) the fin profile was tapered and, 3) fin sidewalls were heavily attacked, creating a severe side wall roughness (SWR).

The CD SEM measurements revealed that during the BARC opening and PR trim step the CD loss was larger on a 90 nm than on a 124 nm pitch (cfr. Figures 2.8 and 2.10). By tuning the BARC opening, the PR trim and the DARC opening steps, we managed to

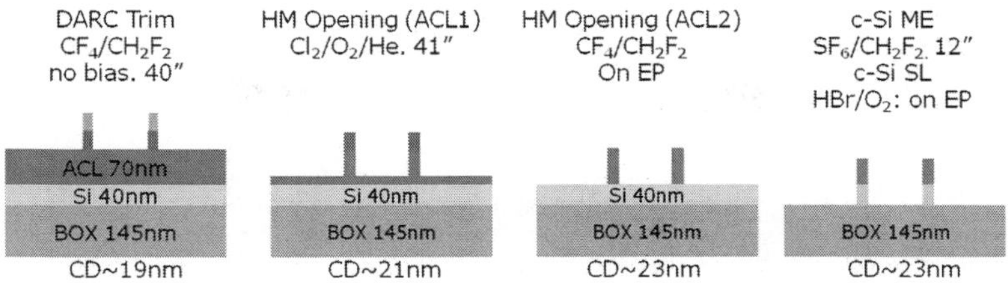

Figure 2.8. Schematic representation of the patterning stack after lithography, BARC opening, PR trim and DARC opening (124 nm fin pitch). See also Color Insert.

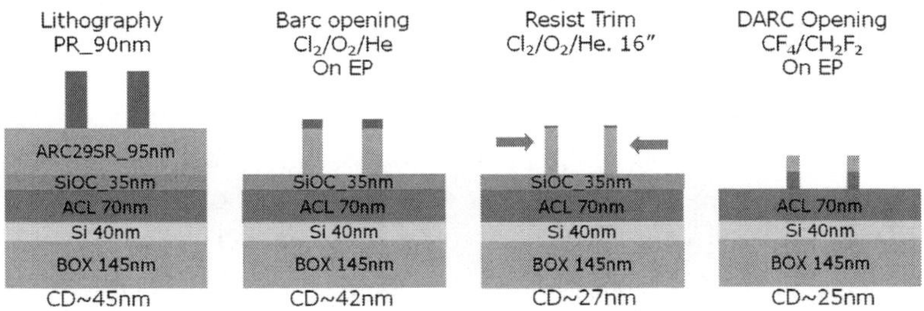

Figure 2.9. Schematic representation of the DARC trim, HM and c-Si patterning (124 nm fin pitch). See also Color Insert.

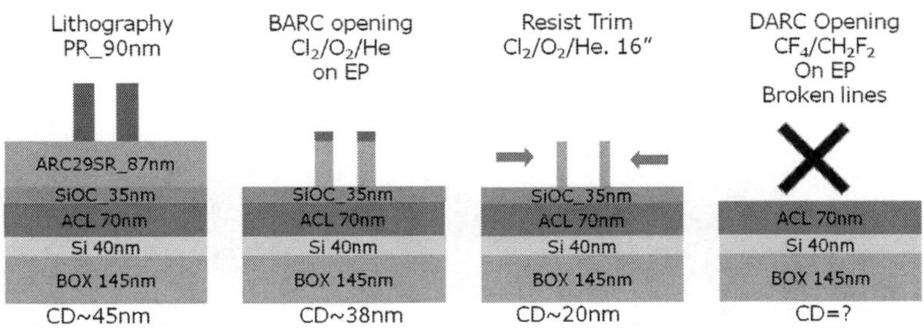

Figure 2.10. Schematic representation of the patterning stack after lithography, BARC opening, PR trim and DARC opening (90 nm fin pitch). The CD values were determined by CD SEM. See also Color Insert.

pattern ~19 nm lines after DARC opening. However, after the HM patterning, using ACL1 and ACL2 etching steps, the fin CD increased from 19 to 28 nm, ending up in c-Si lines with CDs far from the 17 nm target (Table 2.4). The fin CD increased during these ACL1 and ACL2 steps due to sidewall polymer deposition.

Table 2.4. Effect of the polymerizing chemistries on the fin CD after HM patterning

	CD increment during the HM patterning	
Step	124 nm pitch	90 nm pitch
ACL1	2 nm	4 nm
ACL2	2 nm	7 nm
Total	4 nm	11 nm

Note: The fin CD increases almost three times more on the 90 nm than on the 124 nm pitch after the HM patterning.

Moreover, the top-down SEM and XTEM inspections showed a partially tapered fin profile and sidewall roughness, which are indicators of an uncontrolled silicon dry etching process (Figure 2.11). Studying the effect of the softlanding step, we were able to verify that the SWR was directly proportional to the time that the BOX was exposed to the softlanding plasma chemistry after endpoint. We have observed that increasing the overetch time in the softlanding step (after endpoint) from 3 to 7 s impacted the SWR considerably (Figure 2.12).

We have found that these three issues are strongly correlated with each other; this means that by solving one of these problems the others might be partially solved or attenuated. For sakes of

(a) (b)

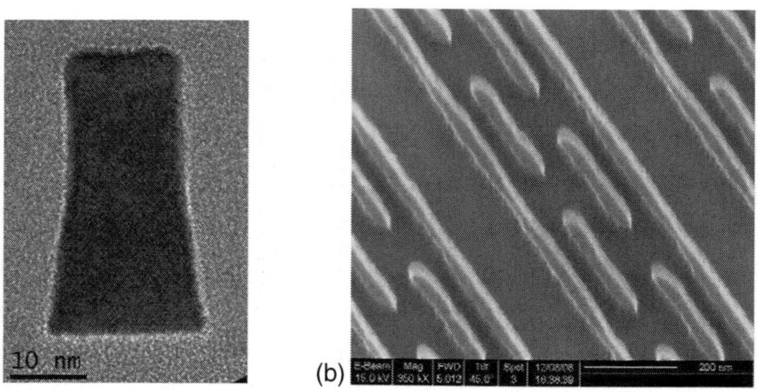

Figure 2.11. (a) TEM cross section after full dry etching fin patterning; the c-Si fin has a bottom tapered shape. (b) Top view SEM inspection after full dry etching fin patterning.

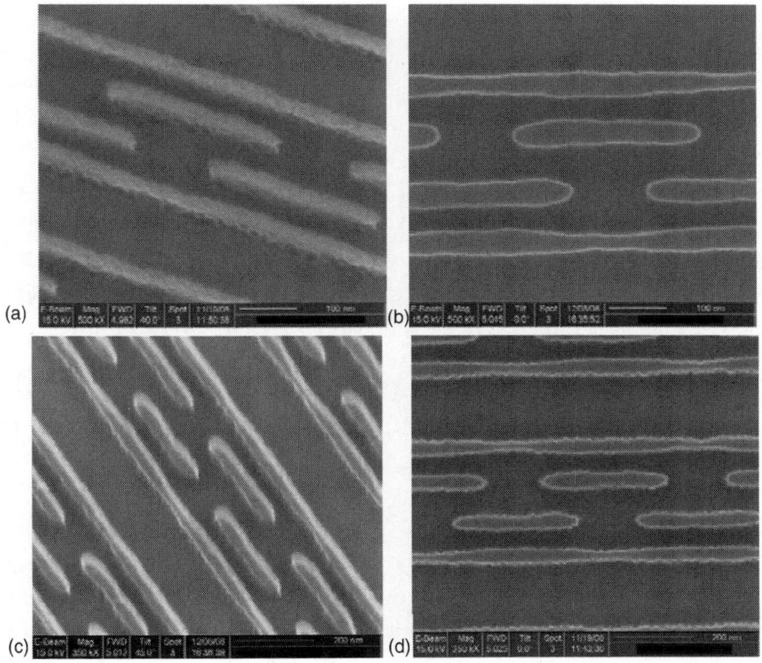

Figure 2.12. Top view SEM inspection after full dry etching fin patterning. (a) and (b) The BOX was exposed to the SL chemistry during 3 s after endpoint. (c) and (d) the BOX was exposed to the SL 7 s after endpoint.

simplicity we decided to discuss them separately in this order: CD tuning, SWR and profile optimization.

2.3.2.1 Fin critical dimension control

As it was previously mentioned, after the BARC opening and tuned PR trim steps, the CD was reduced from 45 to 19 nm, only two nanometers far from the target. However, after the HM patterning, the fin CD increased from 19 to 28 nm, ending up with CDs 11 nm wider than the 17 nm target. It was almost impossible to reach the CD target through the optimization of the HM patterning approach used on the previous 32 nm nodes. Sequential CD SEM measurements indicated that both HM etching steps contribute to this CD increment. 35% of this CD increment was attributed to the Cl_2/O_2

chemistry used during the ACL1 step. This might be understood based on what has been already reported: that etching carbon based layers with Cl_2/O_2 produces a thick sidewall layer of non volatile products such as CCl_x [11]. Nevertheless, the major CD increment (65%) was attributed to the ACL2 step because it is carried out using a highly polymerizing chemistry (CF_4/CH_2F_2) [9, 10].

In order to reach fins with CDs of 17 nm, we decided to avoid polymerizing gases during the ACL HM patterning. Therefore, we switched to a more lean HBr/O_2 chemistry, which mainly results in the formation of very volatile by-products such as CO or CO_2 [12]. The only drawback of etching the ACL in one step is that the DARC (SiOC) has to be removed in a dedicated process without affecting the CD. Therefore, either the initial DARC should be thinner or it has to be thinned down during the etching process.

In view of the above outlined issue, it was decided to reduce the SiOC thickness to 25 nm (going thinner would be adverse for reflection control during the lithography exposure). Finally the ACL patterning was carried out in one single step using HBr/O_2 preserving the CD after PR trim and HM opening. Through these changes it was possible to reach the 17 nm CD target after the HM opening. However, after the c-Si etching the SEM CD measurements revealed a severe line edge roughness (Figure 2.12), which was created by isotropic etching of the sidewalls during the softlanding step. The origin of this problem and how it was solved is presented in the next section.

2.3.2.2 Control of the sidewall roughness

Before optimizing the CD, we found that the SWR problem was partially originated by the ACL non-uniformity thickness. The ACL non-uniformity thickness across the wafer is presented in Figure 2.13. It can be observed that the ACL is 5 nm thinner in the center than at the edge of the wafer. These 5 nm can be crucial for patterning only 40 nm of c-Si. Although the etching process was optimized for having a non uniformity below 5% during the ACL1 step (Figure 2.13), the ACL non-uniformity was impacting the c-Si patterning. From the etching sequence shown in Figure 2.5, it can be seen that the ACL1 step was set up on time; consequently the

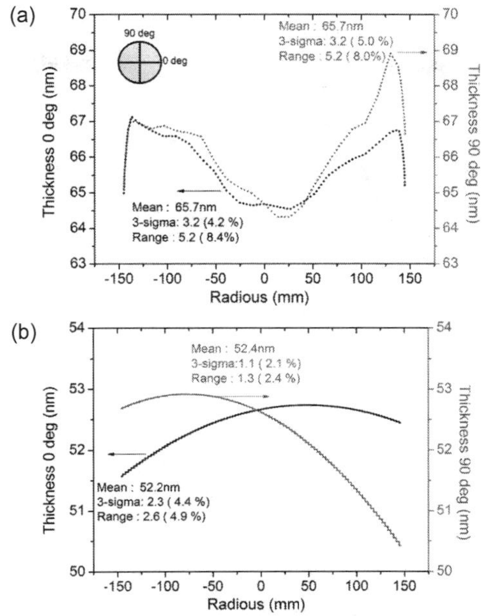

Figure 2.13. Cross section at 0 and 90 degrees of the ellipsometry thickness measurement. a) Uniformity after PECVD ACL deposition, where the center is 5 nm thinner than in the edge of the wafer. b) Uniformity of the dry etching process during the ACL1 step; the etching rate is 78.4 nm with a 3sigma of ~2 nm. See also Color Insert.

non-uniformity of the incoming ACL is transferred from the ACL1 step into the ACL2 step. This last step is not selective to silicon since it is based on fluorine chemistry and therefore the non-uniformity is transferred to the c-Si fin patterning (ME and softlanding steps). Before the CD optimization, we founded a more severe SWR in the center than in the edge of the wafer.

As it was mentioned before, the ME step removes ~80% of the c-Si, where we do not expect a significant contribution to the SWR. We found that the critical step is the softlanding which is based on HBr/O_2 chemistry at 65V bias. The etching time during this step is accurately controlled by endpoint. In order to tune the profile, we applied few extra second after endpoint detection. Actually, these few over-etching seconds were crucial for pulling back the bottom sloped c-Si profile (see Figure 2.6). We detected that instead of correcting the profile this over-etching created a severe SWR. Our interpretation of this problem is explained as follows.

It is generally accepted that the spontaneous reaction of Br with Si is negligible since the assistance of energetic ions is needed for the reaction to proceed [13–16]. The ion assisted chemical reaction of Si with Br has been widely adopted because of its high anisotropy, if this is true then the question here is why the sidewalls are attacked under this plasma conditions when the BOX is exposed. The thermodynamic equilibrium suggests that the spontaneous reaction of Si with Br is possible since the enthalpy of formation of the $SiBr_4$ is −109.3 kcal/mol and the reaction products are highly volatile and stable at room temperature (RT) [15, 16] Furthermore, at "high plasma density" conditions, the $SiBr_4$ desorption is not rate limiting because of the high vapor pressure of $SiBr_4$ (↑$SiBr_4$ gas, °P 10 Torr at RT) [15, 17]. Then the spontaneous reaction is not limited by etching products desorption, but by the Br adsorption and diffusion due to its atomic size and $SiBr_4$ formation [15]. Therefore, the fin sidewalls are not supposed to be etched by Br during the softlanding, because after the c-Si ME the sidewalls are covered with a CxFy polymer layer [18]. This passivation layer should prevent the Br adsorption and diffusion into the c-Si layer.

If the sidewall passivation is not thick enough for withstanding the ion impact of deflected ions during the softlanding, then it can be heavily eroded. The passivation erosion and the c-Si isotropic etching can happen by the combination of two possible mechanisms during the softlanding:

(a) As it will be discuss later, we suppose that a segment of ions cannot reach the bottom of the fins due to an electron shading effect [16]. This means that the negative charging of the inner upper sidewalls (ACL) deflects the ions travelling in its vicinity towards the silicon sidewalls (Figure 2.14). On the other hand, a segment of the incident ions flux is deflected towards the sidewalls due to the positive charge of the new expose area (BOX) [16, 19].
(b) In the presence of this ion bombardment, the oxygen and hydrogen atoms can easily etch the carbon passivation layer. As a consequence, the Si sidewalls are exposed to the Br and H

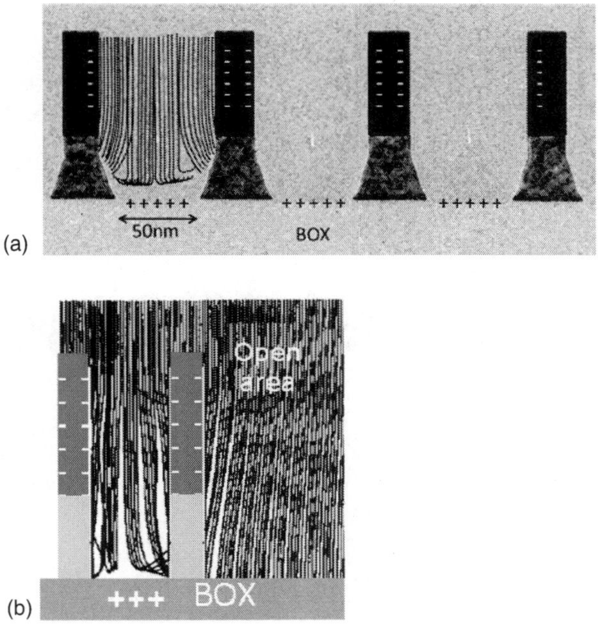

Figure 2.14. Schematic representation of the BOX charging between fins during the softlanding step. (a) The ions are deflected towards the side walls provoking the SWR and tapered profile and (b) and ideal ion deflection towards the bottom of foot of the fins giving a straight profile.

species. In this case under the effect of the deflected ions, the small H atoms can penetrate into the sidewalls and accelerate the isotropic c-Si etching by Br species [17, 20]. We believe that our observations are consistent with the results from Chaung [21], who suggests that in absence of ion bombardment the chlorine atoms covered the silicon surface preventing the H atoms from penetrating into the lattice. It is quite important to mention that the threshold energy for ion enhance etching in HBr is approximately four times higher than the threshold energy for Br_2 plasmas (10 eV and 44 eV, respectively) [17]. The lower threshold energy may be due to the fact that the H atoms penetrate into the film and accelerate the etching. Therefore, ions with energy of 10eV can accelerate the etching of the c-Si fin sidewalls by Br species.

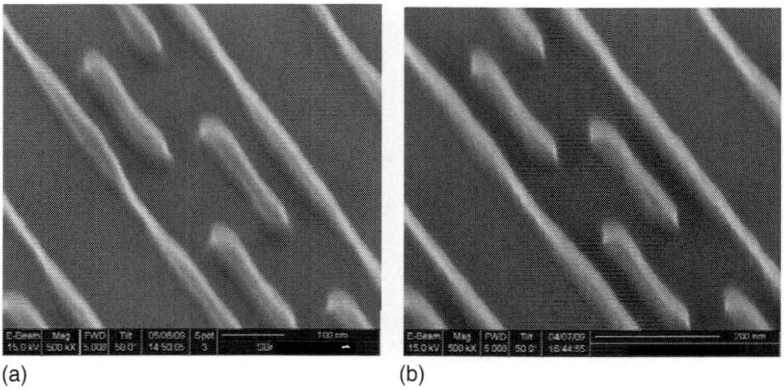

Figure 2.15. Top view SEM image after c-Si fin patterning. (a) Inspection after SL, the process optimization shows smooth side walls after the SL step. (b) Inspection after full dry etching (OE included), the side walls remained smooth.

Once the possible mechanism was understood, the SWR was straightforward solved. The severe SWR in the center of the wafer was reduced when the CD was optimized. This means that the ACL HM was patterned in one single step with high selectivity towards the c-Si. The improved uniformity avoided the premature exposure of the BOX to the HBr/O_2 chemistry during the softlanding mainly in the center of the wafer. Apart from this, the ME was optimized in order to create a thicker sidewall passivation, which can withstand the ion deflection during the softlanding step. After the optimization of the ACL patterning and the c-Si ME, the sidewalls of the fins are smooth as shown in Figure 2.15. Once the SWR was solved, we observed that the fin profile was tapered.

2.3.2.3 Fin profile optimization

In Figure 2.11, we presented the fin profile, which exhibits a bottom tapered shape. We have to mention that the same plasma condition of ME, softlanding and OE steps gave straight fins profiles in larger fin pitches [5–7]. The ME in the current process etches ~80% of the 40 nm c-Si and the profile after this step has a bottom tapered shape (Figure 2.16). The softlanding plasma conditions (8mtorr/350W/–65V/HBr/O_2) have been designed for correcting

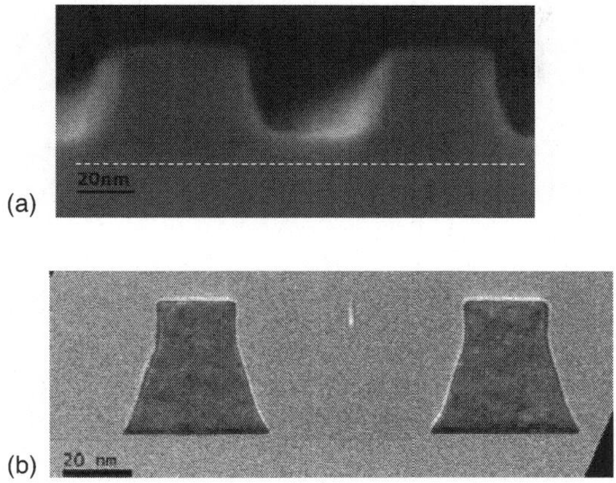

Figure 2.16. (a) SEM cross section after ME, ~85% of the c-Si is removed. The dot line represents the BOX. (b) TEM cross section after the SL on endpoint with 3 s of OE time. The profile after c-Si ME is tapered and after the softlanding the profile is almost the same. This suggests that the softlanding is not correcting the fin profile.

this bottom tapered profile (also called foot). The ion deflection in the softlanding step is the key parameter for correcting this "foot". It is based on the principle of the notching effect, where the charging of the newly exposed dielectric surface deflects ions and subsequently the ions trajectories diverge towards the bottom of the fins [16, 19] (Figure 2.14b).

When the softlanding is extended for 2–3 s after end-point, the profile is corrected due to the notching effect. Nevertheless, according to TEM cross-sections taken after the softlanding, the fin profile had a middle/bottom tapered shape (Figure 2.16). This suggests that the notching effect does not take place at 90 nm pitch using our standard softlanding conditions. These results are not surprising since Nozawa *et al.* [19] experimentally demonstrated that the notching effect is abruptly reduced as the open area decreases. Nozawa explained that "as the open area decreases, the electron shading of the features becomes more significant, and then the electron supply to the sidewalls decreases thereby leading to an increase in the fin potential which brings a decrease in the notching". In Figure 2.17, we present a SEM cross-section of the fins after a long softlanding (10 s in the "notching" zone) in order to determine if the

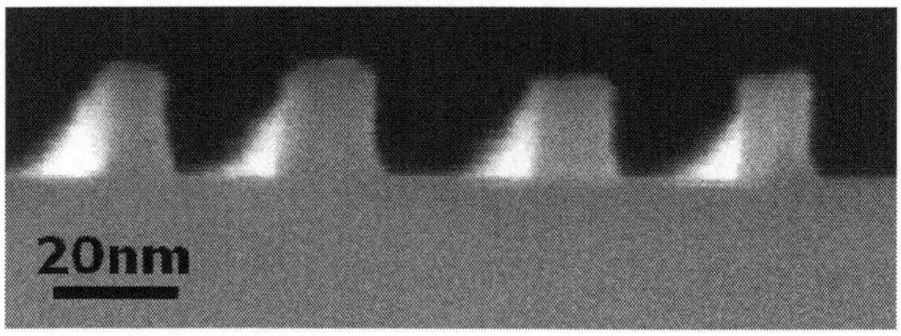

Figure 2.17. Cross SEM of the c-Si after 10 s of SL on the notching zone.

notching effect could happen at extended times at this small pitch. The XSEM revealed that we were unable to create a notch using our standard softlanding plasma conditions, instead it seems that the ion were deflected towards the middle of the fins provoking profile deformation and sidewalls damage.

Since the foot of the fin structures cannot be corrected by the softlanding due to a lack of ion deflection, we stopped the softlanding on endpoint. And, we used the OE (HBr/O_2) step to tune the profile; the advantage of this step is that it is carried out at high pressure and high bias (three times larger than the bias in the standard softlanding) resulting in a very high selectivity towards the BOX and providing high energetic ions that do not deflect prematurely towards the sidewalls'. The higher bias during the OE step enables ions to reach the foot of the fins and correct the profile. In Figure 2.18, the TEM cross-sections illustrate the notch capabilities of the OE step. After the softlanding the profile looks highly tapered. After 10 s of OE step time, the profiles look considerably straighter but still with a visible foot. After 15 s of OE the profile looks straight. If the OE time is extended with 5 s more the notch is clearly visible. These results suggest that the plasma conditions used in the OE step allows the ions to be deflected towards the bottom of the fins instead of towards the sidewalls.

Once this etching process was redeveloped, we were able to fabricate a high yield sub-0.1 μm^2 6T-SRAM cells using high-k/metal gate FinFET devices.

Summarizing, for patterning straight fins with a target CD of 17 nm and with smooth sidewalls, it was necessary to redesign the original stack (decrease the DARC thickness) and redevelop the ACL

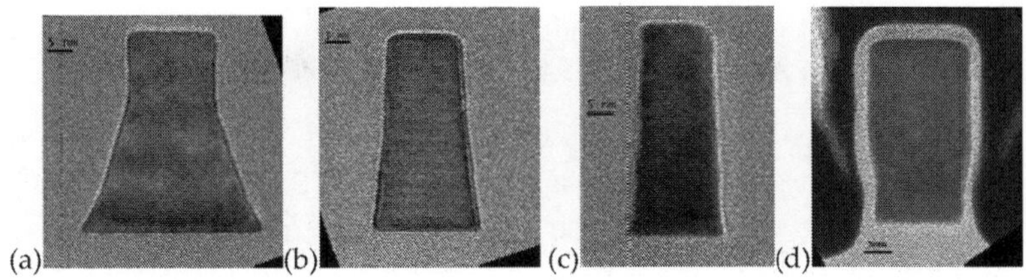

Figure 2.18. TEM cross sections images after soft-landing with different over etching times: (a) 0 s OE, (b) 10 s OE, (c) 15 s OE and (d) 20 s OE.

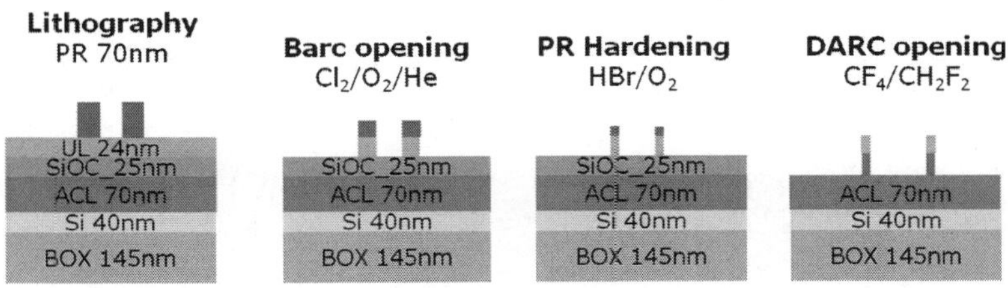

Figure 2.19. Schematic representation of the patterning stack after lithography, BARC opening, PR hardening and DARC opening (90 nm fin pitch).

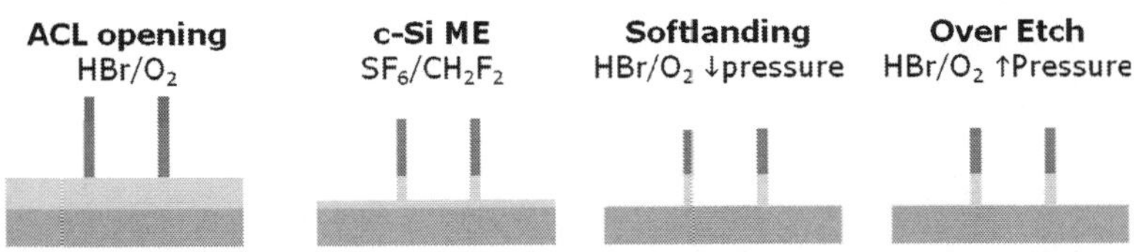

Figure 2.20. Schematic representation of the ACL and c-Si (ME, Softlanding and Over-etching) (90 nm fin pitch).

HM, ME, softlanding and OE steps as shown in Figures 2.19 and 2.20. In order to preserve the CD after DARC opening the two steps ACL opening process were replaced by one step process using an HBr/O_2 plasma chemistry, selective towards c-Si. Straight profiles and the smooth sidewalls were achieved by a good sidewall passivation during the ME and a better control of the ion deflection during softlanding and OE steps.

2.3.3 *Process for Fin Patterning for a Sub-22 nm and 16 nm Node 6T-SRAM Cell (EUVL)*

Above, we presented the dry etching for patterning fins on a 32 nm node (124 nm fin pitch) and a 22 nm node (90 nm fin pitch) cell. We have observed that at these dimensions the dry etching process window was dramatically narrowed. The progress of full field extreme ultraviolet (EUV) scanners makes the exposure of a 16 nm node, in single patterning, possible. As pathfinder for patterning a 16 nm node SRAM cell, imec's EUV alpha demo-tool (ADT) exposed a 80 nm pitch SRAM cell (22 nm node; 0.072 μm^2) allowing dry etching to explore and develop a new patterning strategy for the future 64 nm pitch cell (16 nm node) [22]. The EUV photo resist has different etch resistivity and thickness compared to a 193(i) PR, bringing new challenges for dry etching. In this section we present the dry etching process development for patterning fins on SOI with 15 nm target critical dimension (CD).

One drawback of EUV lithography is the PR budget which is reduced after exposure down to ~50 nm. Figure 2.21 shows the evolution of the lithography stack (PR+BARC or UL), it can be observed that as the fin pitch is scaled down, the PR budget is dramatically reduced.

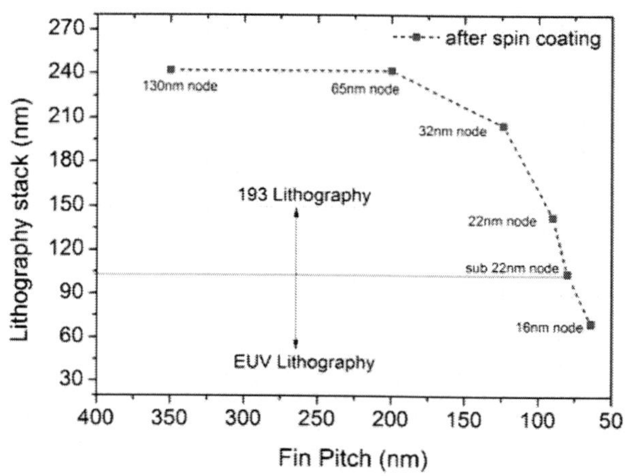

Figure 2.21. Evolution plot of the lithography stack after spin coating. For 193(i), the stack consist of BARC and PR and for the EUVL, the stack consist of UL and PR.

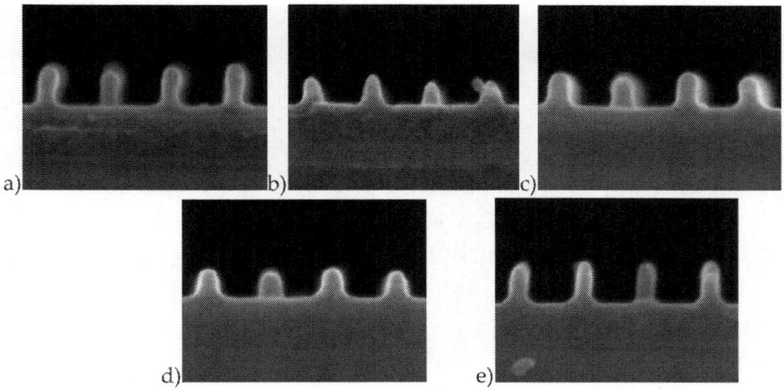

Figure 2.22. PR XSEM pictures of PR height: (a) after exposure (~52 nm), (b) after Cl_2/O_2 UL opening (~42% height reduction), (c) after 30 s of Ar PPT (~23% height reduction), (d) after 30 s HBr PPT (~42% height reduction) and (e) after CH_2F_2/O_2 UL opening (is preserved during transfer). (Scale 100 nm). All these processes were applied to the EUV PR separately.

A low PR budget has implications on the etching process, i.e., the opening of the 24 nm of UL using Cl_2/O_2 or HBr/O_2 chemistries, as we have done it for the previous nodes, seems not to be an option, since the reduced PR height creating a narrow process window for further steps (Figure 2.22b). On the other hand, for the 193i PR nodes, before the DARC opening, we used to apply plasma pretreatment (PPT) using Ar or HBr, which makes the PR more etch resistant. We have observed that during this PPT the PR height decreases due to cross-linking and graphitization effect [11].

After the issues mentioned above, we did not consider to apply any of the PR PPT, because even at short times (<30 s) of PPT the EUV PR height was decreased by ~35% (Figures 2.22c,d). Hence, by avoiding a typical PPT and using a $CF_4/CH_2F_2/O_2$ chemistry for opening the UL, the EUV PR height budget is preserved as much as possible for transferring the pattern into the HM1 (Figure 2.21e). However, even using a high selective chemistry towards the PR for opening the UL, the PR budget is still marginal for patterning 25 nm of SiOC (this thickness was used in the previous 22 nm node, Figure 2.19). One of the main advantages of EUV over 193i lithography is that the patterning stack can be tailored for dry etching because reflection control on EUV lithography (EUVL) is not an issue anymore. Since the thickness of the layers involved on the patterning stack can now be determined by the needs for dry etching, the narrow process window faced in the 22 nm node is considerably opened. Therefore the thickness of the SiOC or HM1 was reduced to 15 nm.

The HM1 opening was carried out using CF_4 chemistry and the proper amount of CH_2F_2 in order to preserve the PR. For the ACL opening we used a lean Ar/O_2 chemistry avoiding any kind of sidewall passivation during this step in order to reach the 15 nm critical dimension target.

In Figure 2.20, it can be observed that the c-Si patterning for the 22 nm node was done using a ME, softlanding and overetch steps. The ME etches ~80% of the c-Si and the profile after this step has a bottom tapered shape. As mention before, the softlanding plasma conditions were designed for correcting this bottom tapered profile, where the ion deflection is the key parameter for correcting this "foot". We have observed that the c-Si patterning is strongly affected by the reduction of the open space between fins. Figure 2.23 shows the evolution of the open space as the fin pitch is scaling down from a 350 nm to 64 nm pitch. We have also observed that the aspect ratio (AR) of the features after the ME may also have an impact on the c-Si patterning, especially during the SL and OE steps [23].

One way to open our process window for patterning the c-Si was to decrease aspect ratio of the features after ME by reducing ACL thickness from 70 nm to 40 nm (Figure 2.22b). We also found that, for the thinner layer of c-Si (30 nm), the SL was no longer needed since the overetch step could correct the fin profile with a high selectivity towards the BOX. In Figure 2.24, we present the TEM cross sections of the fins after dry etching, strip and wet clean.

This dry etching process was fine tuned on the HM1 opening by adjusting the CH_2F_2 flow in order to maintain a good selectivity towards the EUV PR and was used for patterning fins on a SRAM cell (16 nm node; 0.055 μm^2). Summarizing, for patterning straight fins with a target CD of 15 nm, with smooth sidewalls on pitches smaller than 80 nm, it was necessary to redesign the patterning stack (SiOC and ACL thickness) and redevelop the patterning steps such as UL, HM1 and HM2. In order to preserve the CD after HM1

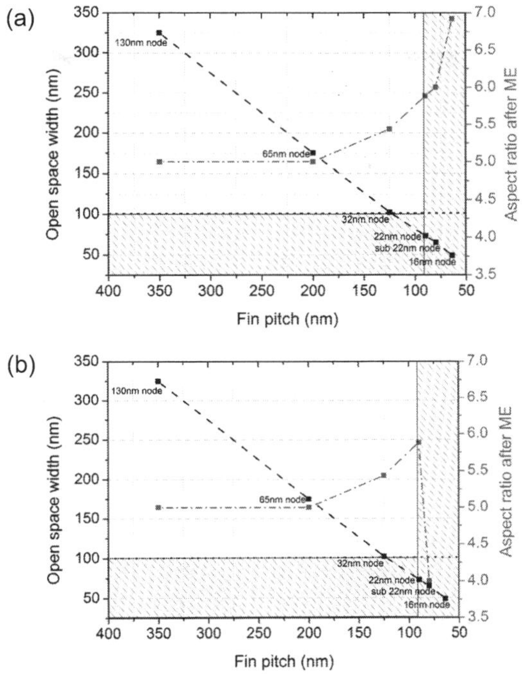

Figure 2.23. Evolution plot of open space between fins as the fin pitch is scaled down. (a) Aspect ratio after ME step (ACL + 80% of the c-Si thickness) maintaining the 70 nm ACL thickness; (b) by decreasing the ACL thickness from 70 to 40 nm, the AR dropped from 6 to 4 for the sub-22 nm node process.

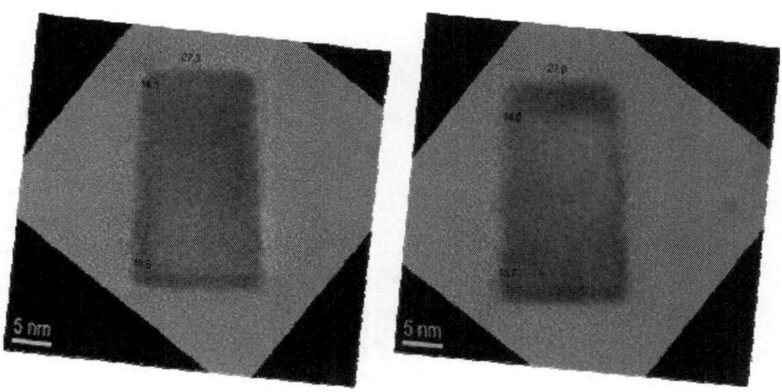

Figure 2.24. TEM profiles of the c-Si fins after dry etching strip and wet clean.

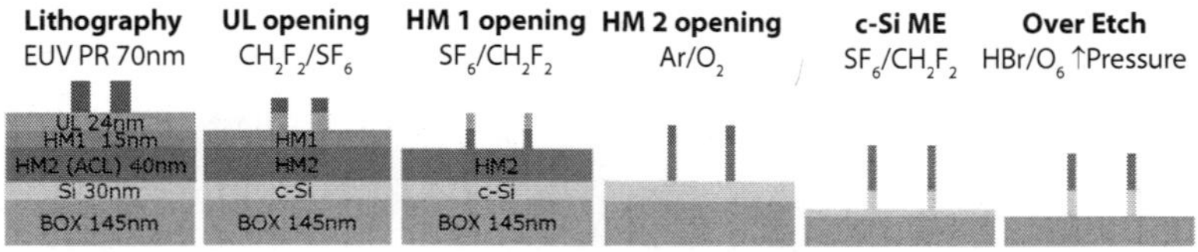

Figure 2.25. A schematic presentation of the final dry etch process.

the ACL opening steps, the use of lean chemistries is needed, i.e., Ar/O_2 chemistry. Straight profiles were achieved by eliminating the softlanding and replacing it by a longer overetch step. This dry etching process reached the CD target of 15 nm with a 3sigma CD uniformity of 3.5 nm. In Figure 2.25, the final dry etching process is sketched.

References

1. M. J. H. van Dal, *et al. ECS Trans,* **13**, (2008), 223.
2. R. J. Shul and S. J. Pearton, *Handbook of Advance Plasma Processing Techniques,* Springer, (2000), pp. 1–32.
3. M. A. Lieberman and A. J. Lichtenberg, *Principles of Plasma Discharges and Materials Processing,* Wiley-Interscience, (2005) pp. 1–22.
4. T. Sugano, *Applications of Plasma Process to VLSI Technology,* Wiley-Interscience, (1985), pp. 25–36.
5. E. Altamirano-Sanchez, *Microelectron. Eng.,* **88**, (2011) 2871–2878.
6. A. Veloso, *et al. IEDM Tech. Digest,* IEEE, 2008, 861–864.
7. A. Veloso, *et al. IEDM Tech. Digest,* IEEE, 2009, 301–304.
8. N. Horiguchi, *et al. Symp. VLSI Tech., IEEE,* 2010, 23–24.
9. S. Arai *et al. Jpn. J. Appl. Phys.* **31**, (1992), 2011–2019.
10. C. K. Park *et al. Microelectron. Eng.,* **85**, (2008), 375–387.
11. E. Paragon *et al. J. Vac. Sci. Technol.* B, **22-4**, (2004), 1869.
12. E. Paragon *et al., J. Vac. Sci. Technol.* B, **23-1**, (2005), 103.
13. S. Tachi and S. Okudaira, *J. Vac Sci. Technol.* B, **4-2**, (1986), 459.
14. C. C. Cheng *et al. J. Vac. Sci. Technol.* B, **14-1**, (1996), 85.
15. J. Pelletier and M. J. Cooke, *J. Vac Sci. Technol.* B, **7-1**, (1999), 59.
16. T. Kinoshita *et al., J. Vac. Sci. Technol.* B, **14-1**, (1996), 1996.

17. A. Steven *et al. J. Vac Sci. Technol.* A, **19-5**, (2001), 2197.
18. O. Luere *et al. Etch Mechanism of Silicon Gate Structures Patterned in $SF_6/CH_2F_2/Ar$* PESM, 2nd International Workshop Leuven, Belgium 2009.
19. Nozawa *et al., Jpn. J. Appl. Phys.* **34**, (1995), 2107.
20. K. M. Tan, *et al. J. Vac. Sci. Technol.* A, **22-4**, (2004), 1500–1505.
21. M. Chuang and J.W. Coburn *J. Vac Sci. Technol.* A, **8-3**, (1990), 1969.
22. E. Altamirano-Sanchez *ECS Trans,* **34(1)**, (2011), 377–382.
23. E. Paragon *et al. J. Appl. Phys.* **105**, (2009), 094902.

Chapter 3

High-*k* Dielectrics and Metal Gate Electrodes on SOI MuGFETs

Isabelle Ferain
Tyndall National Institute, University College of Cork, Ireland
isabelle.ferain@gmail.com

The continuous gate oxide thickness reduction brings the gate stacks to the limit of several atomic layers of dielectric, which causes a dramatic increase in gate tunneling leakage. This gate leakage degradation can be limited by considering gate dielectrics with a higher relative permittivity than SiO_2. In this context, original architectures like the Multiple Gate FETs (MuGFETs) can help to put less stringent requirements on the high-*k* dielectric thickness. In these devices, better channel confinement is obtained by encapsulating the silicon film between two or more gates. Excellent Short Channel Effect control is achieved by reducing the distance between the gates (i.e., thinning the Si film). Therefore, the Short Channel Effect control can be maintained without having to invest considerable effort in thinning the gate dielectric [Lee *et al.* (2007)].

The first section of this chapter covers the processing of high-*k* dielectrics/metal gate electrodes on fully depleted MuGFETs on SOI. The goal is to determine to which extent the integration of such electrodes can help meeting ITRS requirements. A description of

CMOS Nanoelectronics: Innovative Devices, Architectures, and Applications
Edited by Nadine Collaert

ISBN 978-981-4364-02-7 (Hardcover), 978-981-4364-03-4 (eBook)
www.panstanford.com

the gate stack processing is also provided. The second section is dedicated to several methods used for controlling and tuning the work function in MuGFETs with metal gates. In the last section of this chapter a method for work function extraction on SOI MuGFETs is presented. The latter is able to cope simultaneously with the presence of high-k dielectrics and the absence of a bulk contact (SOI). This approach relies on the universality of the dependence between the band structure of a MOSFET and its gate tunneling leakage response.

3.1 Gate Electrodes in MuGFETs

3.1.1 *ITRS Requirements*

For each technology node, standardized values for the threshold voltage V_T are defined for both high performance (HP) and low standby power (LSTP) applications.[1] Obviously, these requirements are independent of the type of architecture considered (standard planar FET or MuGFET) For the 22 nm technology node, $|V_T|$ should reach $\approx$0.15 V for HP applications for both n- and p-type FETs (inversion mode FETs). For LP applications, this requirement becomes $|V_T| = 0.35$ V. These targets are at least 250 mV higher/lower than the experimental V_T measured on undoped MuGFETs with polysilicon gates and an SiO_2-based gate oxide. n-(p-)type MuGFETs exhibit negative (positive) threshold voltages, irrespective of the silicon finger (fin) width W_{fin}.

In order to bring $|V_T|$ closer to the required values on both long and short channel FETs, fin doping may be considered as an option. However it fails in finding an optimum condition (Fig. 3.1) in narrow fins (<20 nm), V_T is almost insensitive to fin doping. In addition, the higher the fin doping, the larger the V_T sensitivity to fin width variations induced by the fin fabrication. Another solution consists in using halo implants. This forces V_T to increase for a limited range of gate lengths. Alas, halo implants also fail in significantly increasing V_T in short-channel FETs, even at gate lengths where the Reverse

[1] http://www.itrs.net/Links/2008ITRS/Home2008.htm.

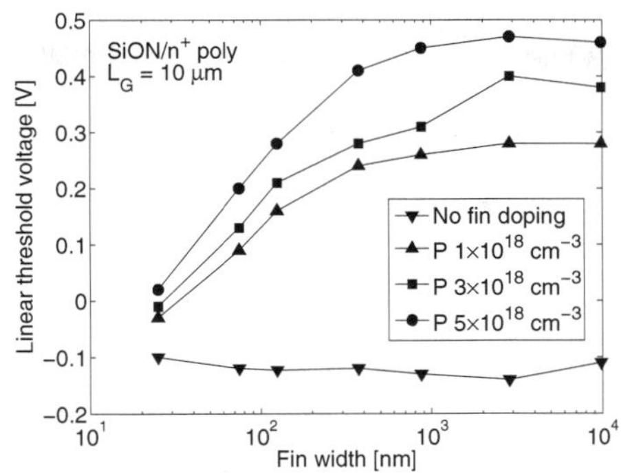

Figure 3.1. Impact of channel doping on $V_{T,Lin}$ as function of fin width, for a n-MuGFET with Silicon oxynitride (SiON)/n^+ polysilicon gate, $L_G = 10$ µm [Collaert *et al.* (2005)].

Short Channel Effect is predominant (Fig. 3.2). For these reasons, the most efficient method for meeting the ITRS requirements is to consider gate electrodes with work functions able to increase $|V_T|$ by 250 to 450 mV. Usually, the range of work functions of interest for planar MOSFETs is defined as 4.65 eV ± 0.55 eV (4.1 eV with a n^+ polysilicon gate, 5.2 eV with a p^+ polysilicon gate). In the MuGFET case, the silicon is undoped but not intrinsic, and a mid-gap work function leads to $\phi_{ms} = -\phi_b$. With the depletion charge

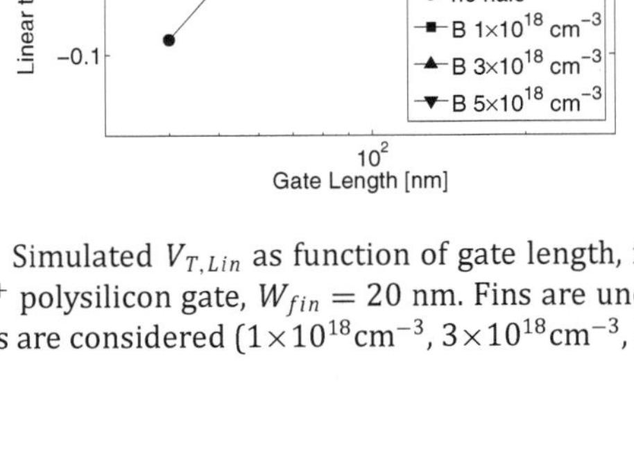

Figure 3.2. Simulated $V_{T,Lin}$ as function of gate length, for a double-gate nFET with n^+ polysilicon gate, $W_{fin} = 20$ nm. Fins are undoped and boron halo implants are considered (1×10^{18}cm^{-3}, 3×10^{18}cm^{-3}, 5×10^{18}cm^{-3}).

being negligible, the threshold voltage of a MuGFET with a mid-gap gate work function can be expressed as:

$$V_T = \phi_b - \frac{\int_0^{t_{ox}} x \cdot \rho(x) dx}{\epsilon_0 \cdot \epsilon_{oxide}} \tag{3.1}$$

which corresponds to a threshold voltage of 0.34 V if the charge stored into the gate oxide is neglected (ρ(x) is the density of charge distributed throughout the oxide.[2]) It must be noted that this expression provides a lower limit to V_T. Note that a surface potential $= 2 \cdot \phi_b$ is assumed but it is actually higher at threshold. Nonetheless, this first-order approximation allows to determine which work functions and thus which metals are the most suitable for HP and LSTP applications:

- $|V_T|$ target for LSTP applications = 0.35 V
  $\rightarrow$ mid-gap gate work function for both n- and p-type MuGFETs;
- $|V_T|$ target for HP applications = 0.5 V
  $\rightarrow$ 4.45 eV gate work function for n-type MuGFETs
  $\rightarrow$ 4.85 eV gate work function for p-type MuGFETs

Although the requirements set on V_T by HP and LSTP applications are the same for both standard planar and MuGFET devices, their conversion in terms of work function requirements differs for these two architectures [De *et al.* (2000)].

3.1.2 *Metal Gates for MuGFETs*

In the present section, narrow fin structures are considered (W_{fin} values of the order of ≈20 nm with a fin height of 70 nm). The gate stack deposition on such structures is divided into several steps. First the gate dielectric, a thin layer of high-*k* material such as $HfSiO_xN_y$ or HfO_2 is deposited. The high-*k* dielectric is deposited on a thin SiO_2 film (also referred to as 'interfacial layer') left after wet chemical processing. Some chemical cleanings leave an interfacial layer whose thickness depends on the wafer orientation if thinner

[2] $\int_0^{t_{ox}} x \cdot \rho(x) dx = Q_{ox} \cdot t_{ox}$ if the charge is uniformly distributed throughout t_{ox}.

Table 3.1. Metal candidates for gate electrodes in MOSFET devices

Elements	Work function (eV)	Elements	Work function (eV)
Hf	3.9	Mo	4.6
Ta	4.25	Ru	4.7
Ti	4.3	Re	4.95
Nb	4.3	Ni	5.15
W	4.55		

than 1 nm [Meuris *et al.* (1995)]. In MuGFETs this can have an impact on the gate oxide thickness uniformity if the upper fin surface and the fin sidewalls are made of two different crystal orientations. A metal layer is then deposited. Unlike planar FETs, metal gates in MuGFETs are kept as thin as possible. This requirement is set by the metal gate etch operation, which is isotropic: the thicker the metal gate, the longer the metal gate patterning and the larger the metal gate undercut under the polysilicon film. In order to limit this undercut, the metal gate thickness is usually limited to approximately 20 nm. After metal gate deposition, a thick layer of undoped polycrystalline silicon is deposited, which smoothens the overall topography.

Several elemental metals exhibit a work function[3] of interest for MuGFET applications (Table 3.1) but metal-like compounds are often preferred. These compounds are usually made of nitrided forms (MoN, TiN, TaN). Since it has been reported that the work function of nitride metal gate electrodes can be adjusted by incorporating various nitrogen contents, they offer more flexibility from a work function tuning point of view [Liu *et al.* (2006)]. Among the nitride metal candidates, titanium nitride (TiN) has been extensively studied as metal gate electrode for MuGFETs. Its bulk properties are well known since it has been long used in microelectronics in back-end of line (BEOL) as a diffusion barrier and also as adhesion layer for tungsten and aluminium interconnects. It presents low resistivity (depending on the deposition technique and conditions) and a mid-gap work function. Moreover, it is compatible with

[3]http://www.hbcpnetbase.com/.

standard CMOS flows from a thermal stability viewpoint. Various deposition techniques are available for depositing thin TiN films but contrarily to the physical vapor deposition (PVD) [Liu *et al.* (2007); Vellianitis *et al.* (2007)], only the metal-organic chemical vapor deposition (MOCVD), the atomic layer deposition (ALD) and the plasma-enhanced ALD (PE-ALD) are expected to ensure conformal metal gate deposition on high aspect ratio Si fins. By 'conformal,' one means that the metal thickness at the top and sidewalls of the fins is the same, even for very tall and narrow fins. In the next paragraphs, an overview of the physical (composition) and electrical characteristics (work function) is summarized for each deposition technique.

3.1.2.1 MOCVD TiN

$Ti[N(CH_3)_2]_4$ (also known as TDMAT or tetrakis (dimethylamino) titanium) is a commonly used organic precursor for the deposition of TiN films. The TiN film is obtained by thermal decomposition of the TDMAT precursor at low temperature ($<400^\circ C$) in order to ensure good step coverage. After deposition, MOCVD TiN films can be subjected to an *in situ* N_2:H_2 RF plasma treatment: it eliminates most of the organic compounds present in the as-deposited film and it crystallizes the TiN film, making it denser and reducing its sheet resistance. Although this plasma step is mandatory for BEOL applications where low sheet resistance is a prerequisite, it cannot guarantee the gate dielectric integrity in FEOL operations. *Ex situ* heat treatments also have a significant impact on the composition of thin MOCVD TiN films. The amount of Ti-C bonds created by the thermal decomposition of the TDMAT precursors can be affected by annealing TiN in N_2 atmospheres [Sun and Tsai (1996); Yun *et al.* (2002)]. Since the work function of the TiN layer depends on its composition, such anneal can modify the TiN work function [Singanamalla *et al.* (2006a)]. Unlike *in situ* plasma treatment, which modifies the TiN crystallites size, *ex situ* slow thermal anneal in N_2 ambient does not significantly decrease the sheet resistance. However, thermal desorption analysis shows that STA is as efficient as plasma treatments in eliminating hydrocarbon compounds without degrading the gate dielectric quality. This elimination of

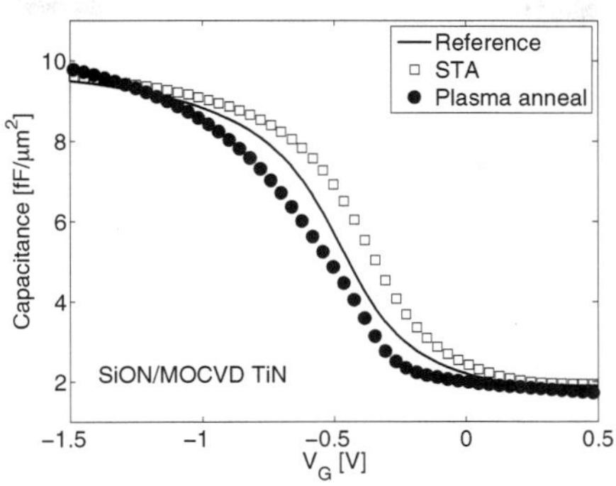

Figure 3.3. Gate capacitance measured on MOS capacitors with MOCVD TiN gates: impact of post-deposition treatments (plasma anneal and STA) [Singanamalla *et al.* (2006a)].

hydrocarbon compounds goes along a V_{fb} decrease with respect to as-deposited TiN samples (Fig. 3.3) [Sun and Tsai (1996)]. This result is consistent with the fact that a reduction in C and N content results into a more metallic TiN film and thus lower metal work function. Carbon and nitrogen have higher electronegativities than Ti and thus higher carbon and/or nitrogen content in the MOCVD TiN film leads to a more p-type work function. On standard planar FETs, it has also been demonstrated that thickness variations of ultra-thin TiN metal gates have a significant impact on the gate work function, irrespective of the deposition method [Singanamalla *et al.* (2006a,c); Choi *et al.* (2005)]. The thinner the TiN film, the more Ti-like the work function will become and the closer the work function will get to 4.33 eV (n-type) (Fig. 3.4). It is attributed to the atomic percentage of Ti at the interface with the gate dielectric and reflects the close relation between work function and composition. It is of importance for very thin metal films where the composition varies significantly until the layer is closed. It has been observed for both MOCVD and ALD TiN thin films. This thickness dependence can have a significant impact on the V_T of MuGFETs where the metal gate must be very thin in order to ensure gate integrity during the gate patterning. The origin of this effect is assumed to be the same for both MOCVD and ALD TiN. It is further explained in the ALD TiN case.

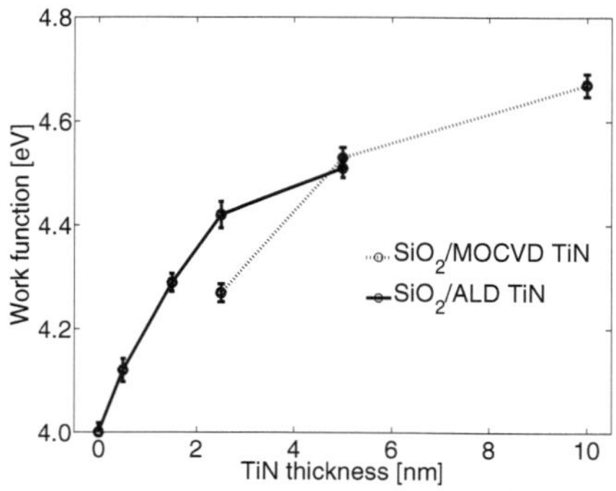

Figure 3.4. Gate work function as a function of the MOCVD and ALD TiN thickness, measured on MOS capacitors with SiO_2/MOCVD or ALD TiN/n^+ polysilicon gates after 520°C Forming Gas Anneal (FGA) and 1050°C spike anneals on all samples.

3.1.2.2 ALD TiN

Like MOCVD TiN layers, atomic layer-deposited TiN films have been developed for advanced interconnect applications. For films thicker than 20 nm, atomic layer deposition (ALD) is a process which guarantees highly uniform and conformal layers. The film thickness is controlled by the number of reaction sequences. The ALD mechanism consists in alternating exposures of a surface to vapors of two chemical reactants. For TiN film formation, one deposition cycle consists in alternating pulses of ammonia (NH_3) and titanium tetrachloride ($TiCl_4$) for instance. The reaction between these precursors is thermally activated and at a deposition temperature <500°C. Similar to the MOCVD technique, which requires enough flux of precursors, the ALD technique requires a minimum amount of deposition cycles in order to guarantee the formation of a continuous and homogeneous TiN film. In the specific case of TiN films thinner than 10 nm, their composition is expected to vary significantly as a function of the film thickness. In order to assess the impact of such variations on V_T, the work function has been estimated for a broad range of ALD TiN thicknesses [Singanamalla *et al.* (2006c)]. A gradual increase in work function is observed when the TiN thickness increases until it reaches ≈5 nm (Fig. 3.4).

This modification is explained mainly by the evolution of the work function as a function of the TiN film thickness and composition, more than by fix charge variations.

The absence of gate depletion (not shown) suggests that even ultra-thin and non-continuous ALD TiN layers can screen the polysilicon electrode from a work function viewpoint. The gate work function reaches then a constant value which is representative of the bulk TiN work function only. Unlike planar MOSFETS, very thin metal gates (from 2 to 20 nm) are usually deposited in a MuGFET process flow. The dependence of the work function on the metal gate thickness is thus critical for these devices.

3.1.2.3 PE-ALD TiN

PE-ALD inherits some remarkable properties from the ALD technique: self-limiting film growth, accurate thickness control and excellent step coverage [Park and Kang (2004); Elers *et al.* (2005)]. PE-ALD TiN deposition is usually carried out with $TiCl_4$, N_2 and H_2 precursors. Lower deposition temperature than ALD is allowed while higher growth rate is achieved. In return, some limitations due to the additional degree of freedom that plasma offers are observed: increased complexity in process control and modification of the gate dielectric composition [Ferain *et al.* (2009)]. It has been observed that the nitrogen profile in the dielectric stack is strongly dependent on the gate treatment: gate dielectrics onto which TiN is deposited reveal a nitrogen profile which varies along with the duration of the PE-ALD process. An extended study of PE-ALD TiN electrodes on MuGFETs is provided in 3.2.4.2.

Two competing mechanisms can explain the work function dependence on the PE-ALD TiN thickness:

- Thick metal gates (thicker than 20 nm): the TiN composition does not vary substantially as a function of the film thickness. Variations in the gate dielectric composition affect the bonding distribution at the metal/dielectric interface [Hobbs *et al.* (2003)], which defines the effective work function.

- Thin metal gates (5 to 2 nm): in this case, variations in the TiN composition are the main factor that contributes to lowering the gate work function, similarly to the ALD TiN case [Singanamalla *et al.* (2006c)].

3.1.3 *Gate Stack Processing*

In order to avoid periodical variations of the gate width after polysilicon patterning, an etch-back operation can be performed directly after the deposition of a thick polysilicon layer [Degroote *et al.* (2006)]. The latter consists in a partial and uniform removal of polysilicon all over the wafer. Although it does not suppress the variations in topography at the polysilicon level, it later contributes to a substantial reduction in thickness variations of the photoresist deposited on polysilicon [Colinge (2008)].

3.1.3.1 Pattern transfer

After deposition of the multiple layered components of the gate stack, the gate area is defined by lithography and patterned. This way of proceeding is referred to as 'direct patterning' or 'gate first approach' since the final dimensions of the gate stack are defined and patterned directly after its deposition. Although it could guarantee better gate stack integrity, a replacement gate or 'gate-last approach' is usually not considered in the case of MuGFET devices. The removal of the dummy gate (usually made of polysilicon) used to define the junction regions and its replacement at the end of the FEOL processing is particularly difficult to remove selectively over the gate dielectric and/or the Si substrate. Therefore, the direct gate etch process is preferred. The purpose of the following sections is to highlight the steps specific to MuGFET patterning.

3.1.3.2 Polysilicon patterning

On MuGFETs, a hard mask is deposited, which consists of a thick oxide, onto which an Anti-Reflective Coating layer is deposited. The latter is covered by photoresist. These three layers form the mask used to define the gate dimensions. A hard mask (oxide, Advanced Patterning Film (APF)) needs to be considered since the photoresist alone would be attacked during the polysilicon etching. After pattern transfer by lithography, both the hard mask and the photoresist can be trimmed in order to define critical dimensions shorter than defined on the mask. This trimming operation is followed by a photoresist strip. At this point, the whole gate stack of planar MOSFETs is generally etched in one anisotropic step. This is no longer applicable to MuGFETs where the polysilicon etch and the metal etch need to be performed separately. With MuGFET devices, the polysilicon patterning is performed as follows:

- Main etch step: anisotropic etching of 80% of the polysilicon, the chemistry involved does not allow selective removal towards metal;
- Soft landing step: polysilicon removal with enhanced selectivity towards metal. Because this operation does not ensure a complete selectivity towards metal, the metal may already be attacked by this operation. Accurate estimation of the optimal duration of this step is therefore critical. This estimation relies on end-point detection based on emission spectrum analysis during polysilicon patterning. This end-point detection needs to be optimized for gate stacks with high-*k* dielectrics. Otherwise, the soft landing step may be too short and leave a 'foot' of polysilicon at the bottom of the polysilicon film (Fig. 3.5(a)), or too long and result in a notch into the polysilicon base. Both effects impose a limitation on the gate length scaling of the device whose ideal polysilicon profile should be straight (Fig. 3.5(b)).
- Over-etch step: this additional polysilicon etching is specific to MuGFETs. Its root cause lies in the large polysilicon thickness variations between the top of the Si fins and the buried oxide level. In dense multiple-fin structures where the distance between fins is in the same order of magnitude as the fin height, the polysilicon thickness at the fin sidewalls is much thicker than on the upper fin surface. Therefore, main etch and soft landing steps are not sufficient to remove the polysilicon left on the sidewalls of the Si fins, outside the gate area. To remove this polysilicon spacer (Fig. 3.6), a short additional anisotropic etch needs

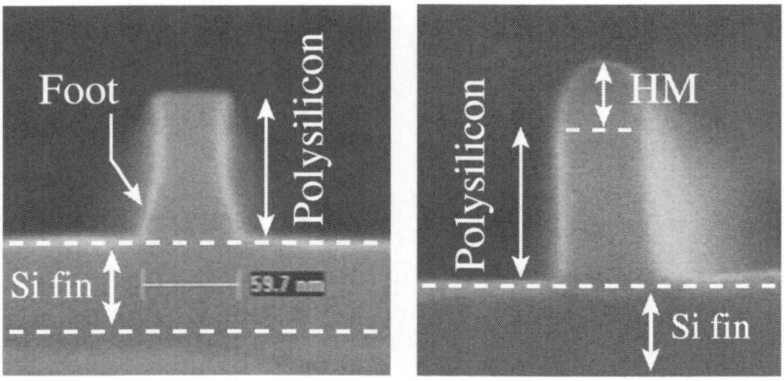

(a) (b)

Figure 3.5. Cutline along the Si fin: (a) polysilicon profile with foot at the bottom, (b) straight polysilicon profile.

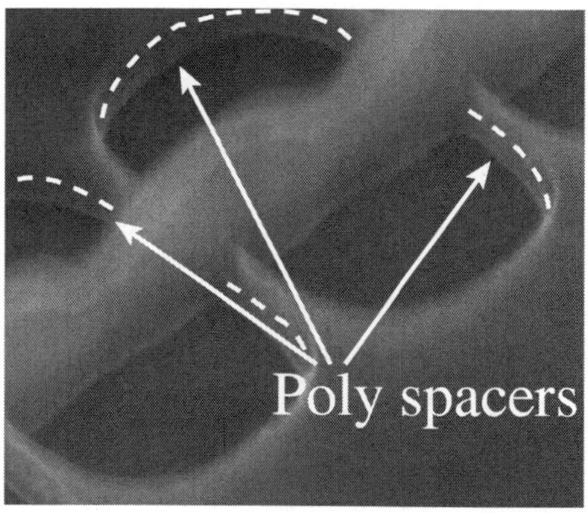

Figure 3.6. HR-TEM micrograph of a multiple-fin MuGFET prior to the polysilicon over etch operation. Markers indicate polysilicon spacers left on the fin sidewalls between the gate and source/drain regions.

to be carried out. Residues of polysilicon compounds left by the patterning can be removed by an organic solvent strip.

3.1.3.3 Hard mask removal

Prior to the metal gate etching, the hard mask removal operation is performed in a diluted hydrofluoric acid (HF) solution. Naturally, the polysilicon gate is also immersed in this HF chemistry. This operation is critical and can affect the gate stack integrity. The diluted hydrofluoric acid solution triggers a galvanic corrosion reaction in systems where the gate stack is formed by materials with very different electronegativities like undoped polysilicon/metal. This reaction is even more enhanced in the MuGFET case where the hard mask is removed when the surface ratio between the polysilicon film and the metal film is favorable to galvanic corrosion. Due to its complexity, this effect and its consequences on the gate's integrity are addressed in 3.1.4.

3.1.3.4 Metal Gate patterning

Chemistries developed for polysilicon gate etch are not necessarily optimal for metal gate etch. In the specific case of TiN gates, BCl_3 and SF_6-based chemistries have been investigated for plasma etching. Both chemistries produce chlorine species which form volatile compounds with the metal. They etch the metal isotropically and can remove $HfSiO_xN_y$ selectively over the Si substrate. An undesired consequence of this isotropy is the lateral removal under the poly gate [Demand *et al.* (2005)]. This undercut must be reduced as much as possible by implementing thin metal layers and by performing a less isotropic etch. For this reason, BCl_3/Cl_2 and SF_6/O_2-based chemistries are preferred since they reduce the lateral metal etch rate by forming a passivating layer on the sidewalls. This layer compensates for the lateral etch and almost straight metal gate profiles can be obtained. Such passivating layers have been shown to be water soluble and are easily removed by water rinse afterwards [Shamiryan *et al.* (2007)].

3.1.4 *Polysilicon Corrosion*

It has already been reported that the immersion in HF-diluted solutions causes the degradation of polysilicon films [Miller *et al.* (2007)]. Due to an electrochemical corrosion process, the polysilicon layers become porous at their surface. This effect is referred to as 'galvanic corrosion' since it results from an oxidation-reduction reaction triggered by the galvanic cell formed by the gate layers and the HF solution. Depending on the severity of such a degradation, the mechanical and electrical properties at the edges of the polysilicon layers can be substantially modified. Therefore, the gate properties are dependent on the gate length of the transistor.

3.1.4.1 Polysilicon corrosion enhancing factors

A galvanic cell is formed when two materials with very different electronegativities are in contact and are immersed into an electrolytic solution. In the specific case of a MOSFET process flow, such galvanic cell is created during the oxide hard mask removal after polysilicon patterning. The contact between two electrodes which show a large electronegativity difference leads to the corrosion of the less electronegative one. The electrolytic solution is formed by the HF chemistry diluted in water with the oxygen dissolved in that solution acting as an oxidizing agent. Once the removal of the oxide hard mask removal in diluted HF is started, the oxygen from this layer dissolves into the solution. The difference in electronegativity between the polysilicon and the metal acts as an external bias which drives this 'oxygen-based' current between the two layers. Since the polysilicon presents the lowest electronegativity in this galvanic cell, the electron current flows from the polysilicon layer to the metal [Garaud *et al.* (2008)]. The magnitude of the corrosion current depends on the concentration of oxygen dissolved in the ionic solution, the polysilicon doping concentration and the type of metal gate, and the surface ratio between the electrodes [Garaud *et al.* (2008); Michaelson (1978)].

The galvanic current is negligible in the case of planar FET structures where the electrode surface ratio is 1:1 during hard mask removal (Fig. 3.7 (left)) [Garaud *et al.* (2008)]. However, the two-step gate patterning in the MuGFET fabrication leads to an unfavorable surface anode/cathode ratio (Fig. 3.7 (right)). Indeed, the Si fins are totally covered by the metal film during the oxide hard mask removal. For a cathode surface significantly larger than the anode surface, the galvanic current can increase by more than one order of magnitude. For this reason, the negative impact of galvanic corrosion is expected to be more significant on MuGFET devices. In addition, if the polysilicon gate is still undoped at this stage of

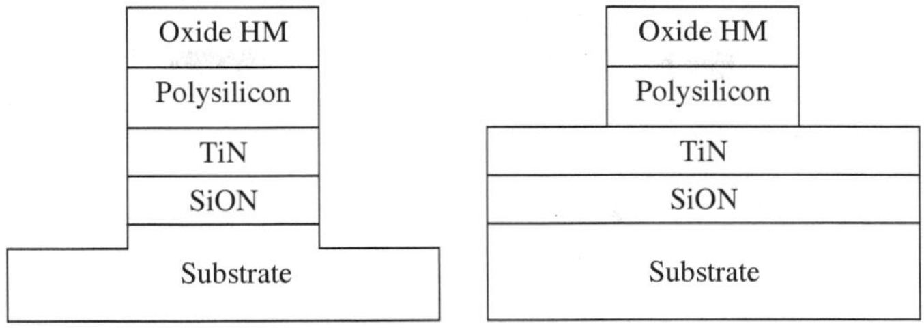

Figure 3.7. Schematics of the gate stack prior to the oxide hard mask removal: (left) planar MOSFETs after complete stack etching, (right) MuGFETs after polysilicon patterning.

the processing, the electronegativity difference between the metal and the polysilicon films is even more important than in a planar FET fabrication where *in situ* doped polysilicon gates are usually considered.

3.1.4.2 Impact on device scalability

In corroded MuGFETs, the edges of the metal gate are no longer covered by polysilicon after hard mask removal. This causes the edges of the metal gate to be etched away during the metal gate patterning operation. As the severity of the corrosion phenomena increases, the amount of short and working devices decreases. The polysilicon corrosion is thus limiting the scalability of MuGFETs. In the next paragraphs, three levels of polysilicon corrosion are compared:

- Sample (a) is a reference device which is 'corrosion free.' The hard mask is removed after spacer formation in a 0.5% HF solution (8 min).
- Sample (b) presents a high degree of polysilicon corrosion. The hard mask removal is carried out prior to spacer formation and the 0.5% HF-diluted solution is air saturated.
- In sample (c), the hard mask removal is performed in a quiescent 0.5% HF-diluted solution with lower oxygen content, prior to spacer formation.

Table 3.2. Effective gate length as extracted from morphological (TEM) analysis

L_{Mask}= 0.25 μm	L_G from TEM analysis
Sample (a)	0.155 μm
Sample (b)	no TiN left
Sample (c)	0.115 μm

In order to extract the effective gate length L_G of the samples, transmission electron microscopy (TEM) imaging was performed on MuGFETs with large fins and short gate length ($L_{Mask} = 0.25$ μm, with L_{Mask} being defined as the length designed on the optical reticle for gate definition). The effective gate length is extracted from the TEM micrographs (Fig. 3.8) and is listed for each sample in Table 3.2. In the most corroded sample, at least 155 nm of TiN is removed as a consequence of the polysilicon degradation. It is thus expected that electrical features like the threshold voltage and the gate leakage will be dramatically affected by the TiN degradation even at gate lengths exceeding 0.25 μm.

3.1.4.3 Impact on threshold voltage

The V_T vs. L_G dependence of n- and MuGFETs is illustrated in Fig. 3.9(a) and 3.9(b), respectively. Two important features must be noted: First, the enhanced galvanic corrosion of polysilicon in Sample (b) causes a strong V_T increase at short gate length, for both n- and p-type MuGFETs. Even long-channel nFETs are affected by this V_T increase. This observation is consistent with the TEM analysis and indicates that such V_T deviation-even on long devices-can only arise from a modification of the metal and gate oxide (not from the polysilicon degradation only); Secondly, the concentration of oxygen dissolved in the electrolytic solution is a key factor in the transmission of the galvanic current. Low oxygen containing HF-diluted solutions (Sample (c)) cause much less degradation of the V_T vs. L_G trend than oxygen containing mixtures dispensed by spray (Sample (b)). Furthermore, a comparable distribution (3σ error) is observed for the reference (Sample (a)) and for Sample (c) (Low oxygen containing solution). This electrical result is in line with the gate oxide thickening and degradation of the Si/gate oxide interface

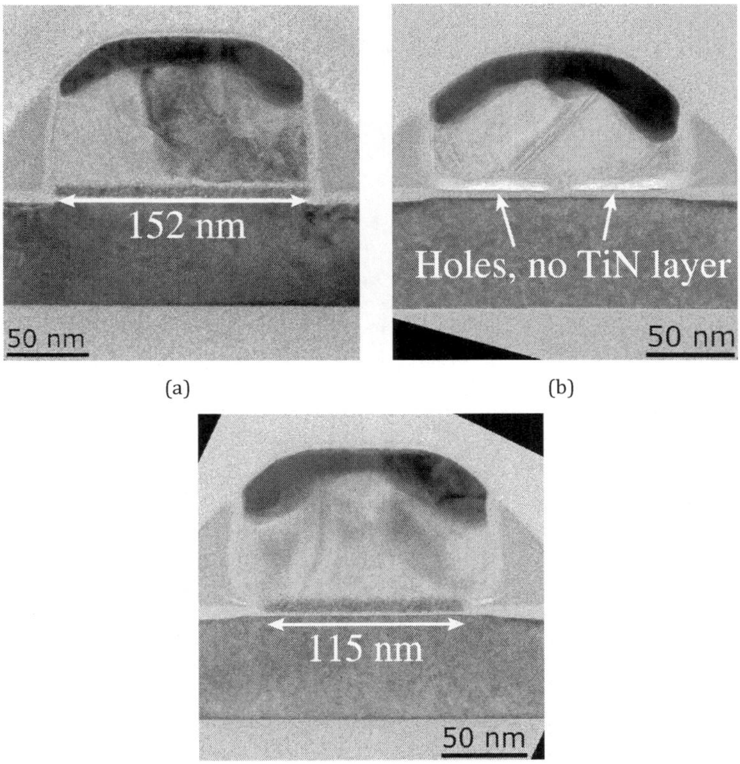

(a) (b) (c)

Figure 3.8. TEM micrographs of MuGFETs: cutline along the Si fin; Sample (a): $L_G = 152$ nm, which is 20 nm shorter than the physical gate length measured after gate patterning (thus including effects of resist trimming and isotropic gate etch), Absence of TiN in Sample (b), indicating that at least 155 nm of TiN is removed, Sample (c): evidence of TiN undercut as compared to Sample (a).

observed by TEM imaging. It suggests that the polysilicon corrosion triggers not only a serious degradation of the metal gate but also of the gate oxide.

Note that the operation of resist stripping is unlikely to cause the removal of more than 155 nm TiN at the gate edge. n-MuGFETs processed either in a unichannel or a CMOS flow suffer from the same degree of corrosion, dependent on the chemistry used for oxide hard mask removal.

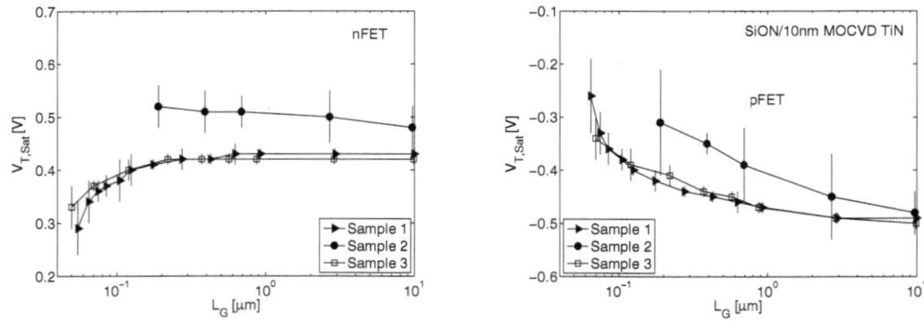

(a) (b)

Figure 3.9. Threshold voltage versus gate length for (a) n- and (b) p-MuGFETs (Sample (a): reference sample without hard mask removal, Sample (b): most corroded sample with hard mask removal in air saturated HF-diluted solution and Sample (c): corroded sample with hard mask removal in low oxygen containing HF-diluted solution).

In order to avoid the polysilicon corrosion and its consequences, three options can be considered: In the first option, the oxide hard mask used for polysilicon patterning is removed after the spacer deposition. In this case, a second spacer deposition is required after hard mask removal to compensate for the recess that it causes. In the second option, the oxide hard mask removal is performed after the polysilicon patterning, in a quiescent and low oxygen containing diluted HF solution. Of course, this limits the degree of freedom for the equipment choice. A last option is to keep the oxide hard mask in order not to expose the polysilicon to the selective epitaxy (SEG) if raised source and drain are implemented. If the polysilicon is completely encapsulated between the oxide hard mask and the spacers, the risk of Si overgrowth is avoided (Fig. 3.10(a)). Otherwise, this overgrowth short-circuits the source/drain and gate regions (Fig. 3.10(b)).

3.2 Multiple-V_T Implementation

3.2.1 *Introduction*

In fully depleted devices such as the narrow MuGFETs, V_T is primarily set by the electrode work function. Mid-gap metal gates

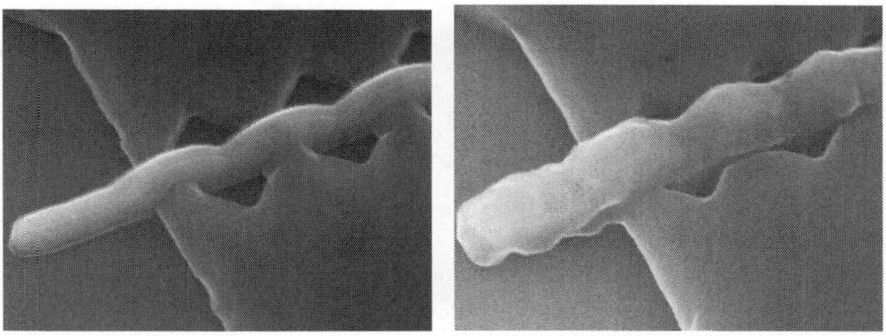

Figure 3.10. SEM micrographs of n-MuGFETs after Si Selective Epitaxial Growth: (a) reference sample with the polysilicon gate still covered by the oxide hard mask during the SEG operation, no additional growth of Si observed on the top surface of the polysilicon film; (b) sample without hard mask during the SEG operation, resulting in a complete Si overgrowth on the gate

allow symmetrical V_T but the absolute value of V_T is too large ($\approx$0.35 V) for HP applications: it causes too low on-state leakage as the power supply voltages scale down. As such, it limits the minimum gate length that one technology node can afford [Chang *et al.* (2000)]. For this reason, CMOS-dedicated solutions are investigated in order to implement, within the same fabrication flow, low (absolute)-V_T with metal gate electrodes. From a conceptual point of view, the dual-metal gate processing is the easiest way to obtain the correct V_T for n- and pFETs [Lu *et al.* (2000)]. It consists in the implementation of metal gates with different work functions, depending on the type of FET: $\phi_m = 4.45$ eV for nFETs and $\phi_m = 4.85$ eV for pFETs. However, in a CMOS process flow, the removal of the first metal layer selectively towards the gate oxide, prior to the second metal layer deposition, is a very sensitive operation as shown in Fig. 3.11. This removal procedure compromises the gate oxide integrity. Different approaches can be developed for modifying V_T with a single metal gate:

- The body of the Si fin can be doped by ion implantations in order to lower ϕ_b, with a limited impact on the depletion charge Q_d;

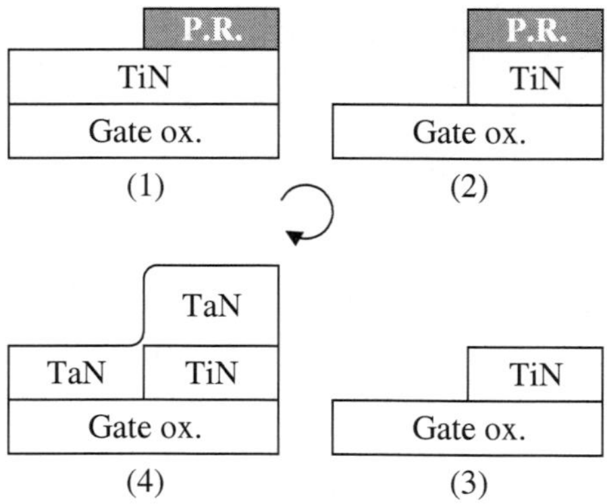

Figure 3.11. Illustration of the fabrication flow for dual metal gate integration. 'PR' stands for 'PhotoResist.'

- Due to the work function sensitivity to the metal/dielectric interface, a modification of the interface either by implantation of As species (for nFETs), by gate dielectric nitridation or by deposition of a rare-earth material-based dielectric cap can be implemented in order to set the correct ϕ_{ms} for n- and pFETs;
- Tuning the metal gate work function ϕ_m by modifying its composition either by inserting a rare-earth oxide or by varying its thickness or by metal inter-diffusion [Matsukawa *et al.* (2007)].

Most of the techniques presented in this section have already been successfully implemented and extensively characterized on planar MOSFETs. However, the MuGFET architecture and the topology of MuGFET-based applications render the implementation of these techniques more difficult. In this section, several solutions for tuning V_T on MuGFETs with a single mid-gap metal gate are presented. For each method, the impact on the device performance (threshold voltage V_T, on-state current I_{on}, off-state current I_{off}, low-field mobility is analyzed and, as far as characterization techniques can enable it, correlated with physical analysis of the gate stack. A fabrication scheme is also proposed for CMOS integration where experimental CMOS material is not available. Naturally, similarities and differences with planar MOSFET-based implementations are highlighted.

3.2.2 *Channel Modification*

Modifying V_T can be achieved either by doping the channel of the MuGFET or by increasing the amount of fixed oxide charge in the dielectric. Obviously, the latter is not an option since it would severely degrade the low-field channel mobility and will also affect the saturation velocity. Naturally, this is detrimental for the intrinsic performance of the device. The impact of channel doping on the device performance has been experimentally evaluated in a CMOS MuGFET process flow where the degree of sensitivity of V_T to W_{fin} variations and to the implantation dose is assessed.

3.2.2.1 Experimental conditions

The fabrication flow considered for this experiment is described in [Collaert *et al.* (2005)]. Prior to the gate definition, boron ion implantation (B) is performed in order to selectively dope the channel of n-MuGFETs (pFET-dedicated Si regions are covered by photoresist). This implant is expected to make the channel region less n-type and thus increase V_T (absolute value). This option enables the implementation of medium V_T ($\approx$0.35 V) in the case of MuGFETs with low work function gate electrodes ($q \cdot \phi_m$ = 4.1 eV). Since the ion implantation is not performed prior to the Si patterning operation, a double-quadrant implantation with a 7° tilt is considered in order to avoid shadowing by the Si fins themselves. Similarly, a double-quadrant arsenic (As) implantation is carried out after appropriate covering of the nFET-dedicated Si regions by photoresist. Various implantation doses are considered for both As and B implantations: 1×10^{12}, 3×10^{12}, 5×10^{12}, 1×10^{13} and 5×10^{13} cm^{-2}. For the reference, MuGFETs are processed without any ion implantation in the channel. All MuGFETs are subjected to a final rapid thermal anneal at 1050°C.

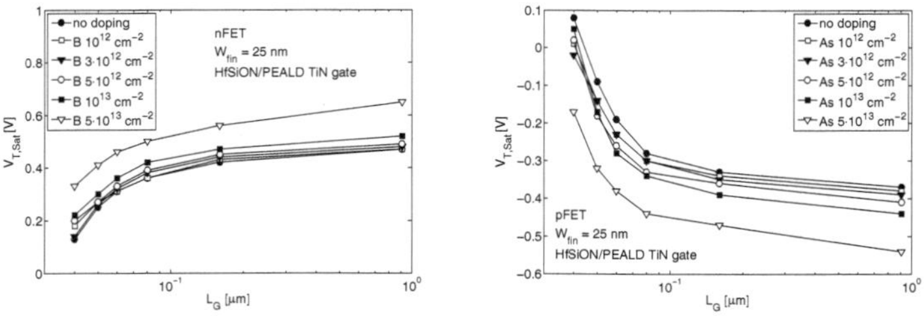

(a) (b)

Figure 3.12. Saturation threshold voltage measured on narrow (W_{fin} = 25 nm) MuGFETs as a function of the gate length: (a) nFETs, (b) pFETs.

3.2.2.2 V_T and W_{fin} dependence

The $V_{T,Sat}$ behavior as a function of gate length is illustrated in Fig. 3.12 for n- and p-MuGFETs. On long-channel nFETs, for instance, Fig. 3.12(a) a very limited V_T increase is seen even when the highest boron dose is implanted (maximum ΔV_T ≈180 mV). There are two reasons for this: First, the carrier concentration in the Si substrate after activation, N_{sub}, is lower in narrow Si fins than in planar Si substrates when the same implantation dose is considered. This can be attributed to several effects: reflection of the implanted species at the Si/ambient interface, back-scattering from within the Si fin and target re-sputtering when the ions collide with the Si outer interface [Duffy (2008)]. Second, a V_T dependence on the Si fin width has been reported [Francis *et al.* (1994)]. This can also explain the reason why a lower ΔV_T is achieved in narrow fin structures as compared to planar ones, even with the same N_{sub} (Fig. 3.13):

$$\Delta V_T = \frac{q \cdot N_{sub} \cdot \Delta W_{fin}}{2 \cdot C_{ox}} \qquad (3.2)$$

3.2.2.3 Device performance

Although channel doping is not a viable option for tuning V_T in narrow MuGFETs, medium implantation doses can still be used for fine-tuning V_T. As such, it is interesting to note that channel doping does not result into any performance loss for doses up to 1×10^{13} cm^{-2}. This observation is consistent with the fact that channel

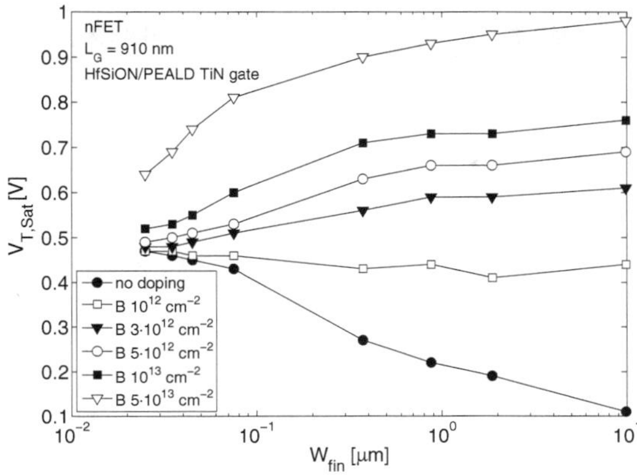

Figure 3.13. $V_{T,Sat}$ as a function of the fin width on long ($L_G = 910$ nm) MuGFETs for various channel implantation doses.

doping does not interfere with the Capacitive Equivalent Thickness, which remains the same for all samples. In addition channel doping degrades the low-field channel mobility at low inversion charge (due to enhanced coulomb scattering in the channel) but does not degrade it substantially at high inversion. However a significant performance degradation is observed for high doses. It is attributed to dopant segregation at the Si interface after the final activation. It has been reported for both boron and arsenic species [Shima *et al.* (2001); Steen *et al.* (2007)] and can possibly explain why the gate capacitance characteristic is degraded in MuGFETs subjected to the highest implantation dose (illustrated for nFETs in Fig. 3.14(a), also observed for pFETs (not shown)). Indeed, dopant segregation may result into a degradation of the Si/SiO_2 interface quality, which, in return, results in reduced gate capacitance and lower channel mobility even at high inversion charge (Fig. 3.14(c)). This is not observed in quasi-planar (very large fins), which confirms the importance of the role played by the ratio between the interface surface and the Si volume (Fig. 3.14(b) and Fig. 3.14(d)). Substantial modification of V_T by significantly increasing the carrier concentration into the substrate is therefore not compatible with the targeted performance. This is also illustrated in Fig. 3.15 where a degradation in performance is observed with the highest

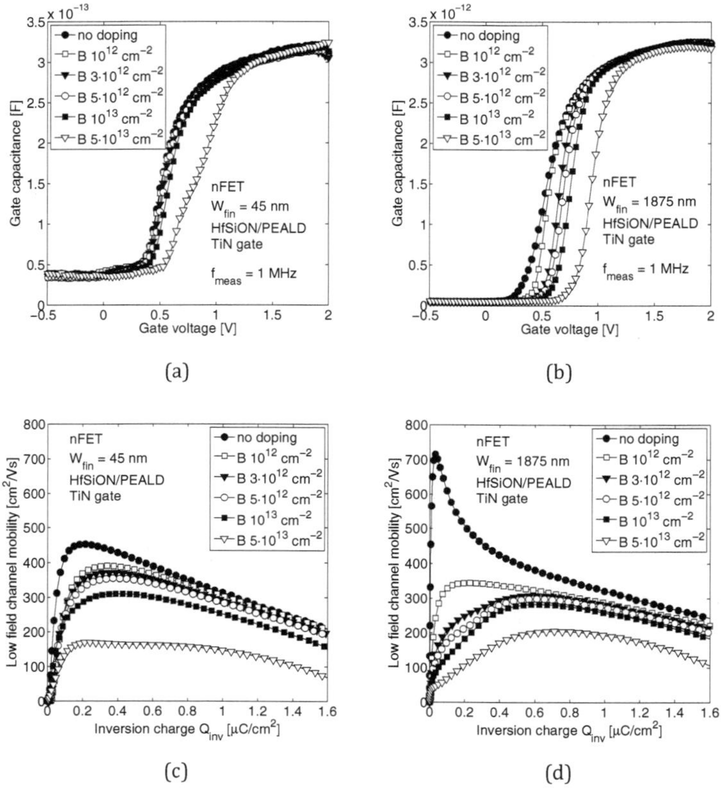

Figure 3.14. Impact of boron implantation doses: gate capacitance measured on (a) narrow (W_{fin} = 45 nm) and (b) quasi-planar (W_{fin} = 1875 nm) n-MuGFETs; low-field channel mobility as extracted from split CV measurement on (c) narrow and (d) quasi planar n-MuGFETs.

implantation dose. Note that amorphization of the fin is unlikely since the implantation doses used for this experiment are much lower than those used for junction implants [Duffy *et al.* (2007)].

3.2.2.4 Advantages

Ion implantation is a commonly used operation with well-know species (boron, arsenic). As such, it limits the costs in terms of process development; it does not require the development of additional photolithographic masksets ('CMOS-toolset compatible').

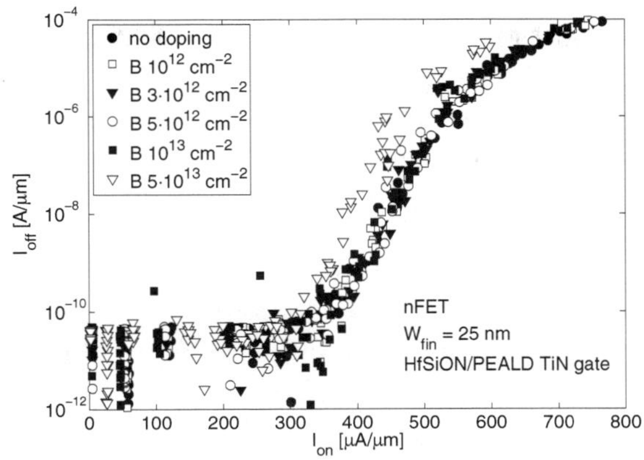

Figure 3.15. Intrinsic transistor performance for narrow ($W_{fin} = 25$ nm) MuGFETs for various channel implantation doses.

In addition, in the case of medium implantation doses, it does not endanger the gate stack integrity since the implantation is performed prior to the gate stack definition.

3.2.2.5 Limitations

The impact of channel doping with boron or arsenic on V_T is almost negligible in narrow Si fins (also observed with fluorine implantations [Xiong *et al.* (2007)]). As the Si fin width decreases and the device enters the fully depleted regime, the electrostatic control of the gate over the channel is enhanced. The threshold voltage and the transconductance of narrow MuGFETs are no longer affected by carrier injection into the Si substrate. Significant V_T variations (hundreds of mV) require a carrier concentration in the Si substrate, which endangers the intrinsic performance of the MuGFET devices.

3.2.3 *Metal/Oxide Interface Modification*

3.2.3.1 Interface dipole model: introduction

For almost three decades, the importance of the gate electrode/oxide interface quality in the definition of V_T has been emphasized [Hickmott (1980)]. Models, referred to as the 'Bond polarization model' or 'Interface dipole theory,' have been proposed in order to highlight the role played by local dipoles created by the contact between the metal and the gate oxide. These dipoles are defined as a local charge transfer (abrupt change in electron density) from the metal into the gate oxide (or vice-versa). They are a consequence of the ionic nature of the bonds formed at the interface, due to the mean electronegativity difference between the constituent elements of the metal and of the gate oxide. It has been demonstrated that the Pauling electronegativity (property of isolated atom) is correlated to the vacuum work function of elemental metals (property of atoms in elemental solid) [Gordy and Thomas (1956); Michaelson (1978)]. Depending on the nature of the bonds formed at the metal/oxide interface and on the electronegativity of the bonded elements, an increase or decrease in the effective gate work function is expected: if the metal (gate dielectric) surface is more electronegative (electropositive) than the gate dielectric (metal) surface, the Fermi level of the gate shifts towards the Si conduction band. In other words, the effective work function decreases. Based on this model, several approaches have been developed in order to create dipoles on purpose at the metal/oxide interface.

3.2.3.2 Implantation-based interface modification

Implantations of foreign species into the metal gate and their diffusion down to the metal/oxide interface is one of the techniques used for creating such dipoles. Depending on the electronegativity of these species and on the materials used as a metal and a gate oxide, a specific dipole orientation is obtained [Pauling (1932)]. Naturally, the mean electronegativity of the gate (prior to the implantation) also plays a role in the definition of the bonds created at the metal/oxide interface. Depending on the initial metal and gate oxide, the implantation of a specific impurity can thus result into different dipole orientations and, as a consequence, into different effective work function. Obviously, this technique can be perceived as a very convenient and litho-friendly way to obtain CMOS solutions with single mid-gap metal gates in planar MOSFETs [Singanamalla *et al.* (2006b, 2007a)]. However, most of the experimental results reported in the literature refer to relatively thick metal gates (>10 nm), which are not recommended in a MuGFET fabrication flow.

3.2.3.2.1 Application to MuGFETs

A feasibility study has been performed on MuGFET devices [Witters *et al.* (2007)]. The latter have been fabricated according to the process flow described in [Collaert *et al.* (2005)]. The gate stack considered for this experiment consists of 10 nm MOCVD TiN deposited on 2.3 nm of HfSiON. Prior to the arsenic implantation, the metal gate electrode is covered with 10 or 15 nm of Plasma-Enhanced CVD oxide. Arsenic is implanted at both sides of the fins by a 45° tilt implantation. The PE-CVD oxide layer is then removed in 0.5% HF solution and followed by the polysilicon deposition. A reference wafer with 5 nm MOCVD TiN on HfSiON and no As implantation has also been included in the experiment.

3.2.3.2.2 Gate oxide integrity

The implantation conditions and subsequent anneal are chosen based upon SIMS measurements on blanket wafers to maximize the amount of As at the HfSiON/TiN interface while avoiding arsenic penetration into the channel. On MuGFETs, an implantation at an energy of 6 keV and an arsenic dose of 2×10^{15} atoms/cm^2 is tested. 10 nm and 15 nm PE-CVD oxide caps have been considered in order to limit the amount of As into the Si substrate. Fig. 3.16 illustrates the SIMS profiles of these two implantation conditions. Unlike the experiments performed on planar MOSFETs, the gate oxide leakage metric is strongly modified after As implantation. Fig. 3.17 shows that an oxide cap thicker than 10 nm is required with these implantation conditions. The evolution of the cumulative plot suggests that the As distribution within the gate oxide (and thus the gate oxide degradation and leakage increase) is tightly bound to the oxide cap thickness variations when this oxide cap is 10 nm thick.

3.2.3.2.3 V_T modification and W_{fin} dependence

Compared to the reference MuGFETs with a 10 nm (5 nm) MOCVD TiN gate electrode, the As implantation lowers the threshold voltage by 300 mV (100 mV) on both n- and pFETs as illustrated for narrow

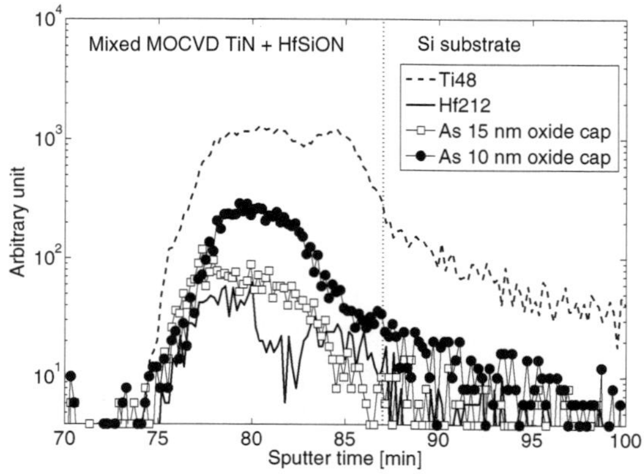

Figure 3.16. SIMS analysis of MOCVD TiN/HfSiON/Si stacks after arsenic implantation (6 keV, 2×10^{15} atoms/cm^2, 45° tilt) through 10 or 15 nm PE-CVD oxide cap, after 1050°C spike anneal and oxide cap removal. The profile of the Ti and Hf elements indicate a strong intermixing between the TiN and HfSiON layers. The observation of a pile-up of As impurities at the metal/gate dielectric interface cannot be observed since this interface is not accurately defined.

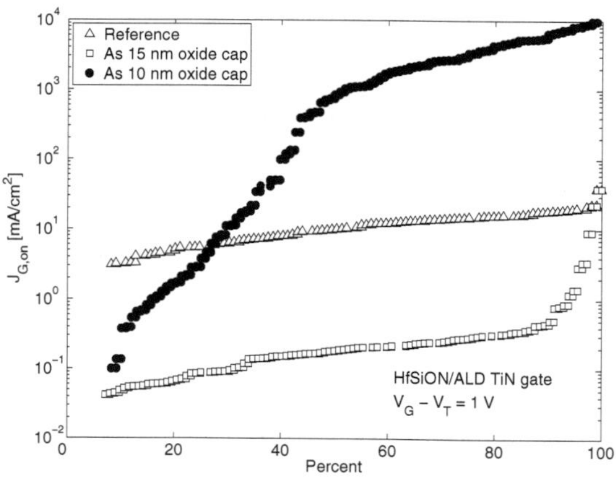

Figure 3.17. Cumulative plot of the gate leakage of n-MuGFETs as a function of the implantation cap thickness (10 nm vs. 15 nm PE-CVD oxide cap). As implantation conditions are: 6 keV, 2×10^{15} atoms/cm^2, 45° tilt, 2 quadrants.

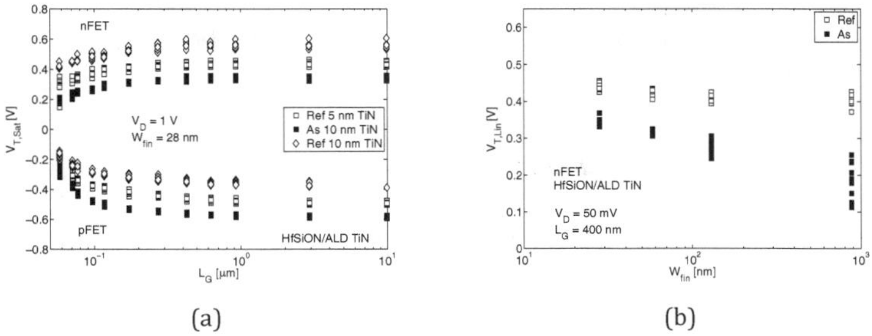

Figure 3.18. (a) $V_{T,Sat}$ as a function of the gate length for n- and p-MuGFETs (W_{fin} = 25 nm): roll-off comparison between the reference samples (5 nm or 10 nm MOCVD TiN) and the implanted sample; (b) $V_{T,Sat}$ as a function of the fin width for n-MuGFETs (L_G = 400 nm); As implantation conditions are: 6 keV, 2×10^{15} atoms/cm^2, 45° tilt, 2 quadrants, 10 nm oxide cap.

Si fins in (Fig. 3.18(a)). Due to the As implantation, the effective work function moves towards the Si conduction band edge (it is also referred to as a more 'n-type'-like work function). Despite differences in gate oxide thickness, the roll-off behavior at short channels is relatively similar for both implanted and unimplanted MuGFETs. Since the top of the Si fin is implanted twice (as compared to the Si fin sidewalls), the threshold voltage of nFETs is lowered further for wider fins, as shown in Fig. 3.18(b). This confirms the impact of the implantation dose on the V_T shift. Only conformal doping techniques could maintain the V_T shift constant over a wider range of Si fin widths. Note that the performance dependence on V_T is not discussed: the gate leakage degradation in implanted MuGFET samples makes the comparison (implanted vs. reference samples) irrelevant.

3.2.3.2.4 Advantages

Modifications of the metal gate properties based on ion implantations facilitate the implementation of multiple-V_T within the same MuGFET fabrication flow. Similar to the channel doping-based method, they do not require any additional maskset development for their integration into a CMOS processing.

3.2.3.2.5 Limitations

The implantation parameters must be defined with great care: the thickness of the buffer layer and the implantation energy must be optimized in order to bring the impurities within the core of thin metal layers, without damaging the gate dielectric. In addition, a post-implantation anneal must be defined, which must drive the impurities to the metal/gate oxide interface, with limited regrowth of the SiO_2 interfacial layer. The implantation dose must also be defined such that the impurity concentration creates a sufficiently large dipole at the metal/gate oxide interface. Moreover, the implantation angle must fulfill two requirements: absence of implantation shadowing by the closest fins (fin pitch dependent) and, as much as possible, uniform doping of the gate electrode.

3.2.3.3 Gate dielectric nitridation

The nitridation of thin gate oxides was initially considered as a solution to prevent boron penetration from the poly gate into the gate dielectric of pFETs with SiO_2 dielectric [Chen *et al.* (1997)]. Meanwhile, another advantage has been demonstrated: nitrided oxides and hafnium-silicates are known to present a higher relative permittivity value than their pure counterparts. Higher permittivity allows thicker oxides (and thus reduced gate leakage) without an EOT penalty [Cubaynes (2004)]. By applying a nitridation process prior to the metal electrode deposition, the dielectric composition at its interface with the metal can be modified. In this case, the composition of the upper part of the dielectric is modified on purpose while the composition of its lower part (interface with the interfacial oxide or the Si substrate) must remain unchanged. Its advantage lies in the fact that the nitridation process can achieve depth-limited modifications of the dielectrics. Its limitation lies in the presence of additional fixed charge into the gate dielectric, which, naturally, modifies V_T but also the effective mobility, μ_{eff}.

3.2.3.3.1 Application to MuGFETs

An experiment has been performed to determine what is the largest V_T shift affordable with a decoupled plasma nitridation (DPN) process and its consequences on the device's performance. For this

Table 3.3. Decoupled plasma nitridation process conditions (room temperature): planar MOSFET samples. The PNA is performed at 900°C, 15 s, 5 Torr.

	RF generator power (W)	Duty cycle (%)	Pulse length (s)	Pressure (mT)
Sample 1	1800	50	90	10
Sample 2	1800	50	90	50

purpose, MuGFETs have been fabricated according to the process flow described in [Collaert *et al.* (2005)]. Their gate stack consists of 0.8 nm of SiO_2 onto which 2.3 nm of MOCVD HfSiO is deposited (40%Hf), with a 10 nm PE-ALD TiN film as gate electrode. Apart from reference samples (no nitridation after the HfSiO deposition), the other samples are subjected to a DPN process. The high-density N_2 plasma is formed by an RF electric field and a N_2 gas.[4] The DPN parameters involved in this experiment are summarized in Table 3.3. Apart from the reference sample (no nitridation of the gate dielectric), two other samples are subjected to the plasma nitridation. For both nitrided samples, the pulsed-RF source parameters stay the same while the effect of the pressure in the nitridation chamber is investigated. After the nitridation, the same post-nitridation anneal (PNA) is considered in order to further stabilize the oxygen and nitrogen profiles in the gate dielectric. Note that the impact of the PNA on non-nitrided samples is not investigated.

3.2.3.3.2 Nitrogen profile characterization

As compared to the commonly used nitridation process, the process conditions used for this experiment are extremely aggressive towards the gate dielectric: the nitrogen profile is expected to extend deep into the gate oxide and the nitrogen concentration is also expected to be higher than for normal nitrided Hf-silicates. For comparison purposes, the nitrogen depth profile has been measured on planar MOSFETs. Their gate oxide made of 2.6 nm MOCVD Hf(40%)SiO on 1 nm SiO_2 is comparable to the gate stack processed on the MuGFETs. The DPN conditions tested on these

[4]The effective power of the pulsed-RF source is characterized by its RF generator power and its duty cycle (Plasma on-time/Total time).

Table 3.4. Decoupled plasma nitridation process conditions (room temperature): planar MOS capacitor samples. PNA is performed at 900°C, 15 s, 0.5 Torr.

	RF generator power (W)	Duty cycle (%)	Pulse length (s)	Pressure (mT)
Sample 3	1750	20	20	8
Sample 4	1750	20	20	50

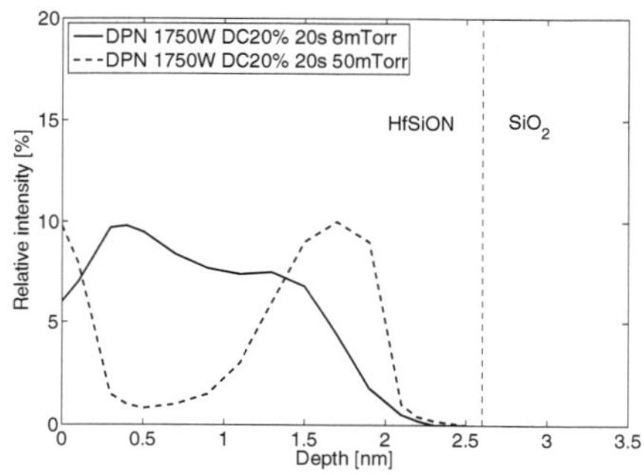

Figure 3.19. Nitrogen depth profile of samples 3 and 4, reconstructed from AR-XPS; the nitrogen concentration relative to the total metal concentration (Hf+SiO) is 24 and 13% for samples 3 and 4, respectively

planar structures are commonly used in a standard MOS fabrication flow (Table 3.4). They are optimized in order to limit the amount of nitrogen introduced in the gate oxide layer (short duty cycle). As such, they provide a lower limit for the nitrogen concentration when compared to the DPN conditions tested on MuGFETs. As illustrated in Table 3.5 and Fig. 3.19, varying the chamber pressure at such low pressure levels results in remarkable changes in nitrogen concentration and profile into the gate dielectric.[5] Since the effective source power is even larger for the MuGFET experiment, it is foreseen that such a nitridation process degrades the low-field channel mobility and the device performance, even though the SiO_2 interfacial layer is not affected by the nitrogen diffusion.

[5]Average HfSiON film thickness = 2.9 nm, average Hf concentration = 40% for both samples.

Table 3.5. Nitrogen profile as reconstructed from XPS analysis on the planar MOS capacitor samples (samples described in Table 3.4). By reducing the plasma pressure, the nitrogen content in the HfSiON layer increases [Rothschild *et al.* (2007)].

	N/(Hf+SiO) (%)	N concentration (at/cm^2)
Sample 3	24	1.5×10^{15}
Sample 4	13	9.6×10^{14}

3.2.3.3.3 V_T and W_{fin} dependence

Long-channel devices present a substantial decrease in threshold voltage ($\approx$400 mV) when subjected to the nitridation at the lowest pressure (illustrated in Fig. 3.20). As such, it meets the requirements for n-MuGFETs. This modification of V_T can reasonably be attributed to two factors: a sharp increase in positive fixed oxide charge (Q_{ox}) and the modification of the metal/gate oxide interface (δD). Although the CET of the nitride samples is increased by 25% (as compared to the reference sample), it is not expected to play a major role in the modification of V_T in MuGFETs [Taur (2000)].

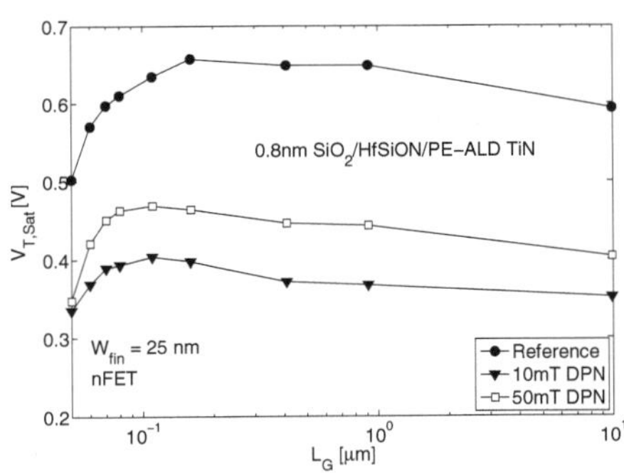

Figure 3.20. $V_{T,Sat}$ dependence on the gate length: comparison between the reference sample and those with heavily nitrided HfSiO gate dielectrics, the V_T lowering goes along with the chamber pressure during the nitridation, i.e., the amount of nitrogen introduced in the HfSiO layer.

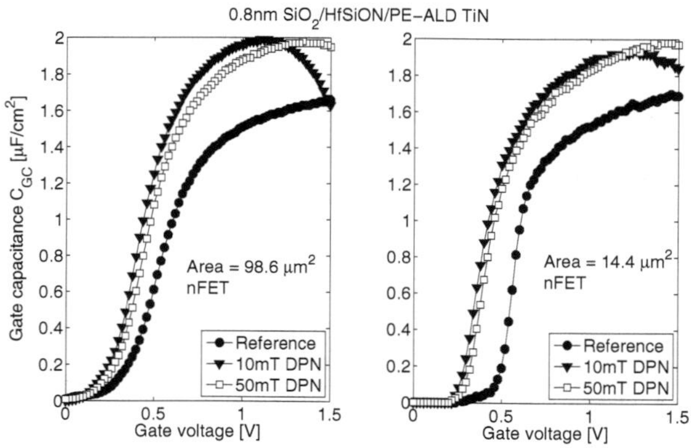

Figure 3.21. Gate capacitance measured on MuGFETs with (left) wide Si fins (W_{fin} = 1875 nm) and (right) narrow Si fins (W_{fin} = 25 nm); for both structures, higher nitrogen content results in reduced CET, as expected; similar CET values are obtained for both quasi-planar and narrow structures, suggesting the conformality of the DPN process at this scale.

3.2.3.3.4 Device performance

At low inversion charge, the mobility degradation reflects the increase in fixed oxide charge into the gate oxide, which, of course, is more pronounced for Sample 3 (Fig. 3.22). At higher inversion charge, this difference among the reference and nitrided samples tends to disappear as the Si surface roughness is not modified by the DPN treatment. As a result, the nitridation process offers the potential to tune V_T by hundreds of mV with improved performance for nFETs. Nitrided samples present a slightly thicker gate oxide than the reference sample (physical thickness = 2.9 nm). However, the nitrogen incorporation makes the gate leakage increase by almost one order of magnitude with the most heavily nitrided gate oxide (Fig. 3.23, sample 3).

3.2.3.3.5 Advantages

Contrary to implantation-based methods, this technique can define a broad range of V_T and does not degrade the performance. However, this is at the cost of a gate oxide leakage increase.

3.2.3.3.6 Limitations

This technique offers a solution for n-MuGFETs only. To achieve

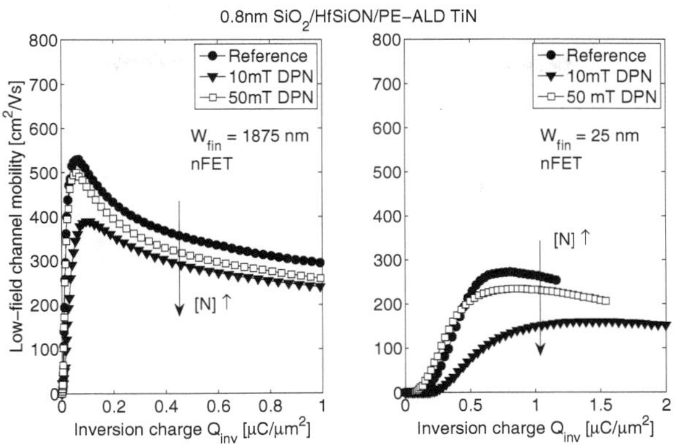

Figure 3.22. Low-field channel mobility extracted on MuGFETs with (left) wide Si fins ($W_{fin} = 1875$ nm) and (right) narrow Si fins ($W_{fin} = 25$ nm); for both structures, higher nitrogen content results in reduced peak mobility, due to the higher fixed charge content in the gate dielectric.

its integration within a CMOS fabrication flow, protection of the pFET devices is required. Of course, photoresist can be used for this purpose. However, its removal after nitridation of the nFET-dedicated gate oxides must ensure the gate oxide integrity.

3.2.3.4 Dielectric capping layers

Another solution for tuning the effective work function of an electrode is to modify the mean electronegativity of the gate oxide layer. To do so, dielectric capping layers are inserted within the metal and the gate dielectric (also referred to as 'base oxide'). They are usually made of rare-earth element-based oxides [Narayanan *et al.* (2006); Lee *et al.* (2006); Jung *et al.* (2006, 2007)]. A method for predicting the expected shift in effective work function due to a dielectric capping layer has been reported [Schaeffer *et al.* (2007)]. It relies on the difference of mean electronegativity between the base oxide and the dielectric capping. The mean electronegativity is defined as the geometric mean and allows to estimate the electronegativity of a multi-component gate dielectric, based on its volume stoichiometry:

$$\overline{EN} = \left(\prod_{i=1}^{N} EN_i \right) \tag{3.3}$$

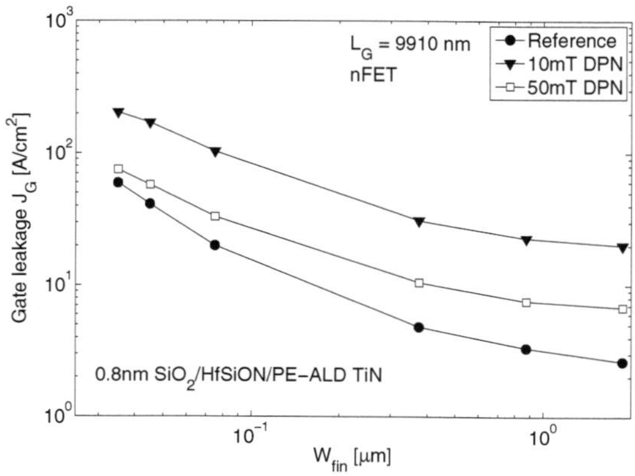

Figure 3.23. Gate leakage extracted on MuGFETs with narrow Si fins (W_{fin} = 25 nm): the gate leakage degradation along with the nitrogen content suggests a relative permittivity increase (limited physical thickness increase).

In Eq. (3.3), EN_i represents the electronegativity of the constituent materials of a metal. The mean electronegativity $\overline{EN}$ has been estimated for the most commonly used dielectrics in this thesis. Results are summarized in Table 3.6 where the Pauling electronegativity of the constituent elements is also noted. According to the literature, the expected shift due to a dielectric cap with respect to HfO_2 can be determined as follows:

- Multi-component materials with an $\overline{EN}$ lower that $\overline{EN}_{HfO_2}$ tend to make the dielectric less electronegative (as compared to the metal gate) and thus, lower the effective work function. This is the case for La_2O_3 and Dy_2O_3 capping layers.
- Similarly, multi-component materials like Al_2O_3 tend to make the dielectric more electronegative (as compared to the metal gate) and thus, increase the effective work function.

However, such a reasoning is no longer valid with SiO_2 as base oxide and HfO_2 as dielectric capping. The model based on $\overline{EN}$ fails in predicting the right work function shift. Indeed, the integration of an

Table 3.6. Pauling electronegativity of common constituent elements and mean electronegativity of common gate dielectrics and dielectric capping layers. Note that the HfSiON composition is not accurately known and a (1:1:1:1) volume stoichiometry is assumed.

Element	Pauling electronegativity	Capping dielectrics	Geometric mean electronegativity $\overline{EN}$
La	1.10	La_2O_3	2.18
Dy	1.22	HfSiON	2.25
Hf	1.30	Dy_2O_3	2.27
Al	1.61	HfO_2	2.49
Si	1.90	Al_2O_3	2.54
N	3.04	$HfSiO_4$	2.66
O	3.44	SiON	2.71
		SiO_2	2.82

SiO_2/HfSiON results in a threshold voltage increase while the $\overline{EN}$-based model predicts a work function decrease. This can possibly be explained by the fact that the $\overline{EN}$ metric does not take into account the interface stoichiometry nor the crystal phases. Moreover, it does not consider the additional oxide charge generated by the dielectric caps. Nonetheless, it illustrates that various aspects (volume and surface stoichiometry, charge, phase) contribute to the definition of V_T.

3.2.3.4.1 Probing interfacial reactions

First, the thermodynamical stability of dielectric capping layers needs to be investigated. A physical characterization has been conducted in order to demonstrate that the metal, the capping layer and the base oxide react with each other at their common interface after a high temperature anneal [Adelmann *et al.* (2007, 2009)]. In other words, the idea of a distinct capping layer between the dielectric and the metal gate is no longer valid after high temperature processing. For this physical characterization, let us consider dysprosium oxide (Dy_2O_3) as dielectric capping layer. This choice is driven by the necessity of implementing low V_T in MuGFETs with a single metal. Indeed, it has been demonstrated on planar MOSFETs that Dy_2O_3 cap layers inserted between the gate dielectric and the metal layer can help lowering V_{fb} [Lee *et al.*

(2006)]. Interfacial reactions are typically expected in the MuGFET processing since the base oxide/Dy_2O_3/metal stack will undergo a high-temperature annealing at 1050°C during the activation anneal after ion implantation. The experiment is performed on large MOS capacitors with a 1 nm thick chemical SiO_2(IMEC clean), onto which either a Dy_2O_3 films is grown by atomic vapor deposition (AVD) or a $HfSiO_4$ film by MOCVD. Four different types of Ta-based gate electrodes are considered: either TaCN-based films deposited both by AVD (Ta_2N, TaCN) or by PVD (TaN, Ta_2C). The stacks are then annealed either at 1000°C for 60 s in N_2 or spike annealed at 1050°C. The resulting structures are analyzed by Time-of-Flight SIMS ('ToF-SIMS') and angle-resolved XPS while the metal densities are determined from X-Ray Reflectivity ('XRR') measurements. The reactivity of the TaCN-based metals is analyzed with AR-XPS compositional profiles (Fig. 3.24). First, the compositional profile of the gate stack made of 3 nm AVD Ta_2N/2 nm Dy_2O_3/1 nm SiO_2 is analyzed after spike annealing at 1050°C. The stack can be well separated into two layers: a TaN layer (with a surface oxide) and a Dy-silicate layer beneath, which has been formed by reaction of Dy_2O_3 with SiO_2 [Adelmann *et al.* (2007); Ono and Katsumata (2001); Adelmann *et al.* (2008b)]. The ToF-SIMS profiles of 10 nm TaCN-

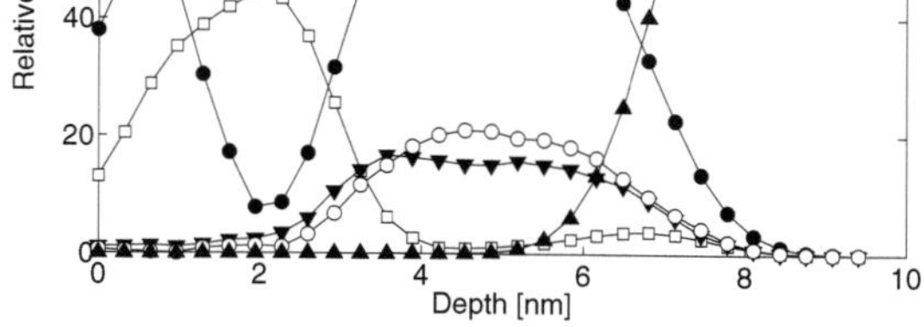

Figure 3.24. AR-XPS composition profile of 3 nm AVD Ta_2N/2 nm Dy_2O_3/1 nm SiO_2 after spike annealing at 1050°C. $DySiO_x$ formation due to reaction of Dy_2O_3 with SiO_2 is observed; however, the interface with TaN appears rather abrupt.

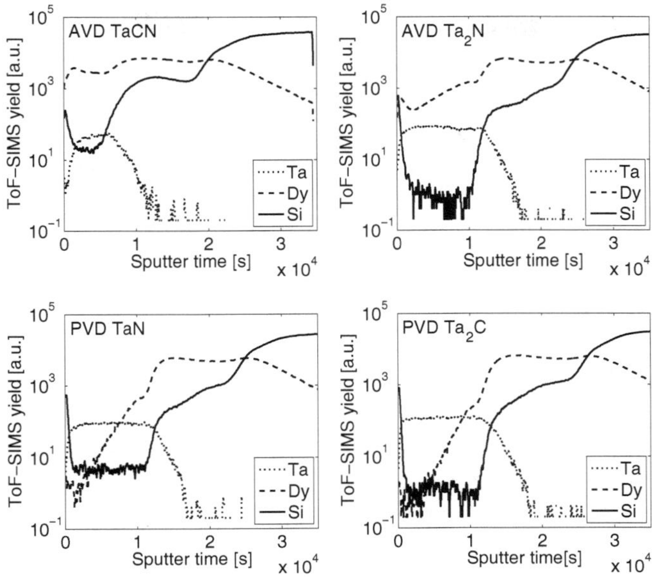

Figure 3.25. ToF-SIMS profiles of 10 nm of AVD TaCN, AVD Ta_2N, PVD TaN, and PVD Ta_2C on 12 nm Dy_2O_3/1 nm SiO_2. All samples have been annealed at 1000°C for 60 s.

based metals/12 nm Dy_2O_3/1 nm SiO_2 after annealing at 1000°C for 60 s demonstrate however, that not all TaCN-based metals are stable in contact with Dy_2O_3 (Fig. 3.25). Strong Dy outdiffusion is evidenced for AVD TaCN (exact composition is $Ta_{0.6}C_{0.3}N_{0.1}$ [Karim *et al.* (2007); Adelmann *et al.* (2008a)]), whereas Dy diffusion is considerably less in AVD Ta_2N and reduced even further in PVD TaN and Ta_2C. The latter two materials can be considered rather stable in contact with Dy_2O_3. An identical trend is observed for Si outdiffusion into the Ta-based materials. The composition of the materials cannot explain the difference in thermal stability of the different TaCN-based materials. Both the variation of C vs. N content as well as the variations in Ta content do not result in a consistent picture. Generally, AVD-grown materials appear to be more reactive than PVD-grown ones. However, it has to be remarked that the observed trends clearly follow the observed trends in material

Table 3.7. Densities of 10 nm of AVD TaCN, AVD Ta_2N, PVD TaN, and PVD Ta_2C on 12 nm Dy_2O_3/1 nm SiO_2 measured by XRR. All samples have been annealed at 1000°C for 60 s.

Metal	Density [g/cm^3]
AVD TaCN	8.0
AVD Ta2N	11.5
PVD TaN	14-16
PVD Ta2C	14-16

density (Table 3.7). This indicates that the diffusivity of Dy and Si in TaCN-based metals is strongly influenced by the density of the material. Another part of the explanation can also stem from the microstructure of the metals. Whereas AVD TaCN is nearly amorphous even after high temperature annealing, AVD Ta_2N and the PVD metals are polycrystalline, as illustrated in the Grazing Incidence X-Ray Diffraction ('GI-XRD') pattern in Fig. 3.26. Thus, as

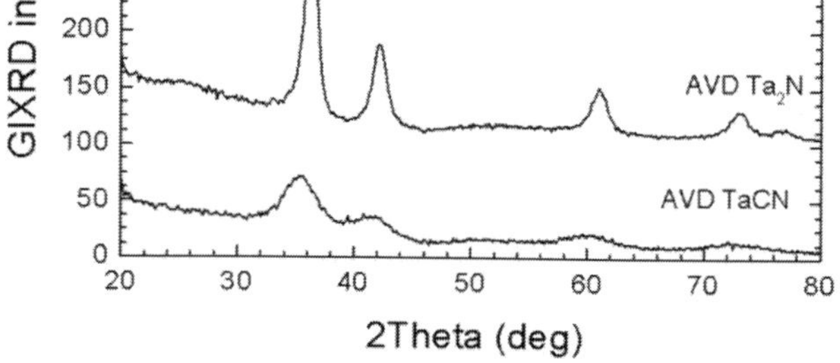

Figure 3.26. GI-XRD ($\omega = 1°$) pattern of 50 nm thick metal films (as indicated) on 10 nm of SiO_2 after spike annealing at 1050°C. The AVD materials show a cubic TaN (rock-salt) structure, whereas the pattern of PVD TaN can be indexed by a mixture of hexagonal and cubic TaN.

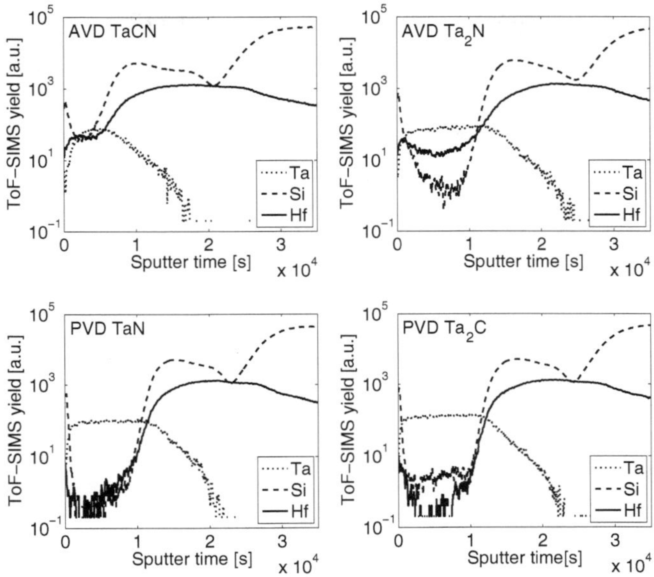

Figure 3.27. ToF-SIMS profiles of 10 nm of AVD TaCN, AVD Ta_2N, PVD TaN, and PVD Ta_2C on 10 nm $HfSiO_4$/1 nm SiO_2. All samples have been annealed at 1000°C for 60 s.

a whole, the data clearly demonstrate the importance of density and microstructure for the thermal stability of metal/Dy_2O_3 stacks. This influence surpasses that of compositional variations in the TaCN-system and thus it becomes difficult to give general thermal stability rules for rare-earth containing gate stacks. Finally, Fig. 3.27 shows the ToF-SIMS profiles of TaCN-based metals on 10 nm $HfSiO_4$/1 nm SiO_2 after annealing at 1000°C for 60 s. The data confirm the trends observed above. AVD TaCN leads to strong Hf and Si outdiffusion. Also, for identical metals, it is generally observed that the Hf profiles decay faster than their Dy counterparts, which indicates that Dy_2O_3 is more reactive in contact with TaCN-based metals than $HfSiO_4$. This physical characterization demonstrates that the gate stack involving Dy_2O_3 cannot be considered as thermodynamically stable since interfacial reactions occur when Dy_2O_3 is in contact with metal gates and gate oxides. The magnitude of the Dy_2O_3 outdiffusion is influenced by the structure of the metal (its phase and its density) and, of course, by the nature of the dielectric capping layer itself. This should be kept in mind if the influence of rare-earth capping layers on device properties is discussed.

3.2.3.4.2 The SiO_2/Dy_2O_3/metal case: application to MOS capacitors

The basic properties of SiO_2/Dy_2O_3/metal gate stacks are investigated on MOS capacitors fabricated on p-type (100) bulk silicon substrates. The gate stacks consist of different thicknesses of SiO_2 base oxide (1.0 to 2.5 nm). An SiO_2 base oxide has been chosen in order to avoid high-*k* specific issues. On this base oxide, AVD Dy_2O_3 caps with a thickness range from 1.0 to 2.0 nm have been deposited. Reference capacitors with 2.0 nm SiO_2 base oxide are left uncapped. Next, 10 nm of metal gate, being either MOCVD TiN or ALD TaN, has been deposited and capped with 100 nm of polysilicon. Some of the MOS capacitors are subjected to an additional heat treatment (800°C, 30 min.) after the gate stack deposition, prior to a spike anneal at 1050°C [Ferain *et al.* (2007)]. The V_{fb} dependence on Dy_2O_3 thickness and metal electrode is given in Fig. 3.28(a). For the same base oxide thickness, TaN electrodes exhibit a higher V_{fb} reduction than TiN ones when inserting an identical Dy_2O_3 layer (same thickness). The V_{fb} dependence on Dy_2O_3 thickness and metal electrode, combined with a TEM micrograph (Fig. 3.29), indicates that Dy_2O_3/metal interdiffusion is the predominant mechanism for V_{fb} reduction while the outdiffusion of Dy_2O_3 into SiO_2 is responsible for EOT reduction and gate leakage improvement by Dy-silicate formation (Fig. 3.28(c)). TiN electrodes achieve higher V_{fb} reduction than TaN within the same Dy_2O_3 thickness range. From the physical characterization performed in 3.2.3.4, it can be assumed that the V_{fb} modification depends on the metal (TiN vs. TaN) but also on the deposition method (MOCVD vs. ALD). In terms of optimum condition for further implementation on MuGFETs, the thickness ratio $Dy_2O_3/SiO_2 = 1{:}2$ (point '1') is an optimum in terms of EOT reduction and process margin Fig. 3.28(b) with acceptable gate leakage enhancement. By 'process margin,' one means that there is limited base oxide regrowth after additional heat treatment.

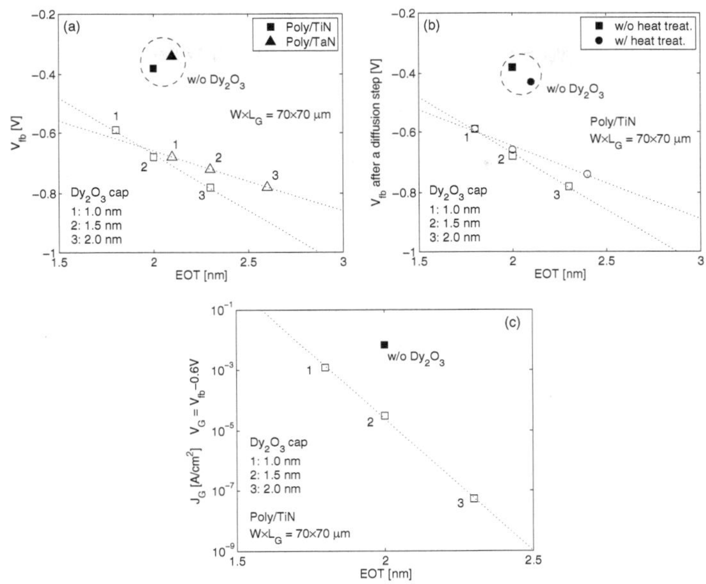

Figure 3.28. MOS capacitors with 2 nm SiO_2/Dy_2O_3/metal (MOCVD TiN or ALD TaN) gate stacks: (a) V_{fb} as a function of EOT, dependence on the Dy_2O_3 thickness and metal electrode, (b) V_{fb} as a function of EOT, dependence on the Dy_2O_3 thickness and additional heat treatment (800°C, 30 min.), (c) gate leakage dependence as a function of EOT, Dy_2O_3 thickness dependence suggesting the formation of higher-k dielectric by intermixing of Dy_2O_3 with SiO_2.

3.2.3.4.3 The SiO_2/Dy_2O_3/metal case: application to MuGFETs

The optimum thickness ratio estimated for Dy_2O_3 and SiO_2 is implemented on MuGFET devices. Both performance and reliability aspects are assessed. For that purpose, MuGFETs have been fabricated with a unichannel process as described in [Collaert *et al.* (2005)]. Their gate stacks are the same than those processed on MOS capacitors for studying the basic gate stack properties. All MuGFETs are annealed at 1050°C. As illustrated in Fig. 3.30(a), the V_T vs. L_G dependence shows that the 1:2 ratio for Dy_2O_3/SiO_2 meets the low nMOS V_T target on short gate MuGFETs (≈260 mV as illustrated in Fig. 3.31). Still, the V_T lowering on long gate

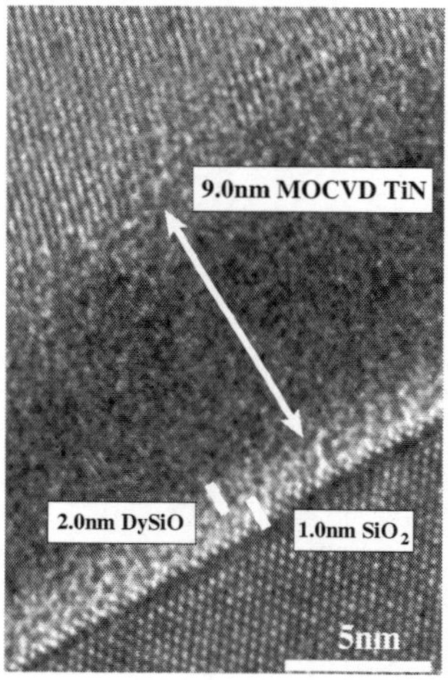

Figure 3.29. HR-TEM micrograph of a TiN/1 nm Dy_2O_3/2 nm SiO_2 gate after S/D activation showing evidences of TiN/Dy_2O_3 and Dy_2O_3/SiO_2 mixing (SiO_2 and TiN thickness reduction)

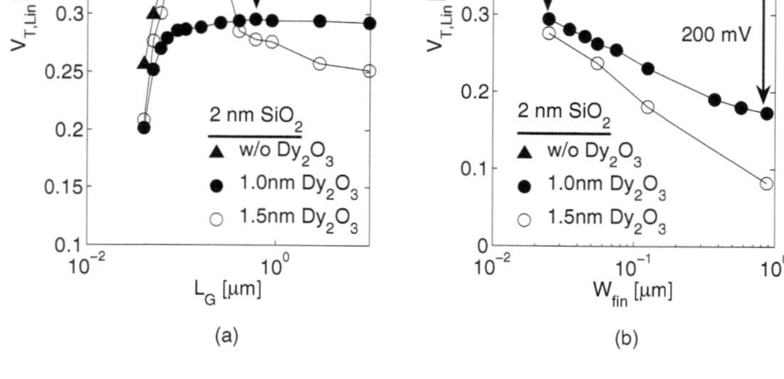

Figure 3.30. MuGFETs ($W_{fin} = 25$ nm, 2 nm SiO_2 base oxide, MOCVD TiN gate electrode) and their V_T dependence on the Dy_2O_3 thickness as function of (a) gate length, (b) fin width.

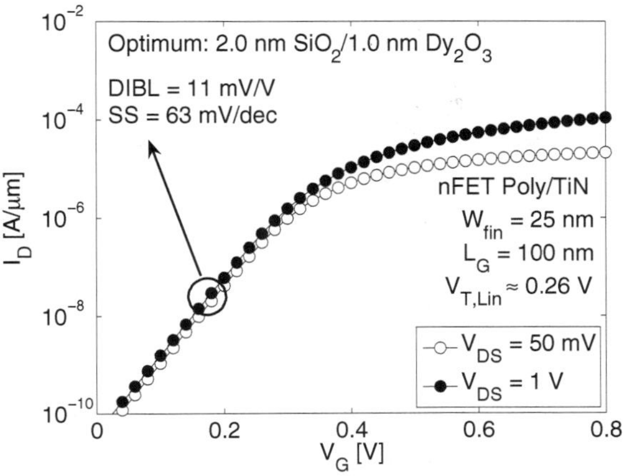

Figure 3.31. $I_{ds}(V_G)$ dependence on MuGFETs and $Dy_2O_3/SiO_2 = 1{:}2$ ratio (optimum ratio with an MOCVD TiN gate electrode).

MuGFETs is less than in long quasi-planar devices (Fig. 3.30(b)) and is attributed to insufficient conformality of the Dy_2O_3 deposition.

Compared to the reference (no Dy_2O_3 cap), MuGFETs with 1 nm Dy_2O_3 cap show lower V_T, better inversion capacitance (Fig. 3.32(b)), comparable low-field channel mobility at high inversion charge (Fig. 3.33(a)) and no performance loss (Fig. 3.33(b)). The improvement in CET is explained by the formation of Dy-silicate (higher relative permittivity than the SiO_2). The apparent absence of performance improvement (despite better CET than the reference and comparable mobility) results from a simultaneous shift in I_{on} and I_{off}: at a given gate length, the MuGFETs with Dy_2O_3 cap present a higher I_{on} but also a degraded (higher) I_{off} than the reference devices (Fig. 3.33(b)). This results in a shift in performance on the initial I_{on}-I_{off} curve. Note that the gate capacitance measurements confirm the lack of conformality of the Dy_2O_3 deposition by the AVD technique. Although some CET improvement is still observed in narrow fin devices with 1 nm Dy_2O_3 (Fig. 3.32(b)), the V_T shift is reduced as compared to quasi-planar MuGFETs (Fig. 3.32(a)). Note also that a thicker Dy_2O_3 cap results in larger CET (and thus less effective SCE control) and degraded mobility (Fig. 3.32(b) and 3.33(a), respectively). This can be interpreted in terms of saturation

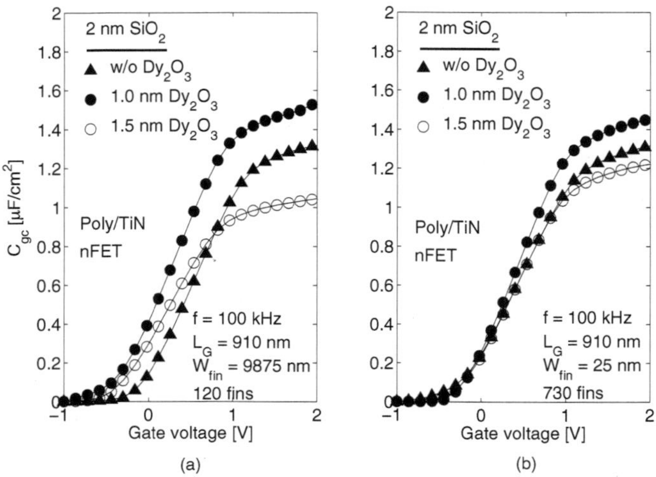

Figure 3.32. Gate capacitance as function of the gate voltage (illustration of the Dy_2O_3 conformality): (a) quasi-planar and (b) narrow Si fin MuGFETs (2 nm SiO_2 base oxide, MOCVD TiN gate electrode)

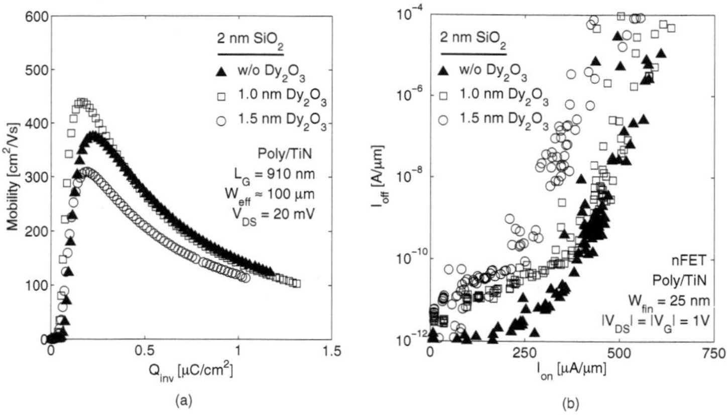

Figure 3.33. MuGFETs ($W_{fin} = 25$ nm, 2 nm SiO_2 base oxide, MOCVD TiN gate electrode): (a) electron mobility dependence on Dy_2O_3 thickness, (b) I_{on}/I_{off} figure of merit.

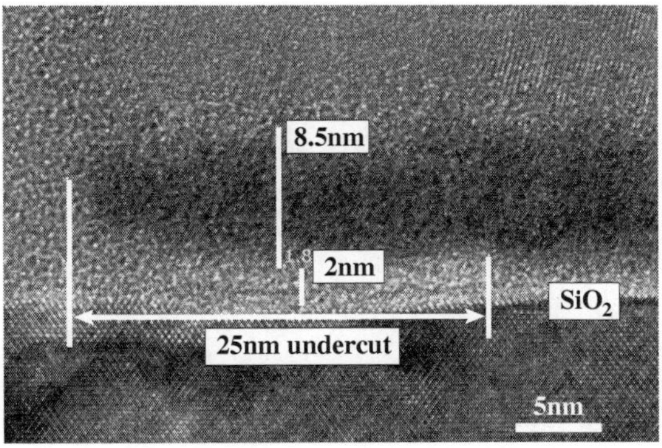

Figure 3.34. HR-TEM micrograph illustrating a lateral gate undercut of a TiN/1 nm Dy_2O_3/2 nm SiO_2 gate after patterning.

of the Dy_2O_3 outdiffusion: the extent of the Dy_2O_3 diffusion into the SiO_2 base oxide is limited by the amount of SiO_2 available for intermixing. It is assumed that thicker Dy_2O_3 film (>1 nm) leads to the formation of a Dy-silicate onto which a distinct (less diffused) Dy_2O_3 remains. This would explain the CET increase and, at the same time, the low-field channel mobility degradation that could be attributed to the high fixed charge content in Dy_2O_3. On TEM micrographs, a lateral gate undercut of the Dy_2O_3 cap is observed (Fig. 3.34). This undercut limits the V_T lowering in short channel devices. Fortunately, this undercut can be eliminated by shortening the HCl-based solution used for etching Dy_2O_3 selectively towards SiO_2 (equipment-related limitation). The $Dy_2O_3/SiO_2 = 1{:}2$ ratio is definitely an optimum in terms of channel mobility as thicker Dy_2O_3 caps or thinner base oxide result into channel mobility degradation (not shown here). This is attributed to the proximity of the Dy_2O_3 to the substrate interface. For implementing multiple-V_T into a MuGFET integration process, the Dy_2O_3 cap has to be removed from devices targeting higher V_T, selectively to the underlying dielectric. To check the feasibility of this process, the blanket removal of Dy_2O_3 has also been tested. As shown in Fig. 3.35, this removal brings V_T back to the level of reference set up by the metal work function. Such a removal is made possible by the absence of Dy_2O_3 outdiffusion at the base oxide and the metal electrode interfaces after the Dy_2O_3

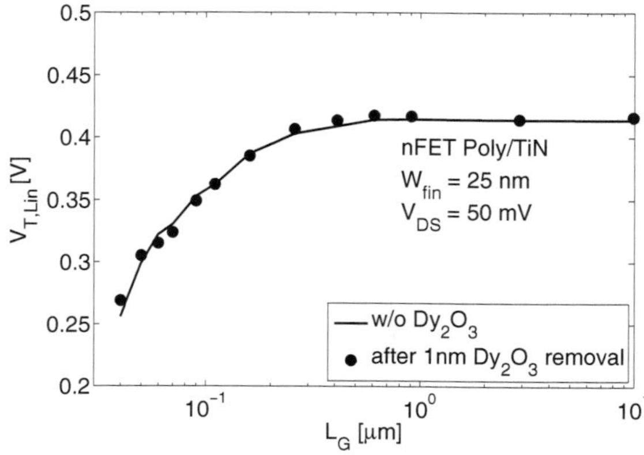

Figure 3.35. Impact of the selective removal of Dy_2O_3 towards the SiO_2 base oxide: $V_{T,Lin}$ as function of L_G of MuGFETs ($W_{fin} = 25$ nm, 2 nm SiO_2 base oxide, MOCVD TiN gate electrode).

deposition. The outdiffusion itself is triggered by high temperature steps (>1000°C) [Adelmann *et al.* (2008b)].

3.2.3.4.4 Advantages

This technique for tuning V_T is efficient over a range of hundreds of mV. As such, it offers the possibility to meet the HP targets. Furthermore, solutions exist for both n- and pFET devices (Dy_2O_3 and La_2O_3 caps for lowering V_T, Al_2O_3 caps for increasing it). In addition, the deposition of such dielectric caps can easily be integrated into a fabrication flow.

3.2.3.4.5 Limitations

First, it must be noted that the deposition technique screened in this section does not ensure the formation of conformal layers. As a consequence, the V_T shifts reported on planar MOSFETs are not necessarily guaranteed on high aspect ratio structures like the MuGFET. In the particular case of Dy_2O_3 caps, an optimum thickness ratio between the dielectric capping layer and the base oxide exists. Based on the physical characterization presented in Section 3.2.3.4.1, this optimum ratio is expected to depend on the choice of the metal gate electrode (material, deposition technique) and also on the nature of the base oxide (SiO_2 or high-k). This optimum ensures decent CET and performance. However, it is not guaranteed that this optimum may fulfill the requirements set on the V_T shift required to reach the HP target. Any ratio above this optimum can offer a larger V_T shift but at the cost of a mobility degradation and of a degraded SCE control. It is also clear that the V_T shift is very sensitive to the overall thermal budget of the device fabrication flow. Moreover, the CMOS implementation is limited by the removal of the dielectric cap selectively towards the base oxide. Indeed, it must guarantee the gate oxide integrity and the choice of dedicated caps for n- and pFETs must ensure similar CET for both types of FETs.

3.2.4 *Metal Gate Modification*

3.2.4.1 Metal-inserted capping layers

The integration of caps (like Dy_2O_3, La_2O_3 and Al_2O_3) within the metal gate itself is another option for tuning V_{fb} (and thus V_T). It modifies the metal/gate oxide interface and, at the same time, moves the fixed charge content of the cap away from the channel. Naturally, an optimum thickness for the rare-earth oxide-based cap needs to be defined, in terms of V_T shift and performance. It is also predicted that the impact on CET of metal-inserted caps will be limited: after a high-temperature anneal, the capping layer must diffuse down to the metal/gate dielectric interface before it starts to interact with the gate oxide. The formation of a higher permittivity silicate is thus more restricted as compared to the case described in section 3.2.3.4. However, this can be seen as an advantage since the selective removal of the rare-earth oxide-based cap should not affect the gate dielectric integrity.

3.2.4.1.1 MuGFET fabrication

An experiment with metal-inserted capping layers has been performed on MuGFETs [Veloso *et al.* (2008)]. It involves both n- and pFETs with different capping layers: Dy_2O_3 and La_2O_3 for nFETs, Al_2O_3 for pFETs. The reference samples have a gate stack consisting of 5 nm of PE-ALD TiN deposited on 2.3 nm MOCVD HfSiO (1 nm of interfacial oxide layer SiO_2). For comparison purpose, MuGFETs with a similar gate stack layer and thin cap layers ($<$1 nm) have also been processed. Caps located at different levels within the gate

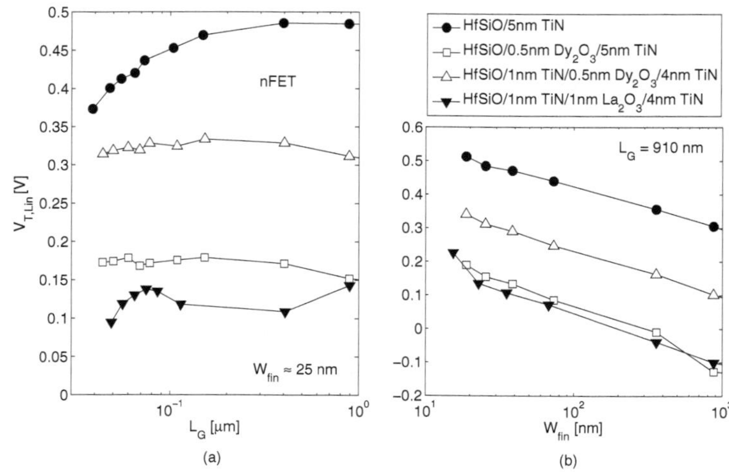

Figure 3.36. n-type MuGFETs: $V_{T,Lin}$ as a function of (a) L_G, (b) W_{fin}, dependence on the capping layer location within the gate stack.

stack have been tested. The cap layers are deposited either onto the HfSiO layer, underneath the metal electrode or in-between two TiN layers depositions with a total metal thickness of 5 nm. In the case of n-MuGFETs, AVD Dy_2O_3 and ALD La_2O_3 are tested while ALD Al_2O_3 caps are being used for the pFET case. In terms of thermal budget, the devices undergo a SEG operation at a 750°C (30 minutes) followed by a 1050°C spike anneal in N_2 for junction activation.

3.2.4.1.2 Threshold voltage: L_G and W_{fin} dependences

The effect of the capping layers on the threshold voltage is illustrated in Fig. 3.36 and Fig. 3.37 for n- and pFETs, respectively. From the V_T vs. L_G dependence, it is observed that the magnitude of the V_T shift depends on the material used as a cap (Dy_2O_3 vs. La_2O_3), which can presumably be linked to its mean electronegativity, its fixed oxide charge content and/or its capacity to diffuse within a given metal. It also depends on the location of the cap: a larger V_T shift is observed when the capping layer is inserted closer to the transistor channel. As such, it is attributed to the fixed oxide charge content present in the capping layer. In addition, improved SCE control is observed for

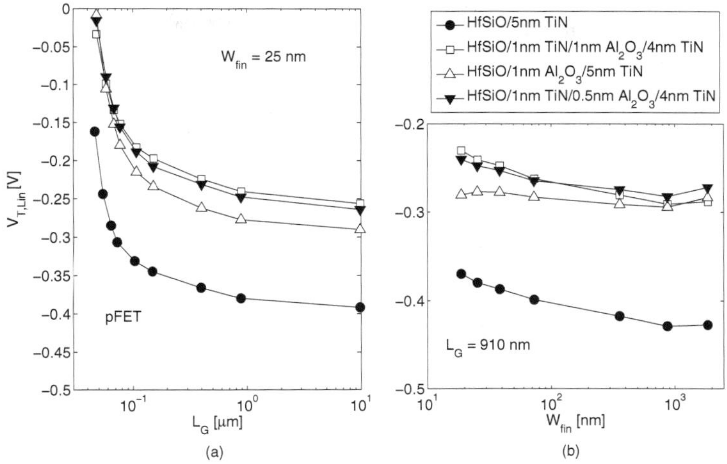

Figure 3.37. p-type MuGFETs: $V_{T,Lin}$ as a function of (a) L_G, (b) W_{fin}, dependence on the capping layer location within the gate stack.

n-MuGFETs with the capping layer inserted within the metal gate electrode. This suggests that thinner CET is obtained by outdiffusion of the capping layer down to the metal/HfSiO interface.

3.2.4.1.3 Performance (mobility) analysis

As compared to the method based on dielectric capping layers, the technique based on metal-inserted caps presents less interest in terms of range for threshold voltage modification and SCE control improvement. However, inserting the rare-earth based oxide within the metal gate electrode presents two major advantages: in terms of μ_{eff} and performance. As the cap is moved away from the channel interface, its fixed oxide charge content has less impact on the low-field channel mobility, as illustrated in Fig. 3.38. Even though the deposition of a capping layer on the gate dielectric does not necessarily result in a performance decrease, a dependence on the nature of the cap is observed. In order to avoid it, the deposition of the capping layer within the metal gate electrode is the best option for guaranteeing similar performance for both capped and uncapped MuGFETs [Veloso *et al.* (2008)]. From a CMOS integration

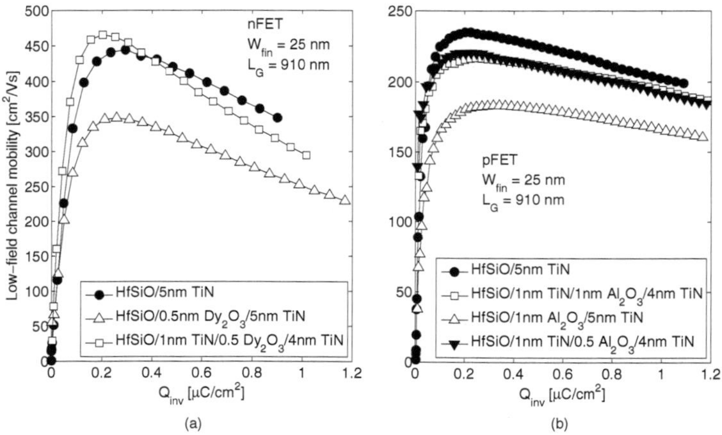

Figure 3.38. Low-field channel mobility measured on MuGFETs (W_{fin} = 25 nm). (a) In the nFET case: as the 0.5 nm Dy_2O_3 cap moves away from the channel interface, μ_{eff} becomes similar for both the reference sample and the sample with the capping layer inserted within the metal electrode; (b) a similar conclusion applies to the pFET case with a 0.5 nm Al_2O_3 cap. Further increase of the capping layer thickness (0.5 nm vs. 1 nm) does not affect μ_{eff} nor V_T (Fig. 3.37).

standpoint, the successful removal of the capping layer selectively towards the metal has been demonstrated [Witters *et al.* (2008)]. This can help to achieve a similar CET for both n- and p-type channel FETs, irrespective of the capping layer involved. After the removal of the capping layer, a thick film of metal is deposited in order to complete the gate electrode (this fabrication scheme is illustrated in Fig. 3.39).

3.2.4.1.4 Impact of vacuum break during the metal electrode deposition

The fabrication of MuGFETs in a CMOS flow may thus require a two-step deposition of the gate electrode. This may have consequences on V_{fb} since thin metal films are involved. Oxidation of the upper metal surface is expected to affect substantially the metal work function, especially in the case of ultra-thin metal films ($\approx$1 to 2 nm). In order to assess the V_T deviation caused by a

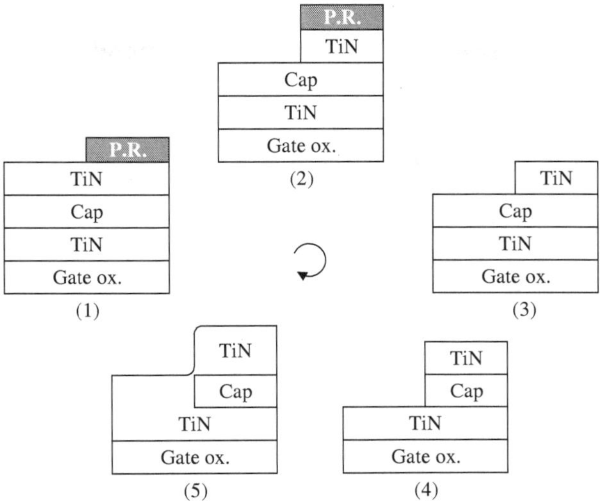

Figure 3.39. Illustration of the fabrication flow for a metal-inserted capping layer integration within a CMOS flow.

two-step metal deposition, MuGFETs involving different types of metal deposition sequences have been considered: two reference electrodes, one made of 5 nm and one made of 10 nm PE-ALD TiN; one metal electrode deposited in two steps, following the sequence: 5 nm TiN deposition, vacuum break, 5 nm TiN deposition; and one metal electrode made of 10 nm deposited at once, then removed completely in a wet cleaning solution, followed by a second deposition of 10 nm TiN. The purpose of the latter sample is to assess whether the removal of TiN selectively towards HfSiO is possible without consequence on V_T. For each sample, the threshold voltage and the I_{on}–I_{off} figure of merit is illustrated (Fig. 3.40). A limited V_T deviation is observed with the electrode subjected to the vacuum break ($\approx$30 mV). It is attributed to oxygen adsorption at the TiN surface, which results in a small increase of the TiN work function, without any consequence on the performance. This is also confirmed by the analysis of the gate capacitance, which reveals an identical CET for both samples. The same conclusion applies to the sample whose electrode underwent a complete metal removal.

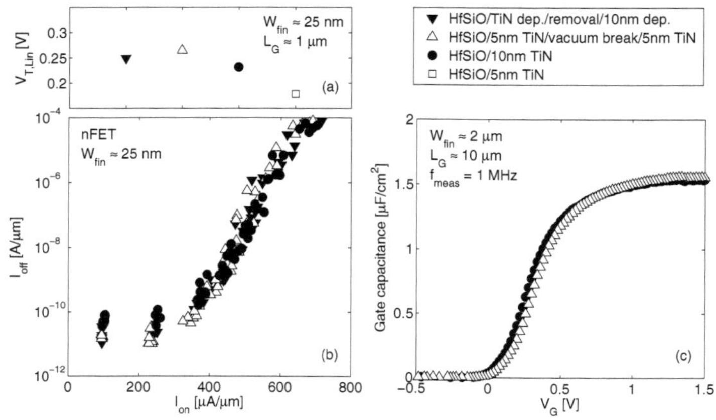

Figure 3.40. Deposition of capping layers within a metal gate electrode: impact of the vacuum break on (a) V_T and (b) the performance of n-MuGFETs ($W_{fin} = 25$ nm), and on (c) the gate oxide capacitance (and thus, CET)

3.2.4.1.5 Advantages

The integration of capping layers within the metal gate electrode keeps the low-field channel mobility, μ_{eff}, and the CET identical to those of the reference electrodes (without capping layer). It also helps to reduce CET variations among n- and p-channel FETs across CMOS designs.

3.2.4.1.6 Limitations

Unfortunately, these advantages are counterbalanced by a lower range for V_T tuning, depending on the nature of the capping layer, its thickness and its location within the metal gate electrode. In addition, the CMOS integration scheme involves the use of a photoresist layer onto the metal gate films. The removal of this resist film must guarantee the metal gate integrity, which is not obvious.

3.2.4.2 Metal thickness-induced V_{fb} shift

In an attempt to modify the metal/gate oxide interface, another option based on the metal deposition technique itself is investigated. It relies on thickness variations of ultra-thin TiN metal gates, which

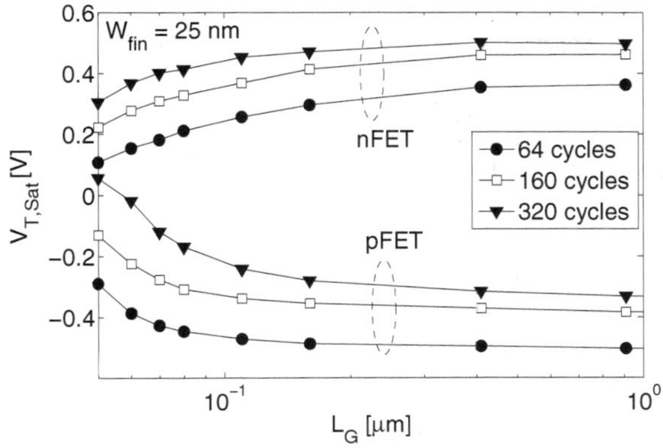

Figure 3.41. Threshold voltage as a function of the effective gate length for n- and p-type channel MuGFETs: impact of the PE-ALD TiN metal gate thickness.

are known to have a significant impact on the gate work function, irrespective of the deposition method [Singanamalla *et al.* (2006a,c); Choi *et al.* (2005)].

The thinner the TiN film, the more Ti-like the work function will become and the closer the work function will get to 4.33 eV (n-type). Since the PE-ALD technique offers very tight metal thickness control, this deposition technique is suitable for studying the impact of varying the TiN thickness on the electrical properties of MuGFETs. In this section, it is shown that the thickness of a PE-ALD TiN metal gate affects the nature of its reaction with the gate dielectric. This, in return, results in modifications of V_T and CET (improved SCE control), which can explain performance enhancement in nFETs without any performance loss in pFETs [Ferain *et al.* (2009)]. Fig. 3.41 illustrates that thin TiN metal gates result into more n-type like work function. On long gate length MuGFETs, up to 140 mV decrease in V_T is observed when the metal gate thickness varies from 10 to 2 nm (320 to 64 cycles, respectively, deposited on a few nanometers of hafnium silicate). Since V_T in MuGFETs is almost insensitive to fluctuations in gate oxide thickness, V_T variations are attributed to variations in the effective work function only [Taur (2000)]. The PE-ALD TiN process has an effect on the gate dielectric as well. Given the V_T differences of the samples, Capacitive

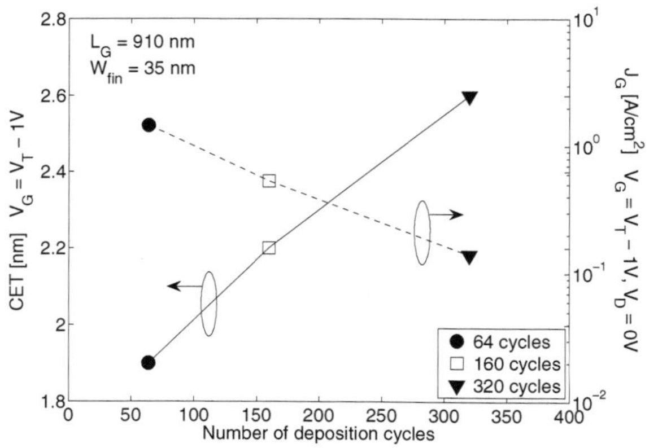

Figure 3.42. CET and normalized gate leakage as a function of the metal gate thickness (expressed in number of deposition cycles). CET and the gate leakage are measured at fixed gate overdrive $V_G = V_T$-1 V for p-MuGFETs.

Equivalent Thickness is extracted at fixed gate overdrive $V_T \pm 1$ V and not at $V_G = 1$ V. A reduction in CET is observed when the metal gate thickness decreases (Fig. 3.42). Both the gate leakage (also measured at fixed gate overdrive) and the drain-induced bias lowering (not shown) confirm the metal gate thickness dependence of CET. At low charge density, there is no significant difference in Coulomb scattering detected when the three different gate stacks are compared. This observation is valid also for quasi-planar MuGFETs (not shown). In terms of fixed oxide charge, the quality of the gate oxide is the same for the three gate stacks. In addition TEM analysis shows evidence of thinner SiO_2 interfacial layer for the gate stack with the thinnest metal gate electrode (Fig. 3.43). This suggests an interfacial oxide regrowth after activation anneal or during the TiN deposition.

3.2.4.2.1 Probing the PE-ALD TiN deposition

Gate stacks identical to those processed on the MuGFET devices (including the gate dielectric) have also been processed on bare Si wafers (it is referred to as 'Batch #1'). After the PE-ALD TiN deposition, all samples undergo a 1050°C spike anneal in N_2 followed by the etch-back of the TiN layer. On each sample,

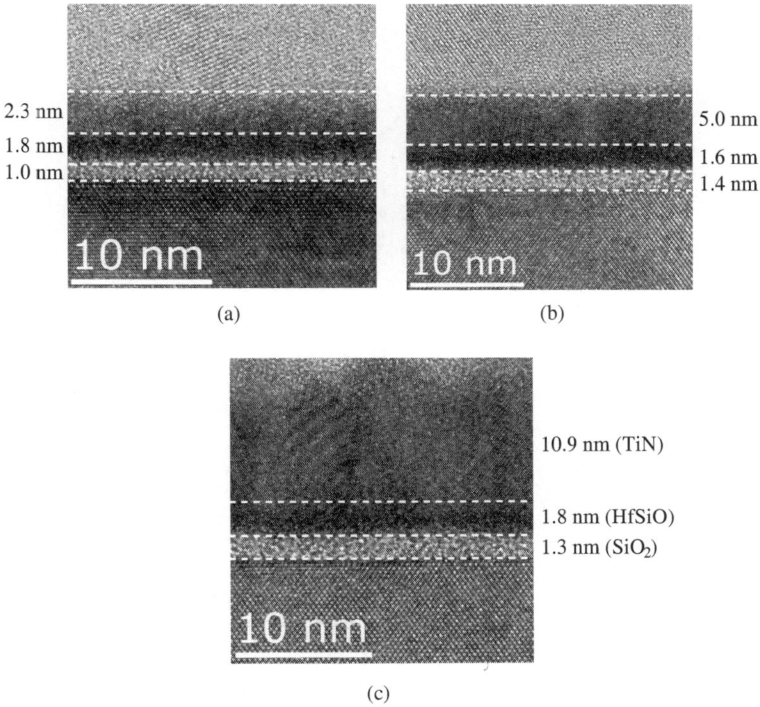

Figure 3.43. TEM micrographs of the gate stacks on MuGFETs: (a) 2 nm, (b) 5 nm, (c) 10 nm PE-ALD TiN.

approximately five monolayers of TiN are left after this etch-back step. Capacitance measurements have been performed on dots patterned after Platinum deposition to form the contacts. These measurements have been carried out at 10 kHz frequency and normalized to account for the dot area. Results are displayed in Fig. 3.44(a). In this figure, a capacitance variation reflecting the metal thickness dependence is observed. Also, a gate voltage shift of the gate capacitance characteristic ($\approx$300 mV) is noted between the samples with extreme metal gate thicknesses. These observations go along with the dependence observed on MuGFETs. The kink in the curves (positive gate voltage) suggests a relatively high density of interface states, which is expected since the samples have not received any FGA to passivate the Si/SiO_2 interface. In order to estimate its impact on the effective work function shift, the

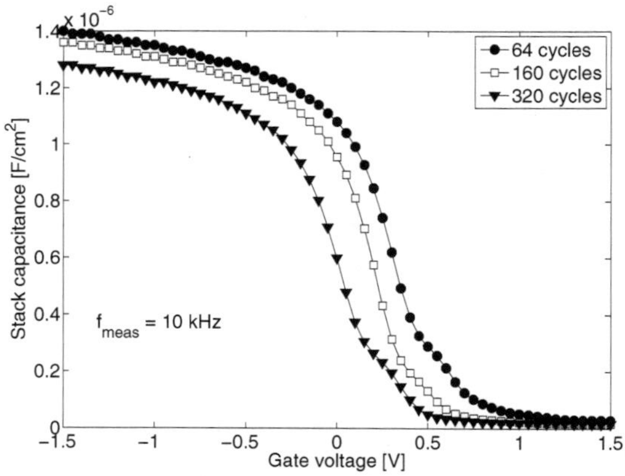

(a)

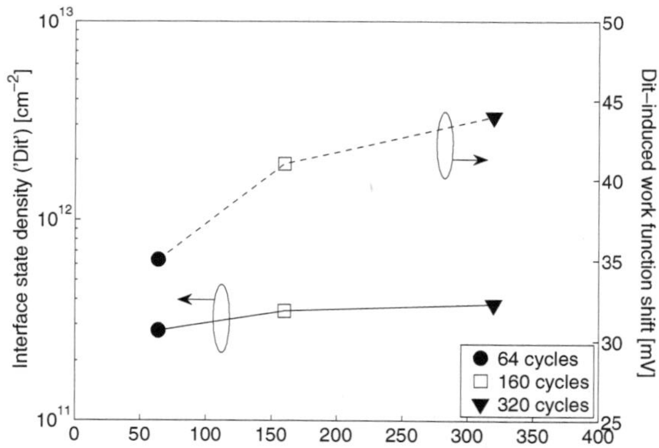

(b)

Figure 3.44. (a) Normalized stack capacitance as measured at 10 kHz, as a function of the PE-ALD TiN thickness (expressed in number of deposition cycles). A 300 mV of flat band voltage shift is observed, which cannot be attributed to interface state density only; (b) Density of interface states and the theoretical work function shift caused by these interface states as a function of the PE-ALD TiN gate thickness.

interface state density distribution has been determined. For this purpose, the Berglund integral is used to link the surface potential to the voltage applied on the gate [Berglund (1966)]. Fig. 3.44(b) illustrates that the interface state density exhibits very little gate stack dependence. It also contributes to a very limited gate voltage shift (maximum 45 mV$\pm$5 mV). The key conclusion from this gate capacitance measurement is that the magnitude of the effective work function shift depends on the initial metal thickness since it defines the composition of the TiN/HfSiO interface. The V_T shift is not attributed to the bulk work function of the metal gate. This conclusion is supported by physical analysis of thick TiN films. For this experiment, 20 nm of TiN have been deposited on 20 nm of SiO_2 (these samples are referred to as 'Batch#2') and submitted to depth profiling by angle-resolved XPS. For a TiN thickness between 15 and 5 nm (i.e., between 2000 s and 700 s of etch time in Fig. 3.45), no significant change in the TiN composition is noted. The work function difference between the 10 and 5 nm metal gate MuGFET samples cannot be attributed to a change in the composition of the metal. The work function dependence is therefore attributed to a modification of the metal/gate dielectric interface. However, this conclusion is not applicable to thinner metal gate electrodes. Indeed, the depth profile (Fig. 3.45) for a TiN thickness of 2 nm is influenced by the composition of the underlying film, i.e., SiO_2 in this case. The TEM micrographs illustrated in Fig. 3.43 present some elements for comparison between thin (2 nm) and thick ($>$5 nm) metal gate electrodes: crystalline features are observed along the whole TiN layer of the thick metal gate electrodes, indicating that these layers are mainly polycrystalline (not observed in the case of the thinnest TiN film, which remains amorphous); in addition, for the thickest metal gate electrode (15 nm), the TiN crystals are elongated in the growth direction indicating a columnar growth. Samples from Batch#1 have also been submitted to Angle Resolved XPS analysis in order to confirm that CET variations are due to a change in the physical thickness of the gate dielectric. In addition to the three gate stacks already mentioned, two reference samples, i.e., without TiN, have been considered. One of these reference samples has been subjected to N_2/H_2 plasma pulses in order to mimic the plasma exposure of the sample before the actual start

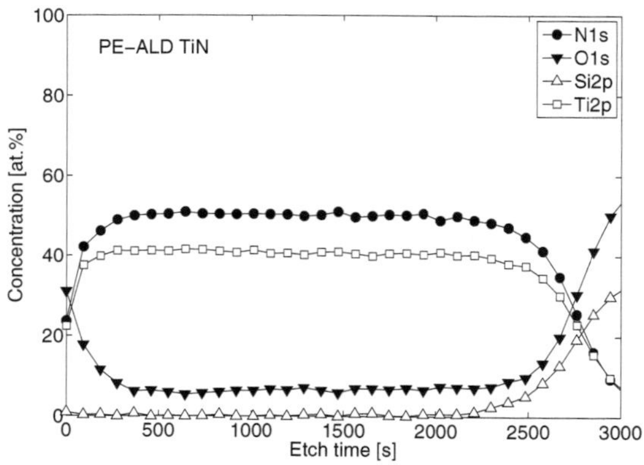

Figure 3.45. Depth profile of 20 nm PE-ALD TiN. Minority Cl and C bonds are not represented.

Table 3.8. Angle-resolved XPS analysis of 2.3 nm $HfSiO/SiO_2$ dielectric stacks: total dielectric thickness w/ or w/o plasma treatment and after PE-ALD TiN deposition

Number of deposition cycles	Total dielectric thickness [nm]	Nitrogen content [%]
Reference (w/o TiN)	3.4	n/a
'Plasma' (w/o TiN)	3.4	3.4
64	3.3	1.5
160 (Reference w/ TiN)	3.3	3.0
320	3.4	4.9

of the TiN deposition ('Plasma' sample). The results presented in Table 3.8 confirm the absence of dielectric etching by the plasma during the metal deposition. This suggests that CET variations are caused by physical modification (thickness and/or composition) of the dielectric, not by significant etching of the dielectric (HfSiO in this case) layer. Both TEM and AR-XPS analysis tend to show that the interfacial layer regrowth is too small for explaining the range of CET variations among the different gate stacks. For this reason, a change in the composition of the HfSiO layer has to be considered. From the same AR-XPS analysis, it has been observed that the nitrogen content in the dielectric stack is strongly dependent on the gate treatment. While the reference sample does not present any trace of nitrogen in the dielectric, the 'Plasma' sample reveals a nitrogen concentration of $\approx 3\%$ with a peak located deep into the dielectric (HfSiO/SiO_2 interface). In addition, the samples onto which PE-ALD TiN is deposited present a nitrogen composition which varies along with the duration of the TiN deposition process (Table 3.8).

3.2.4.2.2 Advantages

Varying the PE-ALD TiN thickness for tuning the threshold voltage of MuGFETs offers numerous advantages. Without requiring strain engineering techniques, it offers substantially higher performance for nFETs without any degradation for pFETs, even on short-channel transistors. In addition, better SCE control can be achieved on low-V_T transistors thanks to a CET reduction.

3.2.4.2.2 Limitations

If the incorporation of nitrogen into the HfSiO film during the PE-ALD TiN deposition is confirmed, this could cause some drawbacks in ultra-thin HfSiO films. Indeed, as the high-k thickness reduces, the nitrogen-induced charge can lower the channel mobility and, possibly the device performance. It can also degrade the device reliability from a bias temperature instability standpoint.

3.3 Flat Band Voltage Extraction in SOI MuGFETs

With ultra-thin gate dielectrics (high-k or not), the chemical and physical properties of the gate electrode/dielectric interface are expected to tune the gate/substrate band alignment and thus the device flat band (V_{fb}) and threshold voltages (V_T). The modification of this interface by the use of dielectric capping layers has already been demonstrated as a route to obtain required V_{fb}/V_T values for n- or pFET planar devices and also on MuGFETs [Kubicek *et al.* (2007); Veloso *et al.* (2008)]. The experimental determination of the band alignment is thus of crucial importance. However, very few experimental techniques are available to directly measure it, despite its significance. In addition, most of these techniques appear not to be suitable for gate work function extraction in MuGFETs on SOI. This would not be an issue as such if the processing of MuGFET devices did not include high-temperature specific steps like SEG. Since such process steps may have an impact on the gate work function, a method for extracting work function directly from SOI MuGFETs is needed. In this paragraph, it is explained why the most common methods used for gate work function extraction appear not to be suitable for extraction of the gate work function on fully depleted floating body FET devices like MuGFETs on SOI.

3.3.1 *Work Function Assessment on MOS Structures*

3.3.1.1 Internal photoemission method

Energy band alignment at insulator/semiconductor or metal/insulator interfaces can be quantified by using Internal Photoemission (IPE) spectroscopy. IPE can characterize a large number of solid/solid interfaces including materials like dielectrics, gate electrodes and substrates (Si, Ge and III-V in general) [Adamchuk and Afanas'ev (1992); Afanas'ev and Stesmans (2007)]. It relies on the photo-excitation of holes and electrons and their transition from one solid to another over the barrier height at their common interface. From a practical point of view, IPE is usually performed on MOS capacitors with a thin (transparent) metal layer. The capacitors are subjected to a monochromatic light illumination in order to stimulate the transition of holes and electrons from the metal to the semiconductor or vice-versa. In addition to the optical stimulation, the samples are biased, which creates an electric field at the interfaces. Depending on the bias set on the metal electrode, different types of IPE transitions will occur, which are detected by measuring the photocurrent. In addition, another current called 'photoconductivity current' (PC) is also collected. It is generated by hole/electron pair generation and their transport within the insulator itself. Based on the IPE and PC currents, a metric Y called 'quantum yield' is extracted, which enables band alignment and bandgap characterization, respectively. Y is defined as the ratio between the number of optically stimulated transitions and the number of excited photons. It can be extracted from the

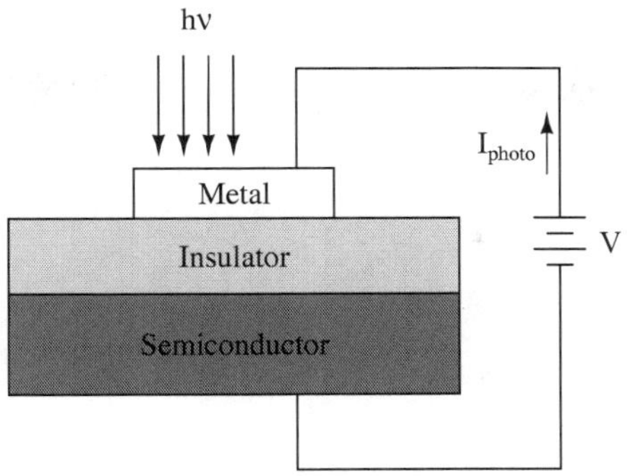

Figure 3.46. Schematic representation of the experimental setup for internal photoemission spectroscopy.

photocurrent I_{photo}, from the absorbed light power P and from the photon energy $h\nu$:

$$I_{photo}\ [\text{electrons/photon}] = \frac{P \cdot Y}{h\nu} \tag{3.4}$$

The type of information (oxide bandgap, barrier height) provided by the quantum yield depends on which transition is considered. The quantum yield based on PC transitions provides information on the oxide bandgap. While the quantum yield based on IPE transitions enables the extraction of the barrier heights defined at a solid/solid interface.

In order to ensure a uniform electrical field at the metal/insulator and/or insulator/semiconductor interfaces, the IPE technique is usually applied on large and thick samples. In addition, a body contact is required for collecting the photocurrent. It is therefore not suitable for extracting the gate work function on devices like multiple-fin MuGFETs.

3.3.1.2 Flat-band voltage vs. EOT method

A second method for work function extraction is the so-called 'V_{fb} vs. EOT' method. It is based on Eq. (3.5), which makes the flat-band voltage dependence on the oxide thickness obvious.

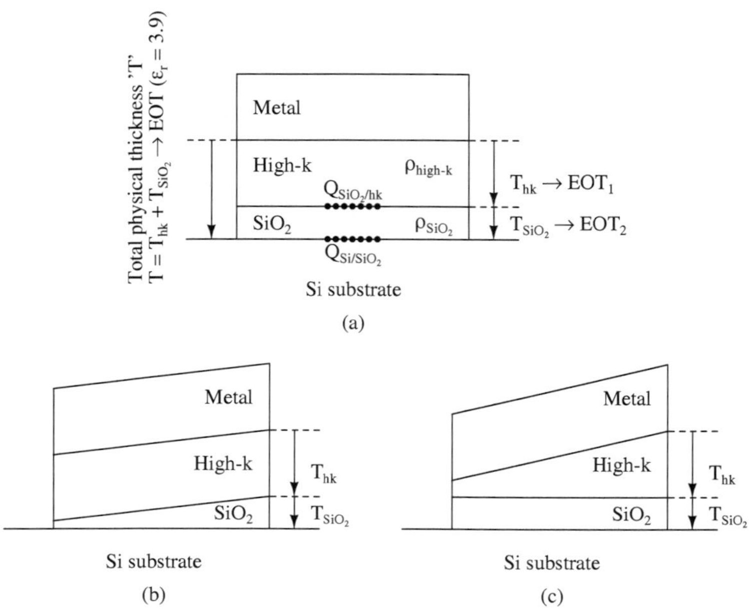

Figure 3.47. (a) SiO_2/high-*k*/metal gate stack structure: charge distribution parameters and their location, (b) Gate stack configuration for SiO_2-induced charge extraction, (c) Gate stack configuration for high-*k*-induced charge extraction.

$$V_{fb} = \phi_{ms} - \frac{\int_0^{t_{ox}} x \cdot \rho(x)dx}{\epsilon_0 \cdot \epsilon_{oxide}} = (\phi_m - \phi_s) + \delta D - \frac{\int_0^{t_{ox}} x \cdot \rho(x)dx}{\epsilon_0 \cdot \epsilon_{oxide}} \quad (3.5)$$

From this method, two coefficients can be extracted: the metal electrode work function from ϕ_{ms} and the gate oxide charge distribution. The method has been extended for gate oxides with multiple layers [Jha *et al.* (2004)]. This extension is essential for bilayer oxides like SiO_2/high-*k* and a brief description of its principles is given for this particular case. The parameters used for describing the charge contribution in the gate oxides are listed in Table 3.9 and illustrated in Fig. 3.47(a). The Equivalent Oxide Thickness of the high-*k* layer is referred to as 'EOT_1' while the SiO_2 thickness is referred to as 'EOT_2' ($EOT = EOT_1 + EOT_2$). Based on the flat band voltage definition (Eq. (3.5)) and given the presence of

Table 3.9. Charge-related parameters for gate oxide characterization.

Symbol	Unit	Origin
ρ	C/m^3	Total charge distribution per unit volume
ρ_{SiO_2}	C/m^3	SiO_2 charge distribution per unit volume
ρ_{hk}	C/m^3	High-k charge distribution per unit volume
Q_{Si/SiO_2}	C/m^2	Surfacic charge at the SiO_2/Si interface
$Q_{SiO_2/hk}$	C/m^2	Surfacic charge at the high-k/SiO_2 interface

the high-k layer, the flat-band voltage can be defined as:

$$V_{fb} = \left[\phi_{ms} - \left(\frac{Q_{SiO_2/hk}}{\epsilon_0 \cdot \epsilon_{SiO_2}}\right) \cdot EOT_1 - \left(\frac{\rho_{hk} - \rho_{SiO_2}}{2 \cdot \epsilon_0 \cdot \epsilon_{SiO_2}}\right) \cdot EOT_1^2\right]$$
$$- \left(\frac{Q_{Si/SiO_2}}{\epsilon_0 \cdot \epsilon_{SiO_2}}\right) \cdot EOT$$
$$- \left(\frac{\rho_{SiO_2}}{2 \cdot \epsilon_0 \cdot \epsilon_{SiO_2}}\right) \cdot EOT^2 \qquad (3.6)$$

The gate work function ϕ_{ms} can thus be extracted if $Q_{SiO_2/hk}$, ρ_{hk} and ρ_{SiO_2} values are known. The estimation of these charge contributions happens in two steps: first, the volumetric charge density in the SiO_2 layer and its planar charge density at the interface with the Si substrate are extracted. If EOT_1 stays constant and EOT_2 varies (Fig. 3.47(b)), Eq. (3.6) reveals a polynomial dependence of V_{fb} on EOT of order two. Q_{Si/SiO_2} and ρ_{SiO_2} can thus be extracted by fitting V_{fb} vs. EOT, by a least-mean square method for instance. Second, the charge contributions due to the presence of the high-k layer and its interface with the SiO_2 layer are also estimated. If EOT_2 stays constant and EOT_1 varies (Fig. 3.47(c)), Eq. (3.6) can be expressed as a function of EOT_2 = EOT-EOT_1. The V_{fb} dependence on EOT is also a polynomial of order two:

$$V_{fb} = \left[\phi_{ms} + \left(\frac{Q_{SiO_2/hk}}{\epsilon_0 \cdot \epsilon_{SiO_2}}\right) \cdot EOT_2 - \left(\frac{\rho_{hk} - \rho_{SiO_2}}{2 \cdot \epsilon_0 \cdot \epsilon_{SiO_2}}\right) \cdot EOT_2^2\right]$$
$$- \left[\left(\frac{Q_{SiO_2/hk} + Q_{Si/SiO_2}}{\epsilon_0 \cdot \epsilon_{SiO_2}}\right) + \left(\frac{\rho_{hk} - \rho_{SiO_2}}{\epsilon_0 \cdot \epsilon_{SiO_2}}\right) \cdot EOT_2\right] \cdot EOT$$
$$- \left(\frac{\rho_{hk} + \rho_{SiO_2}}{2 \cdot \epsilon_0 \cdot \epsilon_{SiO_2}}\right) \cdot EOT^2 \qquad (3.7)$$

In this case, the coefficient of the second order term can be extracted by fitting the V_{fb} vs. EOT dependence. Q_{Si/SiO_2} and ρ_{SiO_2} are known from Eq. (3.6), enabling the extraction of $Q_{SiO_2/hk}$ and ρ_{hk} from Eq. (3.7). Like the IPE technique, this method can also separate the oxide charge contribution from the metal work function. For this purpose, a very limited amount of samples (1 or 2 wafers only) is required for estimating [O'Sullivan *et al.* (2006)]. However, this method suffers from several shortcomings: it requires a body contact to enable complete gate capacitance measurement (from accumulation to strong inversion regime) in order to extract V_{fb}, it requires large gate areas and a broad range of gate oxide thickness values must be considered for varying every oxide layer thickness. In addition, a V_{fb} roll-off on long channel MOSFETs has also been observed at low EOT and increases the uncertainty in V_{fb} [Akiyama *et al.* (2007)]. For these reasons, this method is not the most appropriate for extracting V_{fb} on body-less and narrow structures like MuGFETs on SOI.

3.3.1.3 Fowler–Nordheim transition-based method

Another technique based on the gate leakage current and its dependence on the band structure has been proposed for extracting the barrier height of metal electrodes at the metal/insulator interface of MOS structures [Zafar *et al.* (2002)]. It relies on the gate leakage derivative with respect to gate leakage and does not require any body contact for V_{fb} extraction. Assuming that the affinity of the gate oxide (χ_{ox}) is known, it has been demonstrated that the barrier height (ϕ_m) of a metal electrode can be extracted from a simple gate leakage measurement. This method relies on the transition from direct tunneling to the Fowler–Nordheim (FN) regime when a MOS structure is biased accordingly. Recently, it has been demonstrated that this method for barrier height extraction is also valid with SiO_2/high-k stacks [Wen *et al.* (2006)]. In multiple-layered gate oxides, several transitions can be observed in the gate leakage evolution. Despite its elegance, it is not directly applicable to an arbitrary stack because the voltages needed to observe the transition from direct tunneling to the Fowler–Nordheim regime are quite high (i.e., close to breakdown) or because of the EOT and high-*k* composition dependence. It is particularly critical for gate stacks where the breakdown voltage is only slightly higher than the Fowler–Nordheim transition. In addition, transistor structures are required in order to allow a proper leakage current extraction.

3.3.1.4 Band alignment measurement

Another gate leakage-based technique can also extract band alignment data but at lower voltages than the method proposed in [Zafar *et al.* (2002)] [Pantisano *et al.* (2005)]. In weak inversion, gate leakage current primarily originates from electron tunneling from the inversion layer, while a small fraction is due to EVB tunneling. The EVB tunneling contribution normalized by the gate current contains the desired information on the band alignment and is not affected by EOT in the direct tunneling regime. By comparison of this current ratio (in weak inversion) among different FET devices with metal gate, one can estimate the work function difference between their gates (demonstrated on nFETs only). Unfortunately, this method cannot be directly applied for work function extraction on floating body devices like MuGFETs on SOI: it requires a bulk contact for performing the carrier separation experiment and collecting the EVB tunneling component. In addition, the validity of this method is restricted by the composition of the gate dielectric. As illustrated in Fig. 3.48(a), the portion in weak inversion of the current is substantially reduced as the Hf concentration in Hf-silicate dielectrics increases. This can be explained in terms of band-gap dependence on the Hf content (i.e., dielectric permittivity): the higher the Hf content, the lower the silicate's bandgap. As a result, the ECB tunneling current is expected to increase much faster than the EVB contribution as the gate bias increases (Fig. 3.48(b)). Despite these limitations, the EVB tunneling-based method can provide in-depth understanding of the gate leakage dependence on the energy band structure. This, in return, enabled the development of a gate-leakage derivative-based method for V_{fb} extraction on fully depleted MuGFETs on SOI [Ferain *et al.* (2008)]. Therefore, a detailed analysis of the Valence Band Electron tunneling-based method is provided in the next section before the method for V_{fb} extraction on MuGFETs is presented.

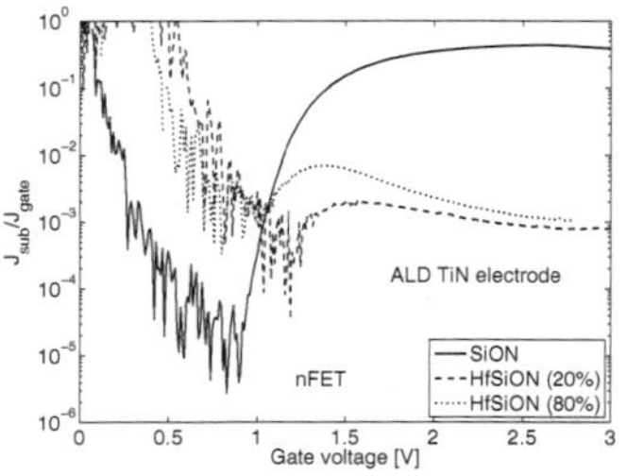

(a)

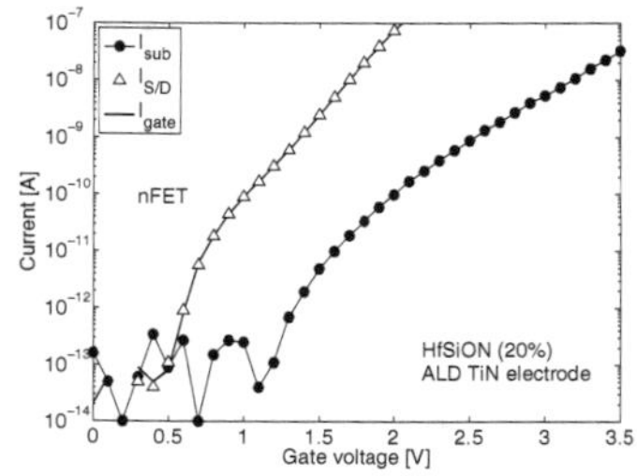

(b)

Figure 3.48. Standard planar n-type MOSFETs biased in inversion: (a) EVB tunneling current normalized by the gate current (standard planar n-type MOSFETs biased in inversion): dependence on the gate dielectric; (b) Gate leakage evolution in the SiO_2/HfSiON(20%Hf)/ALD TiN case.

3.3.2 *EVB Tunneling and Band Alignment (nFETs)*

This section aims to illustrate the universality of the gate conduction mechanism dependence on the band alignment in direct tunneling regime. Different gate electrodes with well known work functions, processed in a CMOS flow on standard planar devices, are considered (Table 3.10). The same channel doping ($N_{sub} = 2 \times 10^{17}\text{cm}^{-3}$) is used for all devices. SiON and HfSiO are the dielectrics considered. On these devices, carrier separation is performed to measure the different current contributions to the gate leakage. Note that only long-channel devices are considered, allowing contributions from gate to source/drain extension overlap regions to be neglected. On these planar FETs, RF Capacitance-Voltage measurements are used to ensure high quality CV results on ultra-thin dielectrics, and thus reliable extraction of V_{fb}, EOT and electric field across the oxide for all samples and biases of interest. From the fitting to the measured data, the voltage drop across the oxide (V_{ox}) is extracted for all samples.

3.3.2.1 EVB tunneling-based metric: definition

The basic principle behind the EVB tunneling-based characterization technique is illustrated in Fig. 3.49(a), 3.49(b) and 3.49(c). Once

Table 3.10. Experimental gate stacks considered (planar nFETs): dielectric and electrode composition, EOT and V_{fb} are extracted from gate capacitance characteristics.

Gate dielectric	Gate electrode	EOT (nm)	V_{fb}(V)
SiON	n^+ polysilicon	1.5	−1.09
SiON	20 cycles ALD TiN	1.3	−0.97
SiON	60 cycles ALD TiN	1.3	−0.80
SiON	100 cycles ALD TiN (2.5 nm)	1.3	−0.74
SiON	200 cycles ALD TiN [Westlinder *et al.* (2003)] (5 nm)	1.3	−0.65
SiON	10 nm ALD TaN [Pantisano *et al.* (2005)]	1.5	−0.37
SiON	10 nm PVD TaN [Pantisano *et al.* (2005)]	1.5	−0.64
SiON + Al_2O_3 [Singanamalla *et al.* (2007b)]	200 cycles ALD TiN	1.6	−0.36
MOCVD HfSiON(50%Hf)	n^+ polysilicon	1.5	−0.83
MOCVD HfSiON(50%Hf)	30 nm Nickel FUSI [Kittl *et al.* (2006)]	0.8	−0.57

the inversion layer is formed, an electron (nFETs) or hole (pFETs) tunneling current supplied by the source and drain junctions flows from the inverted channel into the gate (its density is referred to as $J_{S/D}$). At a gate voltage (absolute) larger than a certain onset, a substrate current (its density is referred to as J_{sub}) is observed, which increases exponentially with gate bias for both n- and pFETs. For nFETs, electrons are tunneling from the Si valence band into the gate while for pFETs, electrons from the gate are tunneling into the Si conduction band [Pantisano *et al.* (2005); DiMaria and Stathis (2001)]. In both cases this onset occurs when the MOSFET is biased such that the voltage drop across the gate oxide V_{ox} is large enough to align the Si valence (nFET) or conduction (pFET) bands with the Fermi energy of the gate electrode ($E_{F,M}$). Both J_{sub} and J_{gate} contain information on the band structure (EOT and $E_{F,M}$) and, as such, are expected to provide information on the effective work function of interest.

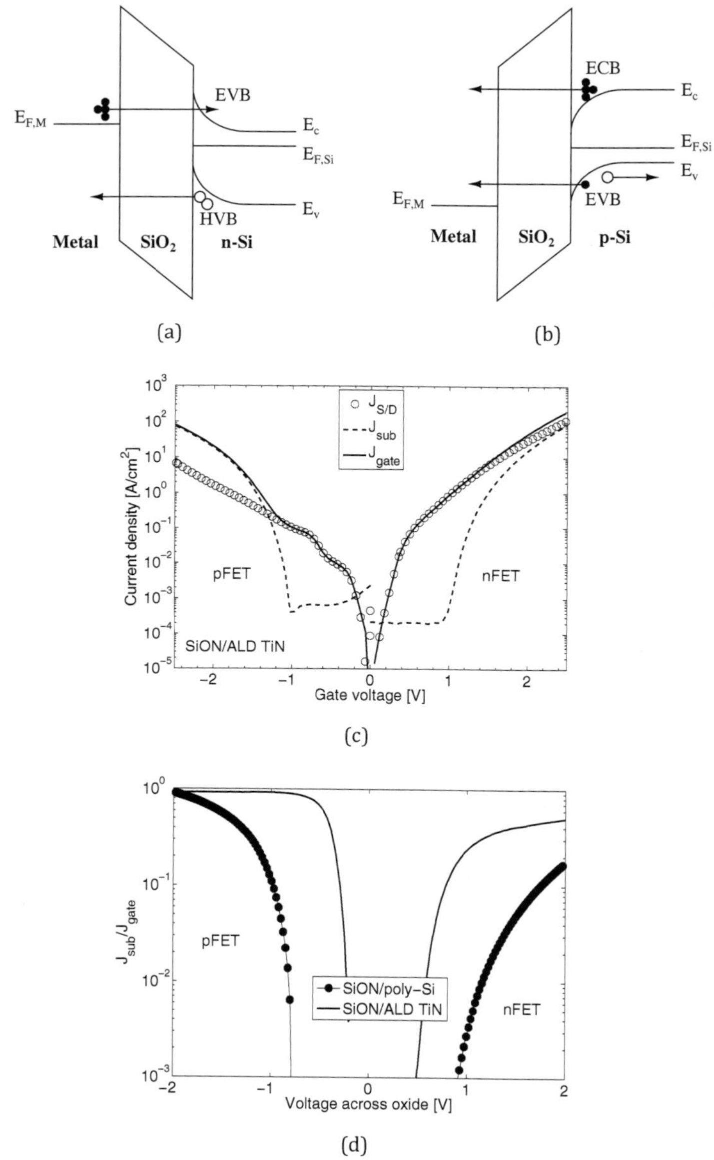

Figure 3.49. (a) and (b) Band diagram of n- and pMOSFET (metal gate) biased in weak inversion; (c) Carrier separation experiment, source, drain and substrate terminals are set at 0 V while the gate voltage sweeps from 0 to + (−) 2.0 V for nFETs (pFETs); (d) Impact of the gate electrode on the J_{sub}/J_{gate} vs. V_G dependence.

3.3.2.2 Metric independence on EOT

Since J_{sub} and J_{gate} individually depend exponentially on the EOT considered, the ratio J_{sub}/J_{gate} is preferred to J_{sub} (Fig. 3.49(d)). It ensures EOT independence of the band alignment metric in the J_{sub} onset region for both n- and pFET devices [Pantisano *et al.* (2005)]. Note the difference between J_{sub}/J_{gate} trends for polysilicon gates and metal gates, respectively. The J_{sub}/J_{gate} ratio reaches its maximum ('1') level at lower V_{ox} with metal gates than polysilicon gates. This is attributed to the higher density of electrons available for EVB tunneling in the metal gate case.

3.3.2.3 Application to n-MOSFETs

J_{sub}/J_{gate} is plotted vs. V_{ox} in order to account for the effect of EOT on the band structure. To do so, the voltage drop across the oxide is measured and the metric for work function extraction is then defined as V_{ox} at J_{sub}/J_{gate} as low as possible (J_{sub}/J_{gate} onset). In the nFET case, V_{ox} is extracted at $J_{sub}/J_{gate} = 1 \times 10^{-3}$ because of the practical limit set by junction leakage. This metric is also referred to as 'EVB tunneling-defined.' Fig. 3.50 illustrates the linear dependence between the EVB tunneling-defined metric and V_{fb}, irrespective of the dielectric composition and of the deposition technique: the work function difference ($\Delta\phi_m$) between the different gate electrodes can be directly estimated by calculating the difference between their respective EVB tunneling-defined V_{ox}. Fig. 3.50 is a key result since it demonstrates the importance of the gate electrode/dielectric interface on the band alignment. From gate leakage point of view, it also demonstrates that fixed charge is of little importance for thin high-*k* gate dielectrics like HfSiO in the direct tunneling regime. In the case of thicker dielectrics involving higher charge content (cf. Fig. 3.48(a)) the linear dependence between the EVB tunneling-defined metric and V_{fb} is no longer valid. This dependence between V_{fb} and gate leakage can be used to benchmark the work function in a very concise way also. With SiON dielectrics, the highest work function is obtained with an Al_2O_3 dielectric cap deposited between SiON and the ALD TiN electrode while the lowest work function is achieved with n^+ poly and thin

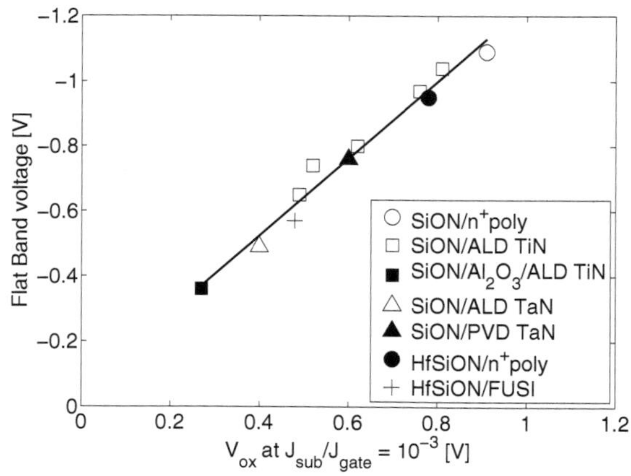

Figure 3.50. Illustration of gate leakage vs. band alignment dependence on nMOSFETs. Multiple data points for SiON/ALD TiN include multiple TiN thicknesses.

ALD TiN electrodes. The V_{fb} shift ($\sim$0.3 V) resulting from the deposition of the Al_2O_3 cap layer is similar to the value extracted from *C-V* measurements and previously reported for the same gate stacks [Singanamalla *et al.* (2007b)].

3.3.2.4 Extension to p-MOSFETs

Results illustrated in Fig. 3.50 are also valid for pFET devices. The gate stacks used in this section are described in Table 3.11. Again considering different EOT values, the ratio J_{sub}/J_{gate} is plotted in order to verify the EOT independence (Fig. 3.51) in the J_{sub} onset region. In the pFET case, the EVB tunneling-defined metric is now defined as V_{ox} at $J_{sub}/J_{gate} = 1 \times 10^{-2}$. The EVB tunneling-defined metric extracted for all pFET samples is summarized with nFET results in Fig. 3.52. The latter further emphasizes two salient features: gate leakage is linked to the band structure: the EVB tunneling-defined metric allows reliable work function extraction in both n- and pFETs, despite the different carriers and mechanisms involved (electrons tunneling from the Si valence band in the nFET case, electrons tunneling from the gate electrode in the pFET case).

Table 3.11. Experimental gate stacks considered (planar pFETs): dielectric and electrode composition, EOT and V_{fb} are extracted from gate capacitance characteristics

Gate dielectric	Gate electrode	EOT (nm)	V_{fb}(V)
SiON	p^+ polysilicon	1.4	0.82
SiON	20 cycles ALD TiN	1.3	0.33
SiON	60 cycles ALD TiN	1.3	0.13
SiON	100 cycles ALD TiN (2.5 nm)	1.3	0.14
SiON	200 cycles ALD TiN [Westlinder *et al.* (2003)] (5 nm)	1.3	0.27
SiON	10 nm PVD MoO [Ohfuji *et al.* (1984)]	2.4	0.56
SiON	10 nm PVD MoON	2.0	0.52
SiON + Al_2O_3 [Singanamalla *et al.* (2007b)]	200 cycles ALD TiN	1.6	0.64

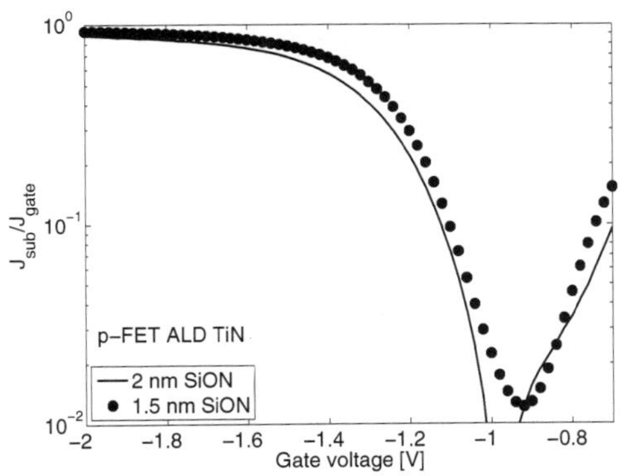

Figure 3.51. J_{sub}/J_{gate} vs. V_G dependence and its EOT independence.

In ultra-thin gate dielectrics, the gate electrode/dielectric interface plays a major role in setting the work function, irrespective of the gate dielectric material (SiON or HfSiO) and deposition technique (MOCVD vs. ALD HfSiO) but also of the gate electrode material (poly or FUSI or metal), deposition technique (ALD vs. PVD TaN) and thickness (ALD TiN variations).

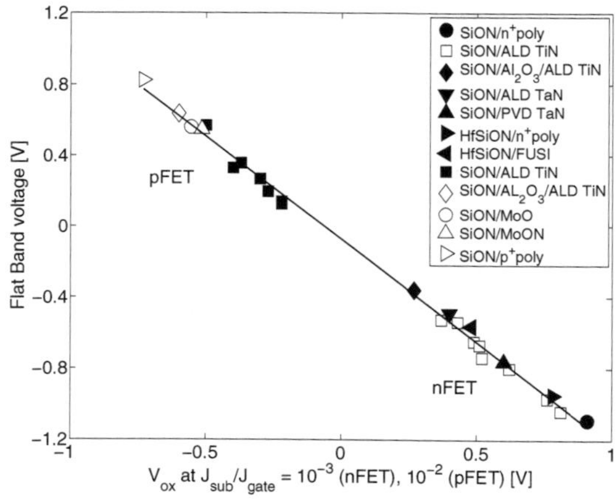

Figure 3.52. Universality of the gate leakage vs. band alignment dependence. Multiple data points for SiON/ALD TiN include multiple TiN thicknesses.

3.3.2.5 Limitations

As this method is based on direct tunneling through the gate stack, it is evident that the physical thickness has to be sufficiently low to ensure this is the case. Apart from this limitation, another due to gate length scaling is foreseen. Since the gate overlap capacitance does not scale down with the gate length, correct estimation of the total gate-to-channel capacitance becomes a matter of concern in short channel FETs. Even though this capacitance can be corrected to account for the gate overlap capacitance, gate length scaling is expected to have a detrimental impact on the accuracy of V_{ox} extraction. In addition, any regrowth at the edges of ultra-thin gate dielectrics will significantly modify the gate conduction mechanism in short channel FETs with respect to long channel ones.

3.3.3 *Gate Leakage Derivative-Based Method*

3.3.3.1 Band alignment and metric definition

For comparison purpose, another metric referring to the gate leakage current and its derivative is collected [Zafar *et al.* (2002)].

The technique relies on the $d(\ln(J_{gate}))/dV_G$ characteristic (later referred to as 'J_{gate}-derivative') of n(p)FETs biased in accumulation (inversion). It is discussed further for the pFET case. The J_{gate}-derivative characteristic presents two maxima as can be seen in Fig. 3.53(a): the first one occurs close to V_T and is attributed to enhanced hole injection from the inversion layer into the gate; the second one appears at larger (absolute) gate voltage. The carrier separation experiment shows that this condition is achieved when the electron injection from the gate (J_{sub}) starts exceeding the hole injection from the substrate ($J_{S/D}$).

The position of the second peak is attributed to the alignment of the gate electrode Fermi level ($E_{F,M}$) with the top of the Si conduction band. The band alignment in this situation is illustrated in Fig. 3.53(b). Now V_{ox} is defined at the second peak of the J_{gate}-derivative characteristic as a metric for work function extraction. This metric is later referred to as the '$J_{sub} = J_{S/D}$-defined' one.

3.3.3.2 Comparison with the EVB tunneling-defined method

Both the EVB tunneling- and $J_{sub} = J_{S/D}$-defined metrics are plotted as function of V_{fb} in Fig. 3.54. Two features are noted at this point. First, the fitted line shows a slightly lower but still acceptable correlation factor ($\rho > 0.9$) with the '$J_{sub} = J_{S/D}$'-defined condition. Indeed, more scattered results are inherent to the $J_{sub} = J_{S/D}$-defined method, as it relies on a derivative function. Second, the two fitted lines are separated by a constant value of 0.15 V on the V_{ox} axis. For a given V_{fb}, the fitted lines are separated by a constant ΔV_{ox}. This distance is expected to correspond to the difference in band bending in the Si due to the metric definitions. On their respective band diagrams (3.53(b) and 3.53(c)), one can see that the metrics are defined at a different voltage drop across the oxide, involving a different band bending in the Si. It is important to note that despite these differences - the EVB tunneling-defined technique relies on band alignment while the technique based on the J_{gate}-derivative is a direct barrier height measurement - both methods allow accurate V_{fb} extraction for thin gate dielectrics. Depending on the application, either may be preferable: the EVB tunneling-defined metric offers slightly higher accuracy but requires a bulk contact.

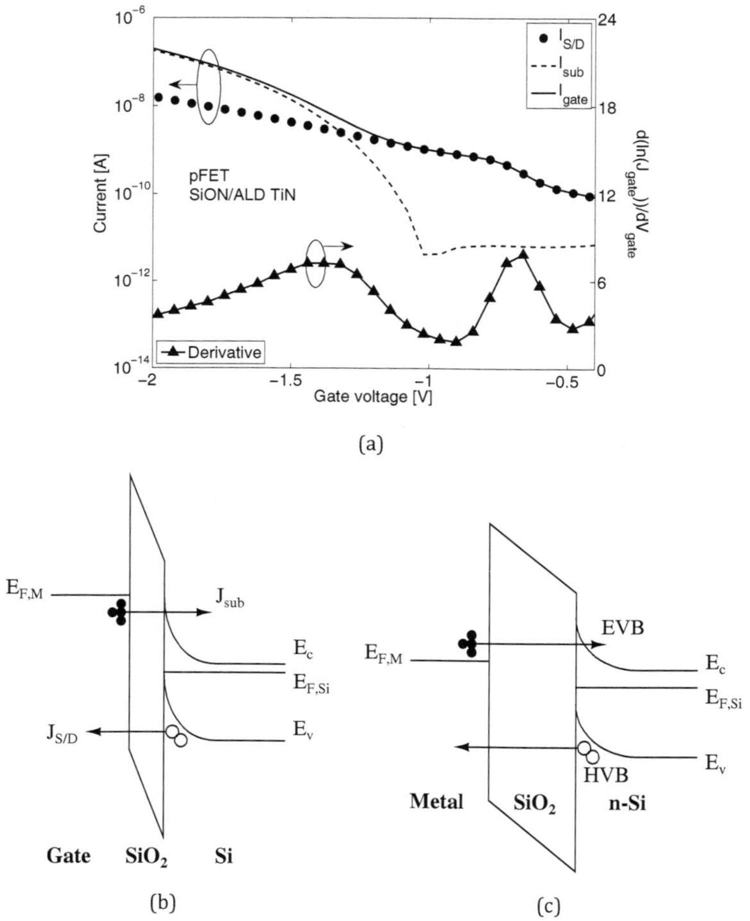

Figure 3.53. (a) Carrier separation experiment on the 5 nm ALD TiN/SiON gate stack (pFET in inversion) and comparison with the J_{gate}-derivative characteristic; (b) Band diagram of pMOSFET (metal gate) biased in strong inversion at $\left|\frac{d\ln(J_{gate})}{dV_G}\right|_{max}$ and (c) for comparison purpose, the band diagram of a pMOSFET (metal gate) biased in inversion at the J_{sub}/J_{gate} onset.

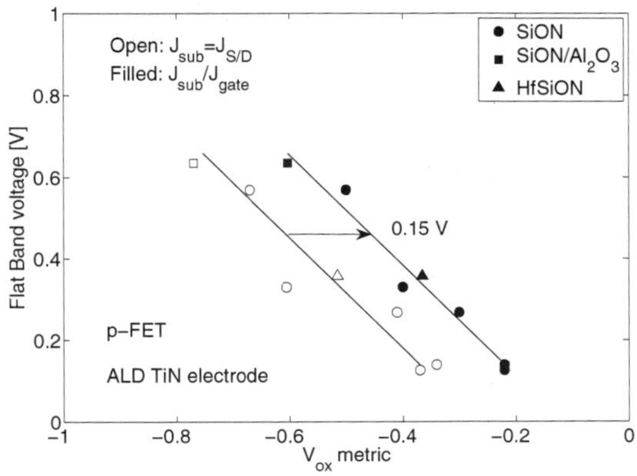

Figure 3.54. Gate leakage vs. band alignment dependence on pFETs: comparison between the EVB tunneling- and '$J_{sub} = J_{S/D}$'-defined metrics. Multiple data points for SiON/ALD TiN include multiple TiN thicknesses.

3.3.4 *The Fully Depleted Floating Body MuGFET Case*

Unlike planar MOSFETs fabricated on bulk Si substrates, the gate capacitance feature of a MuGFET on SOI does not include any accumulation characteristic. It is therefore not possible to accurately estimate the flat-band voltage by modeling the gate capacitance. In this section, it is demonstrated for the first time that both V_{fb} and ϕ_m in narrow MuGFETs on SOI substrates can be successfully extracted by using a leakage-based technique.

3.3.4.1 Framework and constraints

However, two important points regarding the applicability of the V_{fb} extraction techniques in floating body MuGFETs need to be highlighted: first, the absence of a bulk contact makes the extraction of the EVB tunneling contribution impossible. Therefore, the $J_{sub} = J_{S/D}$-defined metric based on the J_{gate}-derivative characteristic is the only viable option for assessing the flat-band voltage. Second, the full silicon depletion does not allow sufficient carrier accumulation and restricts the V_{fb} extraction to MOSFETs biased in inversion. Therefore, pFETs are the only suitable devices for extracting V_{fb} in fully depleted floating body devices since the J_{gate}-derivative of

Table 3.12. Origin of carriers in inversion leakage currents.

Current features	pFET	nFET
$J_{S/D}$	holes are supplied by the p^+ junctions	electrons are supplied by the n^+ junctions
J_{sub}	electrons are supplied by the metal gate	holes are supplied by the substrate

nFETs does not present any optimum feature (see Fig. 3.49(b)). In order to understand why there is no optimum feature on the J_{gate} characteristic of nFET in inversion, it is important to refer to the origins (in terms of carrier suppliers) of each leakage component ($J_{S/D}$ and J_{sub}) for both n- and pFETs (Table 3.12): In the pFET case, the J_{sub} contribution is able to exceed the $J_{S/D}$ one because the density of negative carriers in the gate is much higher than the density of positive carriers in the junctions. Therefore, it is possible for J_{sub} to become larger than $J_{S/D}$ in the inversion regime. In the nFET case, the density of minority carriers in the substrate can never exceed with the density of negative carriers supplied by the junctions. As a consequence, the J_{sub} contribution remains lower than the $J_{S/D}$ one at any gate voltage. This explains the absence of an optimum feature on the $d(\ln(J_{gate}))/dV_G$ characteristic of nFETs in inversion, independent on the type of substrate discussed in the present study (bulk Si vs. SOI). It must be mentioned that any modification of the channel doping (concentration and/or type) and/or work function is not an option to make the V_{fb} extraction possible on nFET devices. The presence or absence of an optimum feature is inherent to the type of FET under study. It also explains the practical limit on J_{sub}/J_{gate} when we define the EVB tunneling-metric: V_{ox} at $J_{sub}/J_{gate} = 1 \times 10^{-3}$ and V_{ox} at $J_{sub}/J_{gate} = 1 \times 10^{-2}$ for n- and pFETs, respectively.

3.3.4.2 Flat band voltage extraction

The MuGFETs used to illustrate the V_{fb} extraction have a nominal fin width of 25 nm and a fin height of 60 nm. They were processed on SOI substrates [Collaert *et al.* (2005)]. Their gate stacks consist of 2 nm SiO_2 and 10 nm of metal gate, being either

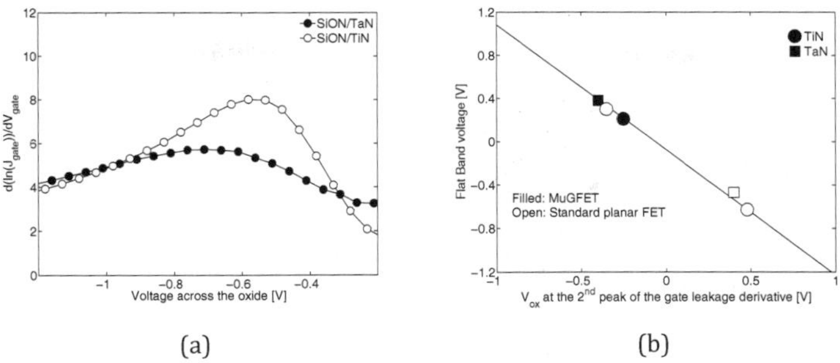

Figure 3.55. (a) Gate leakage derivative-based indicator extracted on narrow MuGFETs, (b) Gate leakage vs. band alignment dependence: comparison between planar FETs on Si bulk substrate and fully depleted MuGFETs on SOI (TaN et TiN metal gates) after appropriate corrections on V_{ox} to account for substrate doping and extraction method differences in MuGFETs.

MOCVD TiN or ALD TaN, capped with 100 nm of polysilicon. Fig. 3.55(a) illustrates the evolution of the J_{gate}-derivative as function of gate voltage. Based on the $J_{sub} = J_{S/D}$-defined condition, $V_{ox} = -0.68$ V and $V_{ox} = -0.53$ V are extracted for the TaN and TiN gates, respectively. This points towards a $\Delta\phi_m$ of 0.15 V between the MOCVD TiN and ALD TaN gate electrodes. For a correct V_{fb} extraction based on (Fig. 3.52), two corrections on V_{ox} are needed: First, V_{ox}-metrics of MuGFETs are re-scaled to account for substrate doping (N_{sub}) difference with respect to planar devices. Differences in N_{sub} between the planar MOSFETs ($N_{sub} = 2 \times 10^{17}\text{cm}^{-3}$) and MuGFETs ($N_{sub} = 1.5 \times 10^{15}\text{cm}^{-3}$) result in a Si bulk potential difference leading to a $V_{ox} = 0.13$ V correction. Second, a $V_{ox} = 0.15$ V correction is added for matching the $J_{sub} = J_{S/D}$ and EVB tunneling-defined metrics (Fig. 3.54). After correction, flat band voltage values are extracted for the MOCVD TiN ($V_{fb} = 0.2$ V) and ALD TaN ($V_{fb} = 0.4$ V) gates on p-type MuGFETs from Fig. 3.52. Their V_{fb} is illustrated on the universal metric curve in Fig. 3.55(b). For the MOCVD TiN gate electrodes, the estimation is very close to the V_{fb} value extracted from planar pFETs. The small difference is attributed to the deposition process (ALD TiN in planar FETs). For the ALD TaN electrodes, planar pFET samples were not available for direct comparison with p-type MuGFETs. However, it should be noted that the V_{fb} difference between ALD TaN and ALD TiN gates on planar nFETs is found to be the same as between ALD TaN gates on p-type MuGFETs and ALD TiN gates planar pFETs. Note that the difference in peak width between TiN and TaN electrodes is not a consequence of substrate doping since it is the same for all MuGFET samples. Therefore it can reasonably be attributed to the electrode material itself. These peak width variations may result from process differences such as nitrogen absorption into the dielectric during gate electrode deposition or small local non-uniformities in the band alignment. The peak width has limited impact on the V_{fb} extraction accuracy and therefore does not endanger its validity.

3.3.4.3 Limitations

3.3.4.3.1 Gate dielectric nature

The gate-leakage based method for V_{fb} extraction on MuGFETs requires the calculation of V_{ox} as a function of V_G. V_{ox} may be difficult to assess in the case of gate oxides with dielectric capping layers for instance (see section 3.2), which may limit the accuracy of V_{ox}.

3.3.4.3.2 Corner effect

In multiple-gate devices, gate current can dramatically increase because of the larger electrical field at the device corners. In order to overcome this major issue, the processing of the MuGFETs includes optimized H_2 anneal for corner rounding right after the fin patterning. This results in nicely rounded corners and helps to prevent a dramatic increase in gate leakage at the corners of the fins [Xiong *et al.* (2004)].

3.3.4.3.3 Crystal orientation effect

In this study, the MuGFET structures present (100) and (110) as crystal orientations for the top and sidewall planes of the fins, respectively. Naturally, this has an impact on the interface state density. Nonetheless, interface states do not interfere with the gate tunneling mechanism. Therefore, the crystal orientation is not expected to interfere with the mechanism onto which the V_{fb} extraction is based. Still, it is worth noting that the gate oxide thickness may depend on the crystal orientation and on the process used for oxide formation [Meuris *et al.* (1995)]. This is the case for ultra-thin gate oxides (<1 nm), which may grow at different rates at the top and sidewall planes of the Si fin. Of course, this may affect the results from V_{fb} extraction but is not an intrinsic limitation of the extraction method itself.

3.3.4.3.4 Metal gate conformality effect

In a similar way, the metal gate conformality may also limit the validity of the gate-leakage based extraction. Indeed, the MuGFET topography may cause different V_{fb} values between top and sidewalls of the fin. This can be due to different metal gate thicknesses (thinner metal gate on the sidewalls) and thus different gate stack compositions between top and sidewalls of the fins. For this reasons, ALD and PE-ALD techniques are preferred for gate stack formation since they allow excellent uniformity for both gate dielectric and metal gate deposition (at least for thicknesses down to 2 nm).

3.3.4.3.5 The Gate Induced Floating Body Effect

As a final comment, the impact of the 'gate-induced floating body effect' (GIFBE) on the V_{fb} extraction is addressed. In partially depleted SOI FETs, the electron injection from the gate into the substrate causes the body to get charged and therefore modifies the body potential. It results in a second peak in the linear transconductance g_m whose magnitude depends on the fin width and gate length. This gate-induced floating body effect may, in return, affect the injection itself [Cassé *et al.* (2004)]. This effect is not a limitation for V_{fb} extraction in MuGFETs with narrow Si fins, which show excellent immunity against GIFBE. However, it is important to remind that this effect may affect the V_{fb} extraction if larger fin structures are tested.

List of Symbols

Symbol	Unit	Description
q	C	Elementary charge $= 1.60218 \times 10^{-19}$
C_{ox}	F/m^2	Gate oxide capacitance
δD	V	Dipole voltage
$E_{F,M}$	eV	Fermi level of the metal gate in a MOS structure

Symbol	Unit	Description
ϵ_0	F/m	Vacuum permittivity $= 8.8541878176 \times 10^{-12}$
ϵ_{SiO_2}	–	Silicon dioxide relative permittivity $= 3.9$
ϵ_{oxide}	–	Gate oxide relative permittivity
g_m	Ω^{-1}	Transconductance of a MOSFET
I_{ds}	A	Net drain-to-source current in a MOSFET transistor
I_{on}	A/μm	On-state drain current in a MOSFET transistor
I_{off}	A/μm	Off-state drain current in a MOSFET transistor
L_G	m	Gate length of a MOSFET transistor
μ_{eff}	m^2/Vs	Effective mobility of electrons and holes
N_{sub}	cm^{-3}	Doping concentration in the silicon substrate
ϕ_b	V	Potential difference between the Fermi level in a semiconductor and its intrinsic Fermi level
ϕ_m	V	Metal work function
ϕ_{ms}	V	Metal/Silicon work function difference
ϕ_s	V	Silicon work function
Q_d	cm^{-2}	Depletion charge
Q_{ox}	cm^{-2}	Oxide charge
t_{ox}	cm	Gate oxide thickness
V_{fb}	V	Flat band voltage
V_G	V	Voltage applied on the gate terminal
V_T	V	Threshold voltage of a MOSFET transistor
$V_{T,Lin}$	V	Linear threshold voltage, drain to source bias $= 50$ mV
$V_{T,Sat}$	V	Saturation threshold voltage, drain to source bias $= 1$ V
W_{fin}	m	Top width of a MuGFET transistor
$q \cdot \chi_{ox}$	eV	Electron affinity of the gate oxide

List of Acronyms

Acronym	Description
ALD	Atomic layer deposition
AVD	Atomic vapor deposition
BEOL	Back end of line
CMOS	Complementary metal oxide semiconductor
DPN	Decoupled plasma nitridation
EOT	Equivalent oxide thickness
ECB	Electron conduction band
EVB	Electron valence band
FEOL	Front end of line
FGA	Forming gas anneal
HP	High-performance
HR-TEM	High-resolution transmission electron microscopy
IPE	Internal photoemission
LSTP	Low standby power
MOCVD	Metal-organic chemical vapor deposition
MOSFET	Metal oxide semiconductor field-effect transistor
MuGFET	Multiple-gate FET
nFET	n-type MOSFET
pFET	p-type MOSFET
PC	Photo-conductivity
PNA	Post nitridation anneal
PE-ALD	Plasma-enhanced ALD
PE-CVD	Plasma-enhanced CVD
SEG	Selective epitaxial growth
SEM	Scanning electron microscopy
SIMS	Secondary ion mass spectroscopy
SOI	Silicon-on-insulator
SCE	Short channel effect
XPS	X-ray photoelectron spectroscopy
GI-XRD	Grazing incidence X-ray diffraction
XRR	X-ray reflectivity

References

Adamchuk, V. and Afanas'ev, V. (1992). Internal photoemission spectroscopy of semiconductor-insulator interfaces, *Progress in Surface Science*, **41**, 2, pp. 111–211.

Adelmann, C., Franquet, A., Conard, T., Witters, T., Ferain, I., Meersschaut, J., Jurczak, M., De Meyer, K., Kittl, J. and Van Elshocht, S. (2009). Interface stability in advanced high-*k*-metal-gate stacks, *Journal of Vacuum Science and Technology B*, **27**, pp. 1021–1025.

Adelmann, C., Lehnen, P., Ragnarsson, L.-A., Conard, T., Franquet, A., Chang, V., Rohr, E., Meersschaut, J., Boissiére, O., Lohe, C., Schram, T., Van Elshocht, S. and De Gendt, S. (2008a). Thermally-stable high effective work function TaCN and Ta_2N films for pMOS metal gate applications, in *Materials Research Society Symposium Proceedings*, Vol. 1073E, pp. 1073–H01–08.

Adelmann, C., Lehnen, P., Van Elshocht, S., Zhao, C., Brijs, B., Franquet, A., Conard, T., Roeckerath, M., Schubert, J., Boissiére, O., Lohe, C. and De Gendt, S. (2007). Growth of dysprosium-, scandium-, and hafnium-based third generation high-*k* dielectrics by Atomic Vapor Deposition, *Chemical Vapor Deposition*, **13**, pp. 567–573.

Adelmann, C., Van Elshocht, S., Franquet, A., Conard, T., Richard, O., Bender, H., Lehnen, P. and De Gendt, S. (2008b). Thermal stability of dysprosium scandate thin films, *Applied Physics Letters*, **92**, p. 112902.

Afanas'ev, V. and Stesmans, A. (2007). Internal photoemission at interfaces of high-*k* insulators with semiconductors and metals, *Journal of Applied Physics*, **102**, p. 081301.

Akiyama, K., Wang, W., Mizubayashi, W., Ikeda, M., Ota, H., Nabatame, T. and Toriumi, A. (2007). V_{fb} roll-off in HfO_2 gate stack after high temperature annealing process — a crucial role of out-diffused oxygen from HfO_2 to Si, in *Symposium on VLSI Technology. Digest of Technical Papers*, pp. 72–73.

Berglund, C. (1966). Surface states at steam-grown silicon-silicon dioxide interfaces, *IEEE Transactions on Electron Devices*, **13**, 10, pp. 701–705.

Cassé, M., Pretet, J., Cristoloveanu, S., Poiroux, T., Raynaud, C. and Reimbold, G. (2004). A specific floating-body effect in fully depleted SOI MOSFETs with ultra-thin gate oxide, *Microelectronic Engineering*, **72**, pp. 352–356.

Chang, L., Tang, S., King, T.-J., Bokor, J. and Hu, C. (2000). Gate-length scaling and threshold voltage control of double-gate MOSFETs, in *Technical Digest International Electron Devices Meeting*, pp. 719–722.

Chen, Y., Liu, I., Gardner, M., Fulford, J. and Kwong, D. (1997). Performance and reliability assessment of dual-gate CMOS devices with gate oxide grown on nitrogen implanted Si substrates, in *Technical Digest International Electron Devices Meeting*, pp. 639–642.

Choi, K., Wen, H.-C., Alshareef, H., Harris, R., Lysaght, P., Luan, H., Majhi, P. and Lee, B. H. (2005). The effect of metal thickness, overlayer and high-*k* surface treatment on the effective work function of metal electrode, in *Proceedings of the 35th European Solid-State Device Research Conference*, pp. 101–104.

Colinge, J.-P. (2008). *FinFETs and other multi-gate transistors* (Springer).

Collaert, N., Demand, M., Ferain, I., Lisoni, J., Singanamalla, R., Zimmerman, P., Yim, Y., Schram, T., Mannaert, G., Goodwin, M., Hooker, J., Neuilly, F., Kim, M., De Meyer, K., De Gendt, S., Boullart, W., Jurczak, M. and Biesemans, S. (2005). Tall triple-gate device with TiN/HfO_2 gate stack, in *Symposium on VLSI Technology*, pp. 108–109.

Cubaynes, F. (2004). *PhD dissertation:Ultra-thin plasma nitrided oxide gate dielectrics for advanced MOS transistors* (Eindhoven University of Technology), iSBN: 90-365-2059-2.

De, I., Johri, D., Srivastava, A. and Osburn, C. (2000). Impact of gate workfunction on device performance at the 50 nm technology node, *Solid State Electronics*, **44**, 6, pp. 1077–1080.

Degroote, B., Collaert, N., Rooyackers, R., Baklanov, M., Boullart, W., Kunnen, E., Jurczak, M. and Vanhaelemeersch, S. (2006). The etchback approach: enlarged process window for MuGFET gate etching, *Microelectronic Engineering*, **83**, pp. 570–576.

Demand, D., Paraschiv, V., Shamiryan, D., Beckx, S., Boullart, W. and Vanhaelemeersch, S. (2005). Dry etch processing of multiple gate FETs with metal gate electrode, in *Proceedings of International Dry Process Symposium*, Vol. 5, pp. 401–402.

DiMaria, D. and Stathis, J. (2001). Anode hole injection, defect generation, and breakdown in ultrathin silicon dioxide films, *Journal of Applied Physics*, **89**, 9, pp. 5015–5024.

Duffy, R. (2008). Trends, challenges in doping, and characterisation of bulk and thin body semiconductor devices, in *2008 Spring MRS Meeting, Symposium E*, p. Tutorial Part 1.

Duffy, R., Van Dal, M., Pawlak, B., Kaiser, M., Weemaes, R., Degroote, B., Kunnen, E. and Altamirano, E. (2007). Solid phase epitaxy versus random nucleation and growth in sub-20nm wide fin field-effect transistor, *Applied Physics Letters*, **90**, p. 241912.

Elers, K.-E., Winkler, J., Weeks, K. and Marcus, S. (2005). $TiCl_4$ as a precursor in the TiN deposition by ALD and PEALD, *Journal of the Electrochemical Society*, **152**, pp. G589–G593.

Ferain, I., Duffy, R., Collaert, N., Van Dal, M., Pawlak, B., O'Sullivan, B., Witters, L., Rooyackers, R., Conard, T., Popovici, M., van Elshocht, S., Kaiser, M., Weemaes, R., Swerts, J., Jurczak, M., Lander, R. and De Meyer, K. (2009). Performance improvement in narrow MuGFETs by gate work function and source/drain implant engineering, *Solid-State Electronics*, **53**, pp. 760–766.

Ferain, I., Pantisano, L., O'Sullivan, B., Collaert, N., Jurczak, M. and De Meyer, K. (2008). Methodology for flat band voltage measurement in floating body MOSFETs, *IEEE Transactions Electron Devices*, **55**, pp. 1657–1663.

Ferain, I., Son, N., Witters, L., Collaert, N., Onsia, B., Kaczer, B., Kauerauf, T., Adelmann, C., Richard, O., Favia, P., Bender, H., Vos, R., Van Elshocht, S., Lehnen, P., San Tamer, K., De Meyer, K., Biesemans, S. and Jurczak, M. (2007). Metal gate technology using a Dy_2O_3 dielectric cap approach for multiple-V_t in NMOS FinFETs, in *Proceedings of the IEEE International SOI Conference*, pp. 141–142.

Francis, P., Terao, A., Flandre, D. and Van de Wiele, F. (1994). Modeling of ultrathin double-gate nMOS/SOI transistors, *IEEE Transactions on Electron Devices*, **41**, 5, pp. 715–720.

Garaud, S., Vos, R., Shamiryan, D., Paraschiv, V., Mertens, P., Fransaer, J. and De Gendt, S. (2008). Galvanic corrosion of stacked metal gate electrodes during cleaning in HF solutions, *Solid State Phenomena*, **134**, pp. 87–90.

Gordy, W. and Thomas, W. (1956). Electronegativity of the elements, *Journal of Chemical Physics*, **24**, pp. 439–444.

Hickmott, T. (1980). Dipole layers at the metal/SiO_2 interface, *Journal of Applied Physics*, **51**, pp. 4269–4281.

Hobbs, C., Fonseca, L., Dhandapani, V., Samavedam, S., Taylor, B., Grant, J., Dip, L., Triyoso, D., Hegde, R., Gilmer, D., Garcia, R., Roan, D., Lovejoy, L., Rai, R., Hebert, L., Tseng, H., White, B. and Tobin, P. (2003). Fermi-level pinning at the polySi/metal oxide interface, in *Symposium on VLSI Technology*, pp. 9–10.

Jha, R., Gurganos, Y., Kim, Y., Choi, R., Lee, J. and Misra, V. (2004). A capacitance based methodology for work function extraction of metals on high-*k*, *IEEE Electron Device Letters*, **25**, 6, pp. 420–423.

Jung, H.-S., Han, S., Lim, H., Choi, Y., Lee, C.-K., Lee, M., You, Y., Chung, Y., Park, J.-B., Lee, E., Baik, H., Lee, J.-H., Lee, N.-I. and Kang, H.-K. (2007). Integration friendly dual metal gate technology using dual thickness metal inserted poly-si stacks (DT-MIPS), in *Symposium on VLSI Technology*, pp. 196–198.

Jung, H.-S., Han, S., Lim, H., Kim, Y.-S., Kim, M., Yu, M., Lee, C.-K., Lee, M., You, Y., Chung, Y., Kim, S., Baik, H., Lee, J.-H., Lee, N.-I. and Kang, H.-K. (2006). Dual high-*k* gate dielectric technology using selective AlO_x etch (SAE) process with nitrogen and fluorine incorporation, in *Symposium on VLSI Technology*, pp. 204–205.

Karim, Z., Barbar, G., Boissiére, O., Lehnen, P., Lohe, C., Seidel, T., Adelmann, C., Conard, T., O'Sullivan, B., Ragnarsson, L.-A., Schram, T., Van Elshoch, S. and De Gendt, S. (2007). AVD and MOCVD TaCN-based films for gate metal applications on high-*k* gate dielectrics, in *ECS Transactions*, Vol. 11, pp. 557–567.

Kittl, J., Pawlak, M., Lauwers, A., Demeurisse, C., Kottantharayil, A., Vrancken, C., van Dal, M., Veloso, A., Kubicek, S., Absil, P., Maex, K. and Biesemans, S. (2006). Work function ni silicide phases on HfSiON and SiO_2: NiSi, Ni_2Si, Ni_31Si_12 and Ni_3Si fully silicided gates, *IEEE Electron Device Letters*, **27**, 1, pp. 34–36.

Kubicek, S., Schram, T., Paraschiv, V., Vos, R., Demand, M., Adelmann, C., Witters, T., Nyns, N., Ragnarsson, L.-A., Yu, H., Veloso, A., Singanamalla, R., Kauerauf, T., Rohr, E., Brus, S., Vrancken, C., Chang, V., Mitsuhashi, R., Akheyar, A., Cho, H.-J., Hooker, J., O'Sullivan, T., B.J.and Chiarella, Kerner, C., Delabie, A., Van Elshocht, S., De Meyer, K., De Gendt, S., Absil, P., Hoffmann, T. and Biesemans, S. (2007). Low V_t CMOS using doped Hf-based oxides, TaC-based metals and LASER-only anneal, in *Technical Digest International Electron Devices Meeting*, pp. 49–52.

Lee, C.-W., Yun, S.-R.-N., Yu, C.-H., Park, J.-T. and Colinge, J.-P. (2007). Device design guidelines for nano-scale MuGFETs, *Solid-State Electronics*, **51**, pp. 505–510.

Lee, T., Rhee, S., Kang, C., Zhu, F., Kim, H., Choi, C., Ok, I., Zhang, M., Krishnan, S., Thareja, G. and Lee, J. (2006). Structural advantage for the EOT scaling and improved electron channel mobility by incorporating dysprosium oxide (Dy_2O_3) into HfO_2 n-MOSFETs, *IEEE Electron Device Letters*, **27**, 8, pp. 640–643.

Liu, Y., Hayashida, T., Matsukawa, T., Endo, M., K. Masahara, O'ushi, S., Sakamoto, K., Ishii, K., Yamauchi, H., Ogura, A. and Suzuki, E. (2007). Nitrogen gas flow ratio controlled PVD TiN metal gate technology for FinFET CMOS, in *Semiconductor Device Research Symposium, 2007 International*, pp. 1–2.

Liu, Y., Kijima, S., Sugimata, E., Masahara, M., Endo, K., Matsukawa, T., Ishii, K., Sakamoto, K., Sekigawa, T., Yamauchi, H., Takanashi, Y. and Suzuki, E. (2006). Investigation of the TiN gate electrode with tunable work function and its application for FinFET fabrication, *IEEE Transactions on Nanotechnology*, **5**, 6, pp. 723–729.

Lu, Q., Yeo, Y., Ranade, P., Takeuchi, H., King, T.-J., Hu, C., Song, S., Luan, H. and Kwong, D.-L. (2000). Dual-metal gate technology for deep-submicron CMOS transistors, in *Symposium on VLSI Technology*, pp. 72–73.

Matsukawa, T., Endo, K., Liu, Y., O'uchi, S., Ishikawa, Y., Yamauchi, H., Tsukada, J., Ishii, K., Masahara, M., Sakamoto, K. and Suzuki, E. (2007). A Ta/Mo interdiffusion gate technology for dual metal gate-first FinFET fabrication, in *Proceedings of the IEEE International SOI Conference*, pp. 143–144.

Meuris, M., Mertens, P., A., O., Schmidt, H., Depas, M., Vereecke, G., Heyns, M. and A., P. (1995). The IMEC clean: a new concept for particle and metal removal on Si surfaces, *Solid State Technology*, **38**, 5, pp. 109–114.

Michaelson, H. (1978). Relation between an atomic electronegativity scale and the work function, *IBM Journal of Research and Development*, **22**, 1, pp. 72–80.

Miller, D., Hughes, W., Wang, Z., Gall, K. and Stoldt, C. (2007). Mechanical effects of galvanic corrosion on structural polysilicon, *IEEE Journal of Microelectromechanical Systems*, **16**, 1, pp. 87–101.

Narayanan, V., Paruchuri, V., Bojarczuk, N., Linder, B., Doris, B., Kim, Y., Zafar, S., Stathis, J., Brown, S., Arnold, J., Copel, M., Steen, M., Cartier, E., Callegari, A., Jamison, P., Locquet, J.-P., Lacey, D., Wang, Y., Batson, P., Ronsheim, P., Jammy, R., Chudzik, M., Ieong, M., Guha, S., Shahidi, G. and Chen, T. (2006). Band-edge high-performance high-*k*/metal gate n-MOSFETs using cap layers containing group IIA and IIIB elements with gate-first processing for 45nm and beyond, in *Symposium on VLSI Technology*, pp. 224–225.

Ohfuji, S., Hashimoto, C., Amazawa, T. and Murota, J. (1984). Oxygen-doped molybdenum films for MOS gate application, *Journal of the Electrochemical Society*, **131**, pp. 446–450.

Ono, H. and Katsumata, T. (2001). Interfacial reactions between thin rare-earth-metal oxide films and Si substrates, *Applied Physics Letters*, **78**, pp. 1832–1834.

O'Sullivan, B., Kaushik, S., Ragnarsson, L., Onsia, B., Van Hoornick, N., Rohr, E., DeGendt, S. and Heyns, M. (2006). Device performance of transistors with high-*k* dielectrics using cross-wafer-scaled interface-layer thickness, *IEEE Electron Device Letters*, **27**, 7, pp. 546–548.

Pantisano, L., Afanasev, V., Pourtois, G. and Chen, P. (2005). Valence-band electron-tunneling measurement of the gate work function: application to the high-*k*/polycrystalline-silicon interface, *Journal of Applied Physics*, **98**, p. 053712.

Park, J. and Kang, S. (2004). Plasma-enhanced ALD of Titanium-Silicon-Nitride using $TiCl_4$, SiH_4, and $N_2/H_2/Ar$ plasma, *Electrochemical and Solid-State Letters*, **7–8**, pp. C87–C89.

Pauling, L. (1932). The nature of the chemical bond. IV. the energy of single bonds and the relative electronegativity of atoms, *Journal of the American Chemical Society*, **54**, pp. 3570–3582.

Rothschild, A., Mitsuhashi, R., Kerner, C., Shi, X., Everaert, J., Dateb, L., Conard, T., Richard, O., Vrancken, C., Verbeeck, R., Veloso, A., Lauwers, A., De Potter, M., Debusschere, I., Jurczak, M., Niwa, M., Absil, P. and Biesemans, S. (2007). Optimization of HfSiON using a design of experiment (DOE) approach on 0.45V V_t Ni-FUSI CMOS transistors, *Microelectronics Reliability*, **47**, 4-5, pp. 521–524.

Schaeffer, J., Gilmer, D., Capasso, C., Kalpat, S., Taylor, B., Raymond, M., Triyoso, D., Hegde, R., Samavedam, S. and White Jr, B. (2007). Application of group electronegativity concepts to the effective work functions of metal gate electrodes on high-*k* gate oxide, *Microelectronic Engineering*, **84**, pp. 2196–2200.

Shamiryan, D., Paraschiv, V., Eslava-Fernandez, S., Demand, M., Baklanov, M., Beckx, S. and Boullart, W. (2007). Profile control of novel non-Si gates using BCl_3/N_2 plasma, *Journal of Vacuum Science and Technology B*, **25**, 3, pp. 739–744.

Shima, A., Jinbo, T., Natsuaki, N., Ushio, J., Oh, J.-H., Ono, K. and Oshima, M. (2001). A model for the segregation and pileup of boron at the SiO_2/Si interface during the formation of ultrashallow p^+ junctions, *Journal of Applied Physics*, **89**, 6, pp. 3458–3463.

Singanamalla, R., Lisoni, J., Ferain, I., Richard, O., Carbonell, L., Schram, T., Yu, H., Kubicek, S., De Gendt, S., Jurczak, M. and De Meyer, K. (2006a). Electrical and material evaluation of the MOCVD TiN as metal gate electrode for advanced CMOS technology, in *MRS Symposium Proceedings*, Vol. 917 E, pp. 0917–E12–02.

Singanamalla, R., Yu, H., Janssens, T., Kubicek, S. and De Meyer, K. (2007a). The study of effective work function modulation by As ion implantation in $TiN/TaN/HfO_2$ stacks, *Japanese Journal of Applied Physics*, **46**, 14, pp. L320–L322.

Singanamalla, R., Yu, H., Janssens, T., Witters, T., Schram, T., Kubicek, S., De Gendt, S., Jurczak, M. and De Meyer, K. (2006b). Effective work function modulation by As implantation in metal gate stacks, in *Dielectrics for Nanosystems II: Materials Science, Processing, Reliability, and Manufacturing*, pp. 49–60.

Singanamalla, R., Yu, H., O'Sullivan, B., Petry, J., Mercha, A., Paraschiv, V., Volders, H., Kubicek, S., De Meyer, K. and Biesemans, S. (2007b). Performance enhancement of poly/TiN/SiON based p-MOSFETs by addition of an aluminum oxide (AlO) capping layer, *Microelectronic Engineering*, **84**, pp. 1865–1868.

Singanamalla, R., Yu, H., Pourtois, G., Ferain, I., Kottantharayil, A., Kubicek, S., Hoffmann, T., Biesemans, S. and De Meyer, K. (2006c). On the impact of TiN film thickness variations on the effective work function of Poly-Si/TiN/SiO_2 and Poly-Si/TiN/HfSiON gate stacks, *IEEE Electron Device Letters*, **27**, 5, pp. 332–334.

Steen, C., Martinez-Limia, A., Pichler, P., Ryssel, H., Pei, L., Duscher, G. and Windl, W. (2007). Characterization of the pile-up of As at the SiO_2/Si interface, in *Proceedings of the 37th European Solid-State Device Research Conference*, pp. 267–270.

Sun, S. and Tsai, M. (1996). Effect of rapid thermal annealing on the electrical and physical properties of metalorganic chemical-vapor-deposited TiN, *Applied Physics Letters*, **68**, pp. 670–672.

Taur, T. (2000). An analytical solution to a double-gate MOSFET with undoped body, *IEEE Electron Device letters*, **21**, 5, pp. 245–247.

Vellianitis, G., van Dal, M., Witters, L., Curatola, G., Doornbos, G., Collaert, N., Jonville, C., Torregiani, C., Lai, L.-S., Petry, J., Pawlak, B., Duffy, R., Demand, M., Beckx, S., Mertens, S., Delabie, A., Vandeweyer, T., Delvaux, C., Leys, F., Hikavyy, A., Rooyackers, R., Kaiser, M., Weemaes, R., Voogt, F., Roberts, H., Donnet, D., Biesemans, S., Jurczak, M. and Lander, R. (2007). Gatestacks for scalable high-performance FinFETs, in *International Electron Devices Meeting*, pp. 681–684.

Veloso, A., Witters, L., Demand, M., Ferain, I., Son, N., Kaczer, B., Roussel, P., Simoen, E., Kauerauf, T., Adelmann, C., Brus, S., Richard, O., Bender, H., Conard, T., Vos, R., Rooyackers, R., Van Elshocht, S., Collaert, N., De Meyer, K., Biesemans, S. and M., J. (2008). Flexible and robust capping-metal gate integration technology enabling multiple-V_t CMOS in MuGFETs, in *Symposium on VLSI Technology*, pp. 14–15.

Wen, H.-C., Choi, R., Brown, G., Boscke, T., Matthews, K., Harris, H., Choi, K., Alshareef, H., Luan, H., Bersuker, G., Majhi, P., Kwong, D.-L. and Lee,

B. (2006). Comparison of effective work function extraction methods using capacitance and current measurement techniques, *IEEE Electron Device Letters*, **27**, 7, pp. 598–601.

Westlinder, J., Schram, T., Pantisano, L., Cartier, E., Kerber, A., Lujan, G., Olsson, J. and Groeseneken, G. (2003). On the thermal stability of atomic layer deposited TiN as gate electrode in MOS devices, *IEEE Electron Device Letter*, **24**, pp. 550–552.

Witters, L., Son, N., Ferain, I., San, T., Singanamalla, R., Kerner, C., Collaert, N., De Meyer, K. and Jurczak, M. (2007). Threshold voltage modulation in FinFET devices through arsenic ion implantation into TiN/HfSiON gate stack, in *Proceedings of the IEEE International SOI Conference*, pp. 31–32.

Witters, L., Veloso, A., Ferain, I., Demand, M., Collaert, N., Son, N., Adelmann, C., Meersschaut, J., Vos, R., Rohr, E., Wada, M., Schram, T., Kubicek, S., De Meyer, K., Biesemans, S. and Jurczak, M. (2008). Multiple-V_t FinFET devices through La_2O_3 dielectric capping, in *IEEE International SOI Conference*, pp. 121–122.

Xiong, W., Gebara, G., Zaman, J., Gostkowski, M., Nguyen, B., Smith, G., Lewis, D., Cleavelin, C., Wise, R., Shaofeng, Y., Pas, M., King, T.-S. and Colinge, J. (2004). Improvement of FinFET electrical characteristics by hydrogen annealing, *IEEE Electron Device Letter*, **25**, pp. 541–543.

Xiong, W., Hsu, C., Cleavelin, C., Ma, M., Patruno, P., Lee, C.-W., Yan, R., Lederer, D., Afzalian, A. and Colinge, J.-P. (2007). Influence of fluorine implant on threshold voltage for metal gate FDSOI and MuGFET, in *Proceedings of the IEEE International SOI Conference*, pp. 35–36.

Yun, J., Choi, E., Jang, C. and Lee, C. (2002). Effect of post-treatments on atomic layer deposition of TiN thin films using Tetrakis(dimethylamido)titanium and Ammonia, *Japanese Journal of Applied Physics*, **41**, pp. L418–L421.

Zafar, S., Cabral, C., Amos, R. and Callegari, A. (2002). A method for measuring barrier heights, metal work functions and fixed charge densities in metal/SiO_2/Si capacitors, *Applied Physics Letter*, **80**, 25, pp. 4858–4860.

Chapter 4

Doping, Contact and Strain Architectures for Highly Scaled FinFETs

Robert Lander
NXP Semiconductors, Central Research and Development, Leuven, Belgium
robert.lander@nxp.com

4.1 Introduction

In spite of massive efforts and investment within the semiconductor industry, gate length scaling has slowed with respect to the demands set out in the ITRS roadmap [1]. This is largely because the gate dielectric thickness has not scaled fast enough. For high performance microprocessor applications this has resulted in severe issues with active power dissipation as the supply voltage cannot be reduced unless the oxide is also scaled. For mobile applications, the other major CMOS technology driver, the poorer gate control of the channel and increased gate leakage has led to an explosion in off-state leakage current levels that severely limit battery life.

A finFET architecture increases the electrostatic coupling of the gate to the channel region and more effectively shields the source-side potential barrier from the drain potential. The impact on the

CMOS Nanoelectronics: Innovative Devices, Architectures, and Applications
Edited by Nadine Collaert

ISBN 978-981-4364-02-7 (Hardcover), 978-981-4364-03-4 (eBook)
www.panstanford.com

device behavior is similar to scaling the oxide thickness but with an important difference: For narrow fin widths the doping in the channel has a much reduced influence on the electrostatic profile. This alleviates several significant scaling issues related to junction formation in planar bulk technologies.

Such a radical change in device architecture also brings new issues, particularly for junction and contact formation, and these are also highlighted, together with potential solutions, in the rest of this chapter.

4.1.1 *Scaling Issues for Planar CMOS Junctions*

The two functions of the junction in a MOSFET are, first, to provide a low-resistance electrical connection between the metal silicide and the inversion layer in the channel and, second, to provide electrical isolation from the bulk majority carriers.

A particular challenge for highly scaled devices is to realize these functions while minimizing the impact of the drain upon the source side potential barrier. So called drain-induced barrier lowering (DIBL) leads to a large increase in off-state leakage current as well as an undesirable sensitivity to uncontrolled variations in gate length. Both these effects are due to the influence of the drain potential upon the potential barrier seen by carriers entering the channel from the source.

In advanced planar CMOS technologies, the junction comprises two distinct regions illustrated in Fig. 4.1. A deep "highly doped drain" region (HDD) isolates the silicide contact from the bulk

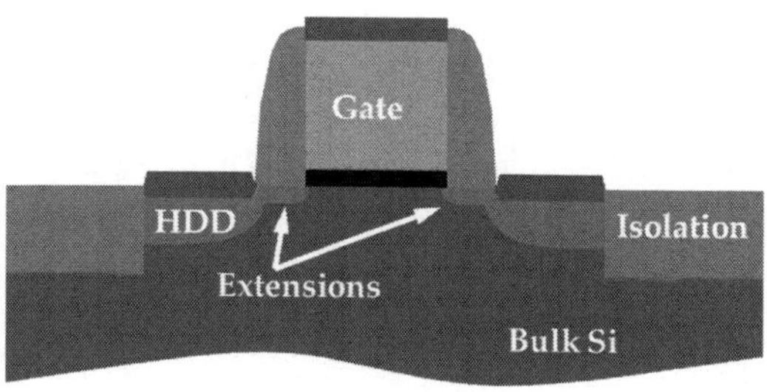

Figure 4.1. Schematic cross section of a planar bulk MOSFET illustrating the extension and highly doped drain (HDD) regions.

majority carriers. The HDD is connected to the channel via a shallow drain "extension" or "low-doped drain" (LDD) region. The depth of the extension region is minimized to minimize DIBL, while the active doping concentration is as high as possible to reduce resistance. The width of the extensions, determined by the spacer width, must be carefully tuned to suppress any DIBL induced by the HDD regions but minimize extension resistance. Some resistance in the extension regions is desirable in order to avoid gate reliability issues caused by hot-carriers. How much resistance is needed is strongly dependent upon the operating voltage (V_{dd}). Both extension resistance and V_{dd} tend to reduce with each new technology node [1].

Even for an infinitely shallow junction the doping concentration in the channel region must be increased with gate length scaling in order to suppress the extension of the drain depletion region toward source. This has several undesirable consequences:

1. Highly doped p-n junctions are susceptible to band-to-band tunneling (BTBT) and, ironically, this is worse for low leakage devices because these require higher V_t's and thus higher bulk doping leading to higher electric fields in the drain junction.
2. The increased ionized impurity scattering in the channel reduces the channel mobility leading to lower drive current.
3. A proportion of the channel doping is mirrored by free charge on the gate which would otherwise be available to modulate the potential of the channel. Hence, higher channel doping results in a degradation of the sub-threshold slope.

Variability has become one of the major obstacles to the extension of Moore's Law. Reducing variations, particularly in threshold voltage, is highly desirable for circuit designers as it is the slowest devices in the distribution that limit the maximum clock frequency at which the various circuit blocks can operate in a synchronous manner. Furthermore, threshold voltage variations degrade the stability of SRAM cells which, in turn, imposes severe restrictions upon the minimum operating voltage [2].

Scaling of CMOS aggravates both the magnitude and impact of device variability for the following reasons. (1) Scaling enables more transistors per chip but this samples more devices from the tail of the distribution. (2) Area scaling demands smaller transistors and so the random fluctuations in the number of dopant atoms in the transistor increases as a fraction of the total dopants. This results in a larger V_t variability [3]. (3) Area scaling has traditionally been accompanied by supply voltage scaling, initially to limit the electric fields that resulted in gate dielectric reliability issues and, in later years, to limit the dynamic power dissipation. This need must be reconciled with the minimum operating voltage required to guarantee functional SRAM, a threshold that is extremely sensitive to parametric variability.

4.1.2 *The FinFET Architecture*

Schematic illustrations of the two most common finFET architectures are shown in Figure 4.2. The SOI finFET is fabricated on a silicon-on-insulator substrate wafer with the electrical isolation between devices provided by the buried oxide (BOX) layer. The bulk finFET is fabricated on a bulk silicon substrate and device isolation is provided by a modified shallow-trench isolation (STI) process. The technological challenges of the STI process have not favored integration efforts with this approach and, thus, many of the examples presented in this chapter are for SOI-based finFETs,

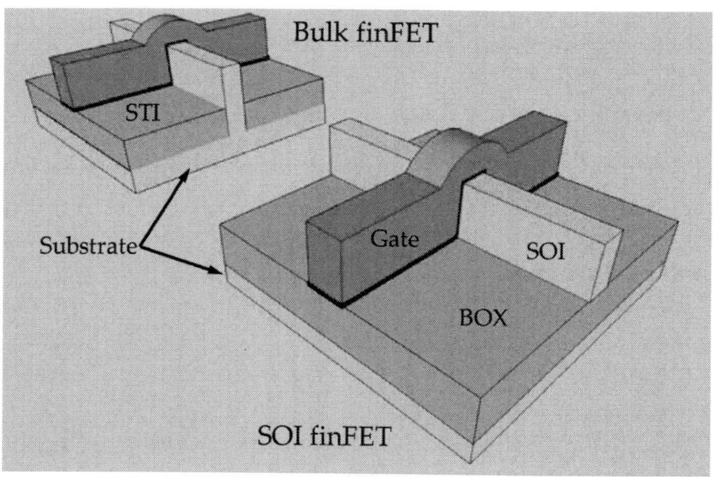

Figure 4.2. Schematic illustration of the bulk finFET and SOI finFET device architectures (shown after gate patterning).

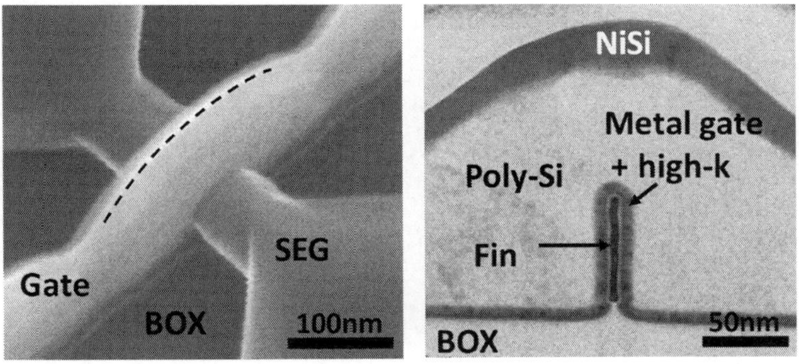

(a) (b)

Figure 4.3. (a) Tilted view SEM image of finFET after selective epitaxial growth and (b) TEM image of finFET cross section in gate plane (see dashed line in (a)) illustrating 5 nm wide Si fin and high-k/metal gate stack. From [5].

although most of the key issues for junction and contact formation are common to both architectures. It should be noted that the first announcement of mass production in a finFET technology was using the bulk finFET approach [4].

An example of an SOI finFET is shown in Figure 4.3. Figure 4.3a is an SEM image after source/drain selective epitaxial growth (SEG) and Figure 4.3b a TEM cross section in the gate plane after salicidation. Visible in Figure 4.3b are the ultra-narrow (5 nm) fin, high-k gate dielectric, metal gate electrode and NiSi layers. Also visible is the recessing of the BOX under the fin due to cleaning steps prior to gate deposition which, for narrow fins, can result in fin collapse. This is a significant disadvantage of SOI over bulk finFETs.

4.1.3 *Performance-Leakage Trade-Offs for Fully Depleted FinFETs*

Shown in Figure 4.4 are schematic cross sections in the horizontal plane illustrating (a) the various resistive components between source and drain silicides that limit the drive current of the device and (b) the various contributions to the leakage current that determine the power dissipation in off-state.

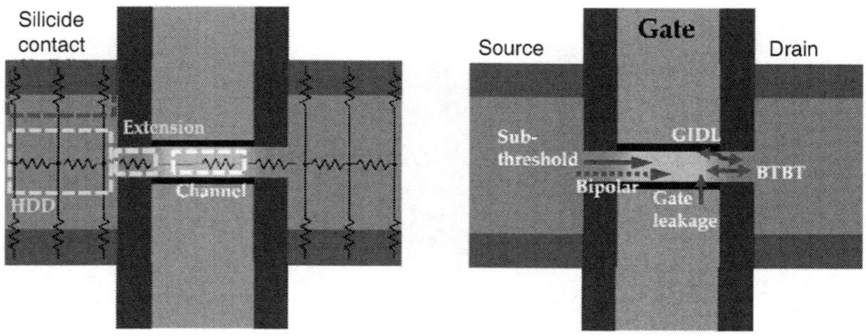

Figure 4.4. Schematic cross section of a finFET in the horizontal (wafer) plane illustrating (a) the resistive components that limit the drive current and (b) the contributions to the leakage current that determine the static power dissipation. For an NMOS device the blue current paths indicate electron conduction and the red paths indicate hole conduction.

The multiple-gate architecture and narrow fin width improve the capacitive coupling between the channel and the gate. This has the desirable effect of suppressing the influence of the drain on the source-side potential barrier and so dramatically reducing DIBL, as shown in Figure 4.5. For sufficiently narrow fins the coupling is so strong that the channel will be fully depleted and doping can even

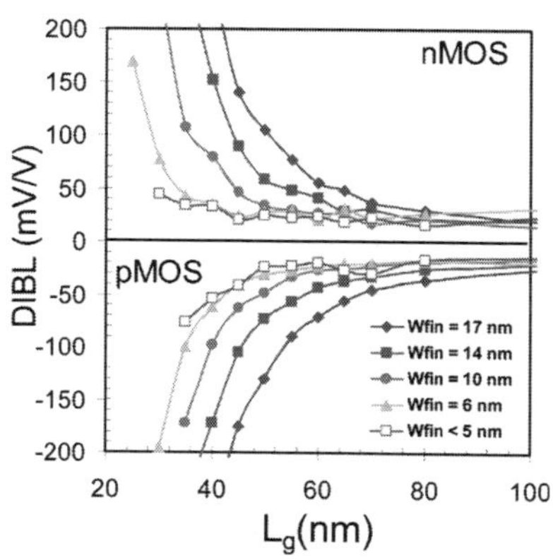

Figure 4.5. DIBL as a function of gate length for nMOS and pMOS finFETs for various fin widths [5]. No intentional channel doping was applied for these devices.

be eliminated entirely without severe leakage issues. Fin widths of 15 nm or less, required for sub-32 nm CMOS technology nodes, will be fully depleted under all operating conditions even up to channel doping levels of $10^{19}\,cm^{-3}$.

Eliminating the channel doping has several advantages:

1. The combination of ionized impurities in the channel and the geometric enhancement of the gate electric field in the corners of the fin results in a parasitic channel at the corners. This channel occupies only a small fraction of the overall device width but has a lower threshold voltage and can greatly increase the overall leakage in the sub-threshold range. Eliminating the doping in the channel eliminates this parasitic channel.
2. A fully depleted architecture benefits from an improved sub-threshold slope because the gate voltage that would otherwise be spent in modulating the charge state of the channel doping is now applied exclusively to modulate the channel potential.
3. The large coupling capacitance between channel and gate reduces the impact of channel dopants, and thus of dopant number fluctuations, upon the threshold voltage. Of course, eliminating the channel doping entirely offers the best possible immunity to dopant number fluctuations. The reduction in parametric variability offered by fully depleted architectures is considered by many to be the single biggest advantage over planar bulk.
4. The carrier mobility in the channel is increased in the absence of channel doping due to the reduction of ionized impurity scattering.

Reducing fin width generally reduces leakage current and parametric variability but there are limits. Mass-production of fins with dimensions below 10 nm is a major challenge for current commercial lithography and etch tools. At these dimensions even small variations in fin width will result in unacceptable parametric variations with consequences for SRAM scalability and logic circuit performance. The mobility of the carriers in the channel will degrade as they are squeezed between the interfaces and, as will be explained in Section 4.3, the extension resistance can increase dramatically for fin widths below 10 nm.

As for planar bulk technologies, it is desirable to have active doping concentrations in the extension and HDD regions as high as possible in order to minimize the resistances in the semiconductor and at the contacts. As for planar bulk, this concentration is limited by the materials and fabrication processes, and by the fraction of these dopants that are permitted to penetrate the channel region, leading to DIBL.

It should be noted that band-to-band tunneling currents are a strong function of the peak electric field and caution must be taken in the device design to avoid excessive enhancement of the gate-drain electric field. This is a particular issue for finFETs because the wrapping of the gate around the top of the fin results in a geometric enhancement of the peak electric field. This leakage mechanism is commonly referred to as "gate-induced drain leakage" (GIDL) and can dominate the drain current in off-state [6].

A problem particular to floating body devices, such as SOI finFETs, is parasitic bipolar amplification. Since there is no contact to fix the equilibrium concentration of the minority carriers in the channel, any current due to GIDL or channel-drain BTBT will inject excess minority carriers into the channel. Note that here we define "minority" as holes for NMOS and electrons for PMOS. The charge associated with these excess carriers pulls down the barrier to majority carriers at the source resulting in a current that can be many times larger than the original BTBT current. Here the source, channel and drain form, respectively, the emitter, base and collector of the bipolar transistor. How much the BTBT current is amplified depends upon how rapidly the minority carrier concentration can return to its equilibrium value which, in turn, depends upon the minority carrier lifetime.

An important performance booster that must be considered is channel strain. Process-induced strain is an innovation that has been introduced relatively recently in planar CMOS technologies in order to minimize the channel resistance. The carrier effective masses, sub-band populations, and scattering rates can be influenced greatly by high levels of strain in the conducting material. Strain alone has little effect upon the leakage currents and so offers improved performance without increased static power dissipation. The optimum strain architecture does depend upon device type (NMOS or PMOS) and independent optimization for both device types can add significant complexity to the process, as will be described in Section 4.6.

4.2 FinFET Device Process Sequence

A significant advantage of finFETs is that the processes and tool requirements remain very similar to those used in planar CMOS technologies. This greatly lowers the barriers to adoption, partly because the materials and processes are already well-understood but also because the extraordinary cost of a modern wafer fab, typically more than $1 billion, demands that it be able to serve several technology generations.

A typical finFET process sequence is shown in Figure 4.6 illustrating the key process steps between gate patterning and self-aligned silicidation. This example is for an SOI finFET but the process steps shown here are common to both SOI and bulk finFETs.

The finFET architecture does bring new issues that are detailed, together with some of the potential solutions, in the following sections and in the order within the device fabrication sequence.

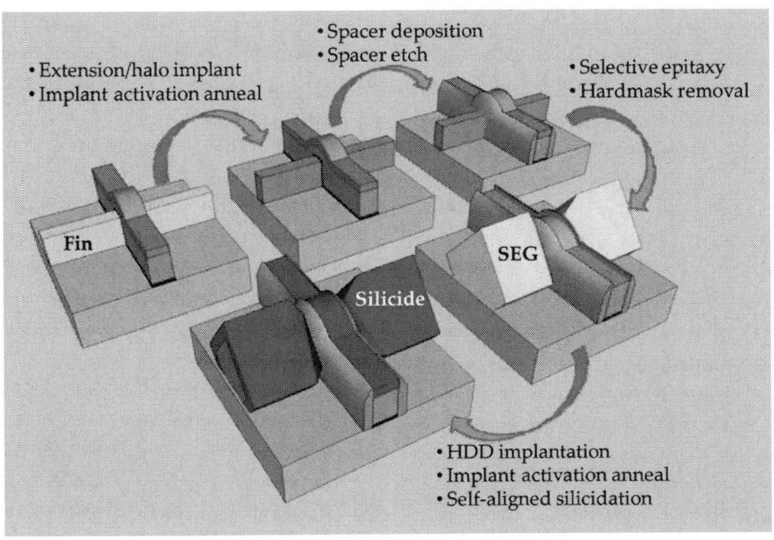

Figure 4.6. Key process steps between gate patterning and silicidation for an SOI FinFET.

4.3 Extension and Halo Formation

The shallowness, profile abruptness and dopant atom density in the semiconductor are limited by the practicalities of the materials and available processes. Introduction of dopants by diffusion from the surface has been used in the past, but for advanced CMOS technologies it is now replaced by ion implantation. This offers independent control of dopant density and depth and is compatible with simpler, photoresist-based patterning schemes. It does, however, result in damage cascades as the energetic ions collide with the atoms in the crystal and displace them from their lattice sites. For heavier ions, such as As or BF_2, at high doses this damage can be so severe as to entirely amorphize regions of the crystal. All damage must be repaired in order to minimize the junction leakage caused by electrical traps associated with crystal defects. Also, the implanted ions must be relocated to substitutional lattice sites for them to become active as dopants. Both of these effects can be achieved by high-temperature annealing above 700°C.

One of the most significant innovations in planar CMOS technology was the introduction of "pocket" or "halo" implants. Instead of doping the channel prior to gate patterning, most of the channel dopants are introduced at the same time as the extensions. This is done using ion implantation at high tilt angles to locate the dopants under the gate beyond the extension region. This approach offers few advantages in terms of DIBL or leakage with respect to the standard approach but it does ensure that the total number of dopants in the channel is less dependent upon gate length. In other words, a shorter device will have a higher channel doping concentration. This counters the impact of uncontrolled variations in gate length upon the threshold voltage and, as described in the previous section, variability has become one of the major obstacles to the CMOS scaling.

Halos can be applied in a finFET technology but the impact of the doping on the potential profile in the channel is limited by the large coupling capacitance to the gate. Where the potential is less well coupled to the gate, for example, between the STI regions beneath the bulk finFET, halos can play an important role.

The processes considered for dopant incorporation and dopant activation are discussed in more detail in the rest of this section, but first we will address the issue of "conformal doping."

4.3.1 *Pitch Constraints and Conformal Doping for Extensions*

For a tall finFET most of the gate width runs down the sides of the fin. The source and drain extension regions must therefore extend along the entire fin height if the source and drain are to access the full device width. This is frequently referred to as "conformal doping" and is considered to be one of the major challenges of junction engineering in finFETs.

Consider first dopant incorporation using a standard planar CMOS approach. Vertical implantation of source/drain dopants would need sufficient energy to penetrate the entire fin height. Unfortunately this will degrade the short channel behavior as the lateral abruptness of the dopants after implant is strongly correlated with the implant depth. A seemingly obvious solution is to implant at a high tilt angle using much lower ion energies but, because area scaling demands that nMOS and pMOS be located very close together, this is of limited use. As shown in Figure 4.7, high tilt implants will not reach the fin due to shadowing by the photoresist masking the complementary device.

Shadowing is less of a concern for logic transistors, where NMOS and PMOS are grouped such that the width of the implanted regions is usually much larger than the minimum fin pitch. The most aggressive n/p pitches are found in SRAM cells where NMOS and PMOS transistors are located in pairs (illustrated in Figure 4.7). SRAM is one of the key building blocks of modern ICs and frequently occupies a large fraction of the overall chip area. Hence, any finFET junction technology must enable n/p pitch scaling.

The issue can be alleviated by implanting the dopants from one side only, as illustrated in Figure 4.7. This approach increases the spacing between the edge of the resist shadowing the implant and the fin to be implanted. Such a single-sided implant is also observed to be beneficial for the device performance [7], as will be explained in Sections 4.3.7.

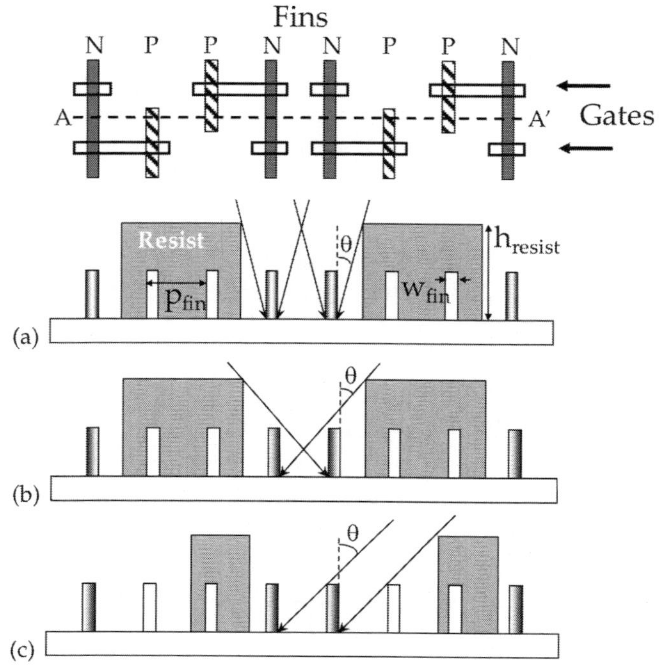

Figure 4.7. Top view of gate (horizontal lines) and fin (vertical lines) layout for dense SRAM together with schematic cross sections (of line A→A′) illustrating the photoresist pattern and limitations on implant tilt angle for three approaches: (a) Standard, (b) 2 × 1-sided and (c) 1 × 1-sided.

Simple geometry tells us that the maximum tilt angle is limited by the resist height (in the first two cases) or fin height (in the third case) and, in all cases, by the fin pitch. The minimum fin pitch is plotted in Figure 4.8 as a function of implant tilt angle together with the targeted fin pitch for the 22 nm technology node [1]. In this case a resist thickness of 130 nm and a fin height of 60 nm are taken.

A limit of around 35° for the 22 nm node is indicated for the 1-sided approaches whereas the standard two-sided approach is limited to 15°. This should be remembered when considering the impact of tilt angle upon the junction performance which will be discussed in the following sections.

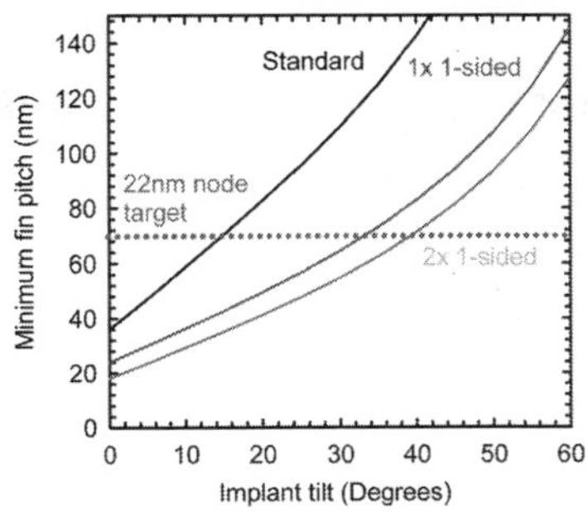

Figure 4.8. Minimum fin pitch required to avoid shadowing during implant vs. tilt angle for the three implant schemes illustrated in Figure 4.7. Also shown is the fin pitch targeted for the 22 nm node. A resist thickness of 130 nm and a fin height of 60 nm are taken. See also Color Insert.

4.3.2 *Dopant Incorporation by Ion Implantation*

The efficiency of ion implantation into narrow silicon fins is a strong function of ion energy and tilt angle. Atomistic modeling of these processes [8], shown in Figure 4.9, indicates that significant fraction of dopants are reflected by the sidewall for low implant energies and low tilt angles. Thus, an implantation limited to a tilt angle of 15° is very inefficient. At higher energies and high tilt angles a significant fraction of dopants is transmitted through the fin. These

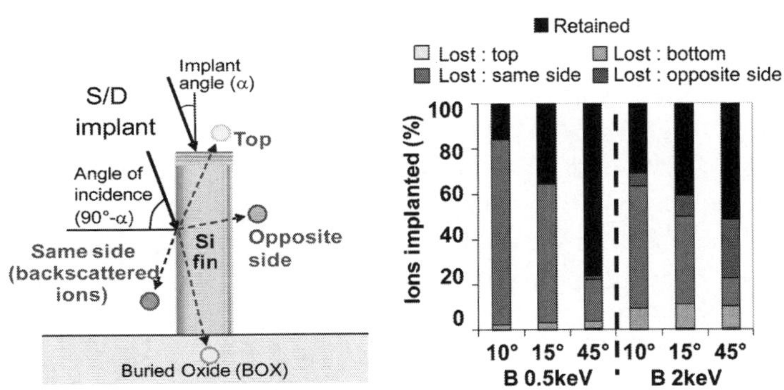

Figure 4.9. Atomistic modeling of implanted dose retained or lost to various directions for a 10 nm Si fin. Backscattering is dominant at low angles while transmission is significant at high angles and energies. Taken from [8]. See also Color Insert.

ions only increase the damage to the crystal without contributing to the conductivity. The increased implant time required to achieve the desired doping concentrations add to the cost of the process and, as will be described below, excessive implant damage is highly undesirable for narrow fin devices.

4.3.3 *Alternatives to Ion Implantation*

4.3.3.1 Plasma doping

Plasma doping (also referred to as plasma-immersion ion implantation) was originally developed as an alternative to conventional ion implantation for ultra-shallow junctions in planar CMOS. It has the advantage that it can achieve high dopant currents (and so faster throughput) for low energies with much reduced ion energy contamination [9]. This is a particularly challenge for conventional ion implantation of light elements such as boron. Plasma doping has been also proposed as a technique to achieve conformal doping in finFETs.

Plasma doping uses a dopant-containing precursor gas as the source. The plasma is induced above the wafer, usually by RF excitation. Ions are accelerated from the plasma toward the wafer by a DC or pulsed DC bias voltage applied to the backside of the wafer. The chamber conditions and gas ratios can be tuned to achieve a relatively short ion mean free path and thus a wide range of incident angles at the wafer surface. The plasma also deposits neutral dopant atoms that are not accelerated by the DC bias and these have an even wider range of incident angles [10].

This technique has been applied to finFETs with some success for PMOS devices [11] (boron is lighter and so more easily scattered to larger angles) but the effectiveness of this technique for dense p/n fin pitches has yet to be proven. It has a notable disadvantage that the proximity of the plasma to the wafer results in a significant sputtering of the resist and wafer surface.

4.3.3.2 Vapor phase doping

In the vapor phase doping (VPD) technique, the dopant atoms are deposited on the surface by thermal decomposition of precursor gases (e.g., B_2H_6, PH_3 or AsH_3). The dopants must then be diffused into the silicon and activated by annealing at high temperature.

This has been suggested as a method to achieve conformal doping in finFETs but to date very few device data have been reported using this technique. It also has the drawback that the polymer-based photoresist layers cannot be used to mask the complementary devices as these are not compatible with the high temperatures required to achieve reasonable deposition rates. Furthermore, it relies upon thermally activated diffusion processes to incorporate the dopants into the silicon which conflicts with the need for abrupt junction profiles in very short channel devices.

4.3.3.3 Epi tip

Epitaxial growth of silicon on source and drain regions is probably required at HDD level (as will be discussed in Section 4.5) but can also be applied at extension level in order to provide conformal doping. Dopants can be incorporated at very high concentrations during the epitaxial growth with the advantage that the growth will occur only on exposed silicon surfaces.

The drawbacks of doped epi (also at HDD level) are, first, the need for separate masking and epitaxy steps for each device type. The masking is more complex as the pattern must be transferred from polymer photoresist into a masking layer that can withstand the high temperatures required for selective epitaxial growth. Second, epitaxy is a costly and complex process compared to ion implant. Finally, applying epitaxy at extension level requires a thin spacer on the gate sidewall to avoid growth on the gate sidewall and electrical shorts to the fin.

Incorporation of multiple spacer and epitaxy steps between gate patterning and silicidation has the potential to deliver a highly optimized doping architecture but, even neglecting cost and complexity, the number of spacer etch steps may be limited by the need to retain the gate hardmask until the final epi step is complete. This will be described further in Section 4.4.

4.3.4 *Dopant Retention*

Short range diffusion of dopants during implant activation can be tolerated and may be necessary to achieve high levels of dopant activation but the high surface area to volume ratio of narrow silicon

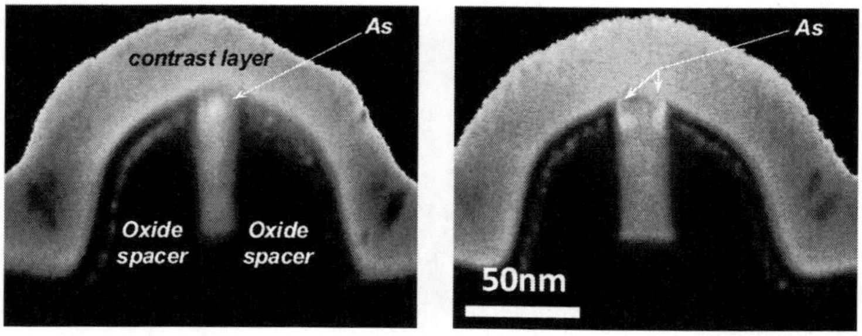

Figure 4.10. HAADF analysis As concentration profile in a Si fin following ion implantation (left) and following anneal (right). The light areas correspond to the location of peak As concentration (analysis performed by Marcel Verheijen, Material Analysis Group, Philips, Eindhoven).

fins makes this architecture particularly sensitive to interfacial segregation of dopants. Once trapped at the interfaces the dopants are no longer electrically active.

This phenomenon has been observed for both As and Sb [12] and an example is shown in Figure 4.10 for a 20 nm silicon fin implanted with As where the As profile is imaged by High Angle Annular Dark Field analysis (HAADF). Prior to anneal, the majority of dopants are located in the centre of the fin. Following high-temperature anneal (1050°C) the As has migrated to the Si/SiO_2 interfaces.

4.3.5 *Dopant Activation*

The conductivity of the junctions is limited by the number of electrically active dopants in the LDD and HDD regions and the overlap with the gate region. The upper limit of the active dopant concentration is determined by the density of dopant atoms and by the fraction of these that are located on substitutional lattice sites. The density of substitutional dopants that silicon can accommodate is termed the "solid solubility." It depends upon the dopant species and it increases with temperature, thus favoring high-temperature post-implant anneals with a rapid cool-down phase. This rapid cool-down freezes the dopants on substitutional sites at concentrations well above their equilibrium solid solubility at room temperature. For this to be effective the subsequent processing must be kept below temperatures that would enable the substitutional dopants to recover their equilibrium concentrations (typically 700°C or above).

A major disadvantage of annealing during or after junction formation is that it drives the diffusion of dopants leading to deeper and less abrupt junctions. For implanted dopants, this effect is aggravated by the presence of large numbers of interstitial Si atoms in the damage cascade. These catalyze the diffusion processes of several important dopant species, notably phosphorous, arsenic, and especially boron. The excess of Si interstitials in the implanted regions continues to enhance the diffusion rate until they recombine at vacant lattice sites or until they diffuse to and annihilate at the Si surface. This effect is known as transient enhanced diffusion and is best avoided by spending as little time as possible above about 700°C.

Thus, rapid thermal annealing at high temperatures (>1000°C) and for short times (<1 sec) has become the industry standard and much effort has gone into the development of anneal tools that can generate such extreme temperature profiles in a uniform and reproducible manner.

The very high surface area to volume ratio of narrow silicon fins should provide a very efficient sink for interstitial Si atoms and is expected to reduce transient enhanced diffusion, although to date the experimental evidence shows only modest improvements in profile abruptness [13]. What has been demonstrated is that damage recovery in thin silicon fins can be far less effective than for junctions formed in planar bulk silicon [8].

As described above, the active doping concentration in the extensions is ultimately limited by the solid solubility of silicon rather than the absolute concentration of dopant atoms. Thus, it is to be expected that the total resistance of the extension regions will scale inversely with fin width. This is indeed observed (see Figure 4.11), but also apparent is that the scaling behavior is dependent upon the implant conditions. This dependence can be attributed to the effect of the fin geometry upon the effectiveness of the damage recovery.

In planar bulk the recrystallization of regions amorphized during implantation begins from the amorphous/crystalline interface and proceeds in a front that moves toward the surface until all the silicon

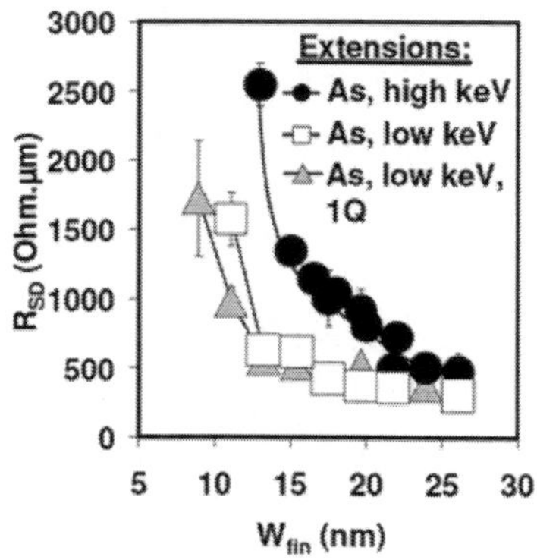

Figure 4.11. Source-drain resistance extracted for finFETs with varying fin width and for several extension implant conditions. Low energy and one-sided (1Q) implants improve R_{SD} especially for narrow fins. R_{SD} was extracted by plotting total source-drain resistance at high gate bias vs. physical gate length and extrapolating to $Lg = 0$ nm.

is repaired. This mechanism is commonly referred to as "solid-phase epitaxy" (SPE). For narrow fins the non-amorphized region can be extremely narrow, confined to the bottom of the fin or even to the channel region under the gate. Furthermore, the disruption of the crystal periodicity at the interfaces slows the SPE growth and allows alternative nucleation mechanisms time to compete with the desired mode of regrowth [14]. These alternative mechanisms have no common template aligned to the channel crystal orientation resulting in twin boundary defects or even polycrystalline regions, as shown in Figure 4.12. These defective regions contain large numbers of electronic traps and have been shown to increase both the series resistance and the variability in drive strength of the devices [24].

Solutions for {110}-oriented sidewalls require a monocrystalline region to be retained during implant that can seed subsequent regrowth throughout the height of the fin. This favors implant species with lower mass that produce less crystal damage (B or P rather than BF_2 or As). Damage recovery can also be improved by widening the fin, at the cost of scalability, reducing the implant energy, at the cost of dose retention (see previous section), or implanting from only one side. Conveniently the last solution is

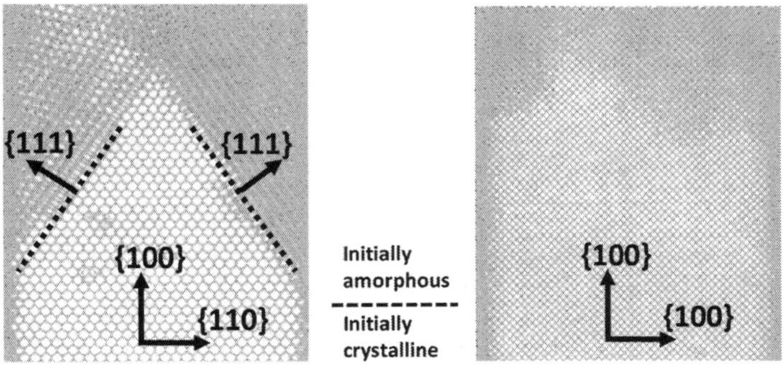

Figure 4.12. Molecular dynamic simulations of silicon recrystallization during anneal for two fin sidewall orientations. For {110}-oriented sidewalls the retarded growth at the sidewalls leads to twin boundary defects. In the case of {100}-oriented sidewalls, the regrowth within the body of the fin is not impeded by the presence of the sidewalls [8, 15].

also a solution for mitigating the pitch constraints described in Section 4.3.1.

The impact of the sidewall interfaces upon the regrowth is dependent upon the crystal orientation. For example, molecular dynamic simulations, shown in Figure 4.13, accurately predict the {111} twin boundary defects observed for a fin with {110}-oriented sidewalls (and shown in Figure 4.12). Also shown is the

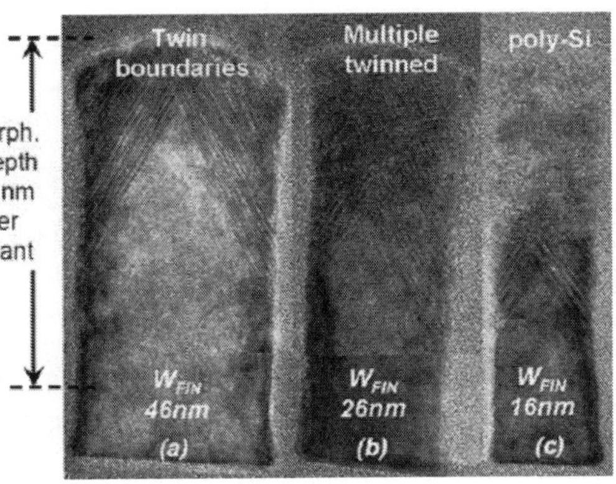

Figure 4.13. XTEM of wide and narrow fins after amorphizing implants and rapid thermal annealing (RTA) at 1050°C showing the poor fin crystallinity for the narrow fin.

defect-free recrystallization predicted for a fin with {100}-oriented sidewalls [15]. The ultimate choice of fin sidewall orientation is also influenced greatly by other considerations, especially carrier mobility (see, for example, [16]), and the best finFET performances to date have been reported for fins with {110} sidewall orientation in spite of the relatively poor recrystallization behavior.

4.4 Spacer Formation

Dielectric spacers are needed to ensure electrical isolation of the gate from the source and drain especially during the salicidation process. The desired spacer architecture is illustrated in Figure 4.14. Spacers are formed by deposition of a thick dielectric layer (or layers) and applying a highly anisotropic etch that leaves a layer of dielectric exclusively on the vertical sidewalls of the device.

Anisotropic etching can be readily achieved with dry etch processes. The electric field in the etch chamber accelerates ions toward the surface, resulting in a sputtering of surfaces directly exposed to the bombardment. The impact of this sputtering upon the anisotropy of the etch can be greatly enhanced by polymers formed from the reaction products. These polymers build up on the sidewalls, because of the reduced sputter rate, and inhibit chemical

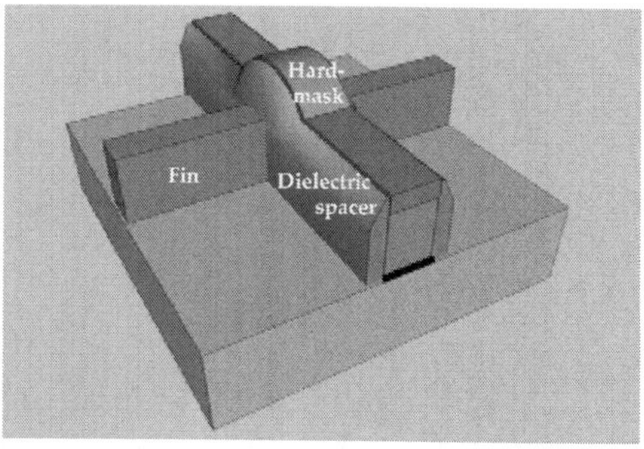

Figure 4.14. Illustration of desired spacer architecture for a finFET. Note that the spacer is present only on the gate sidewalls exposing the fin for epitaxy or contact metallization. Also the hardmask is retained on top of the gate to prevent epitaxial growth on this area.

etching of the underlying layers. The etch chemistries and chamber conditions are normally tuned such that the latter effect is dominant in determining the etch rate of the spacer material. This is done because chemical etching is preferred to physical etching from the point of view of etch selectivity to the buried oxide, gate hardmask, and silicon fin. In this way an etch process can be achieved that is both highly anisotropic and highly selective.

The need for selective epitaxial growth on the HDD regions (described in detail in Section 4.5) imposes several constraints on the preceding process steps. The spacers must be removed from the sidewalls of the silicon fin because those regions must be exposed to the gas phase during epitaxy or no silicon will grow there. This is not trivial as the spacers must remain on the sidewalls of the gate in order to electrically isolate the gate from the source and drain.

One means to achieve this spacer architecture is to make the gate significantly taller than the fin. The width of the spacer after etch is dependent upon the height of the sidewall and so the smaller isotropic component of the etch can be relied upon to remove the thinner fin spacer while leaving at least some of the gate spacer intact.

Several alternative techniques have been proposed. One example being to selectively enhance the etch rate of the fin spacer by ion implantation. The damage to the dielectric caused by the ion bombardment greatly enhances the chemical etch rate. The selectivity to the gate spacer material is achieved by tilting the ion beam parallel to the gates such that only the dielectric on the fin sidewalls is implanted [17].

It is also notable in Figure 4.14 that the hardmask on top of the gate has been retained. This is a preferred approach to avoid excessive epitaxial growth on the gates. The choices of materials for gate hardmask and spacers are thus complicated by the need to etch the latter without attacking the former (during spacer etch) and then the need to remove the former without attacking the latter (prior to silicidation). Solutions exist, as have been shown by numerous publications of functional devices, but the leading companies are usually reluctant to discuss the details of these materials as innovations here are difficult to protect with a patent. Remember that the hardmask material is removed before salicidation so proving infringement of patents from the final product is not trivial.

4.5 Selective Epitaxial Growth, HDD and Salicidation

The architecture of the epitaxial growth and HDD modules is determined, to a large extent, by the need for a low series resistance between the self-aligned silicide and the extension region. For this reason we will first address the requirements and limitations of the salicide module and then consider how these influence the choices for the selective epitaxy and HDD modules that precede it.

4.5.1 *Self-Aligned Silicidation*

The function of the self-aligned silicide (frequently referred to as "salicide") is to provide a stable and low-ohmic connection between the silicon and the interconnect layers above. It also serves to reduce the in-plane resistance of the source, gate and drain regions, which can be significant for operation at very high frequencies [18].

Self-aligned silicidation comprises a metal deposition step followed by an anneal that drives a reaction where the metal is in contact with silicon. The unreacted metal is then removed by a highly selective wet etch chemistry. This approach has been applied in planar CMOS technologies for many generations with only modifications to the choice of reactive metal. Currently the most advanced CMOS technologies use a Ni or Ni/Pt alloy. It should be noted that the gate hardmask must also be removed prior to the salicide module otherwise no silicide will form on the gate. A schematic illustration of the desired salicide architecture is shown in Figure 4.15 and a TEM cross section of an SOI finFET following Ni salicidation is shown in Figure 4.16.

The silicide contact and source/drain resistances are a particular concern for a finFET technology as the silicon surface area and volume beneath the metal silicide are limited. This can lead to both high contact resistance and high spreading resistance in the HDD region.

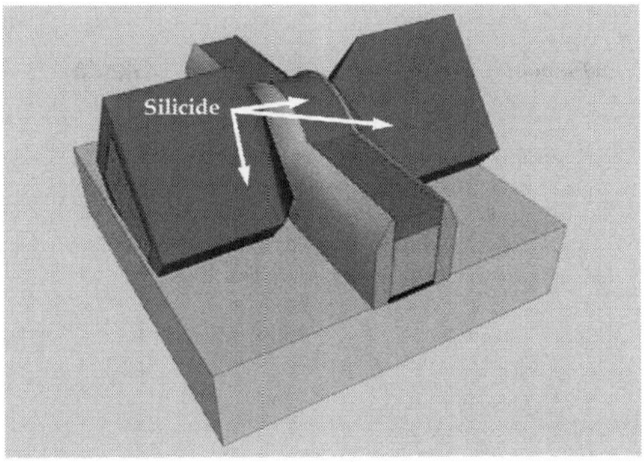

Figure 4.15. Schematic illustration of desired salicide architecture for an SOI finFET.

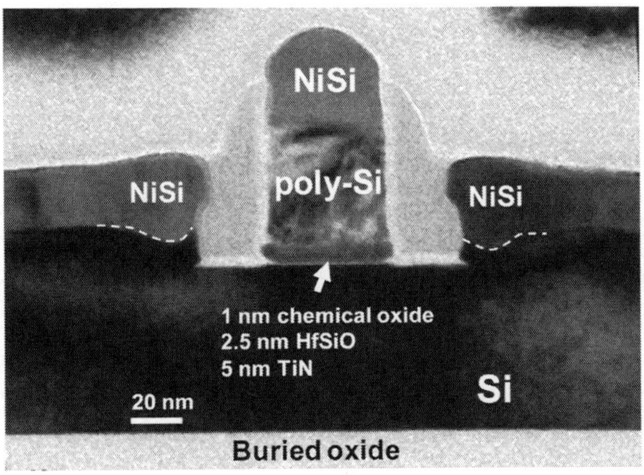

Figure 4.16. TEM cross section image in the gate plane of an SOI finFET illustrating NiSi on gate, source and drain. From [5].

One attractive solution to reduce the contact resistance at the silicide-semiconductor interface would be silicides with work-functions matched to that of the underlying silicon. This greatly increases the diffusion and thermionic emission current across the Schottky barrier but would require separate silicides for nMOS and pMOS devices, adding significant complexity to the process. Much effort has been devoted to the identification of such silicides [19] but, to date, little evidence has been presented of contact resistances much below that achieved with conventional NiSi contacts.

The contact resistance can also be reduced by increasing the doping concentration in the silicon beneath the silicide. The tunneling current across the Schottky barrier is a very strong function of the electric field beneath the metal and, for mid-gap metal work-functions and high doping concentrations ($\gg 10^{18}\text{cm}^{-3}$), this current component dominates over diffusion and thermionic emission. Partly for this reason the implantation and activation conditions of the HDD are tuned to achieve the maximum active doping concentration immediately below the silicide. This concentration is once again limited by the solid solubility of the dopants in the silicon and by the need to limit any degradation of the short-channel behavior of the device.

A phenomenon known as "dopant segregation" has been shown to reduce further the contact resistance of the silicide interface. Certain dopants, notably boron, phosphorous, arsenic, and antimony are rejected from the growing silicide as the reaction consumes the silicon in which they are located. The silicidation reaction temperatures are typically much lower than that required to induce significant dopant diffusion in silicon so a very high concentration of dopants builds up at the silicon/silicide interface. Observations of this effect in silicide-gated MOSFETs indicate that the effective work-function of the silicide can be modified over a wide range. How many of these dopants are electrically active and how they influence the work-function is still debated but a significant reduction of the contact resistance is observed in experiment [20, 21].

Forming a thermodynamically stable NiSi silicide layer requires a thickness of at least 10 nm. This will consume 9 nm of Si during the silicidation reaction. Below 10 nm thickness the silicide will agglomerate during subsequent high-temperature steps. Allowing for around 5 nm dopant depletion beneath the metal it is apparent that, for fins below 30 nm width, the spreading and contact resistances will be severe. Knowing that a fin width of less than $L_g/3$ is needed in order to benefit from the enhanced gate control of the 3D architecture, it can be seen that there is no fin width that satisfies both the requirements of scalability and low series resistance.

This apparent conflict between series resistance and scalability can be resolved by increasing the volume of silicon in the HDD regions by selective epitaxial growth prior to HDD implantation. How this technique is implemented is described in detail in Section 4.5.3.

4.5.2 *The Doping-Less Transistor?*

A more radical solution can be considered if contacts can be formed with silicide work-functions aligned near to the silicon band-edges. This might eliminate the need for selective epitaxial growth or even the need for doping. This doping-less transistor can be considered if (1) the silicide interface can be located sufficiently close to the gate edge, (2) the contact resistance is sufficiently low, and (3) it offers sufficient diode isolation in off-state. Achieving the first requirement demands exceptional control of the silicide growth rate and interface morphology (silicide-silicon interfaces are rough on the nanometer scale). Achieving the second and third requirements demands a near-ideal Schottky contact.

Even if all these requirements can be met then still care must be taken that the proximity of the silicide to the gate does not result in very high electric fields. Band-to-band tunneling resulting from very high electric fields in the drain/gate region is commonly referred to as "gate-induced drain leakage" (GIDL) and can dominate the off-state leakage in finFETs [6].

In practice, the best results for doping-less transistors have been achieved with dopant segregated silicide contacts [22]. In this case the dopants not only influence the effective work-function but probably also improve the contact behavior by providing some p-n diode isolation. Thus the term "dopant-less" is not entirely deserved.

4.5.3 *Selective Epitaxial Growth*

Epitaxial growth is a well-established technique to grow ultra-thin layers on mono-crystalline substrates. The grown layers conform to the underlying crystal structure and the thickness can be controlled almost to the atomic scale.

For finFETs the growth must be selective in the sense that nothing is deposited on the dielectric layers that isolate the gate source and drain (e.g., spacers, BOX or STI). Selective epitaxial growth has particular challenges because the deposition conditions required to avoid growth on the dielectric regions make the epitaxial growth rates especially susceptible to local variations in pattern density and temperature. For this reason selective growth was avoided for many years until 2002 when Intel announced that it would be incorporated into high-volume production in their 90 nm CMOS generation microprocessors. This remarkable development enabled Intel to enhance the performance of their PMOS devices by filling the HDD regions with a compressively strained SiGe alloy and so boosting the hole mobility in the channel.

A cross section of the HDD region of a finFET following selective epitaxial growth is shown in Figure 4.17. The original silicon interfaces are still visible indicating that the epitaxial growth is not perfect. Also visible are the crystal facets formed during epitaxy. The low surface energy of the {111} silicon surface favors facet formation with this surface orientation. The presence of these facets confirms that the epitaxial layers conform to the crystal template of the fin.

The resistance (normalized to 1 μm gate width) between the silicide and the edge of the spacer is also plotted in Figure 4.17

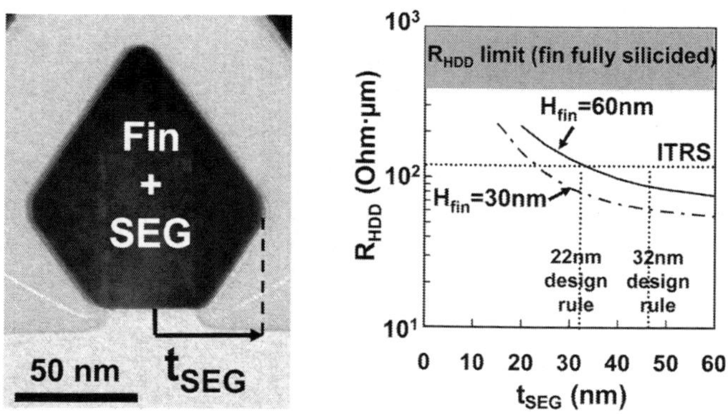

Figure 4.17. Resistance of the HDD regions as a function of the SEG thickness (defined as shown on the left) from 3D device simulations. A 10 nm fin and 13 nm NiSi thickness is taken. A 60 nm high fin can just meet the resistance specification defined by the ITRS [1] at the 22 nm node device pitch.

as a function of the epitaxial thickness. For a planar technology, this parameter would not vary significantly with device width but, because of the geometry of the finFET, this resistance does not scale ideally with fin height. This explains why the shorter fin is less sensitive to resistance in the HDD region (even if the current drive per unit chip area is superior for the tall fin).

The thickness of the SEG is limited by the need to separate devices (this limit is indicated by the design rule for the 22 nm and 32 nm nodes in Figure 4.17). Adjacent SEG regions can be allowed to merge within one device, for example, where multiple fins are needed to provide sufficient drive current for one device. This is also beneficial for area efficiency as fewer vias are needed to the interconnect layers. It does require that different pitches are used for n/n or p/p fin spacing vs. n/p fin spacing. Fixed pitch design has enabled CMOS scaling well beyond what was thought possible with the current generation of lithography tools and any finFET layout that utilizes multiple pitches will encounter significant technological obstacles. One possible approach to reduce the number of vias per device is a local interconnect level below the main METAL1 layer. This adds process complexity and cost but could be achieved without significantly reducing the area efficiency.

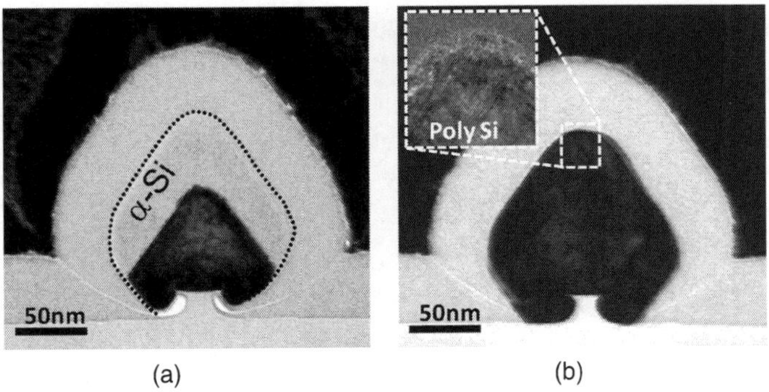

Figure 4.18. Cross section TEM images of HDD region of SOI finFET (a) following As implantation and (b) following subsequent damage recovery anneal. Polycrystalline silicon grains are visible in the high-resolution image. The light layer coating the SEG region was applied to enhance the image contrast [24].

Another parameter that can limit the SEG thickness is the parasitic capacitance between gate and source/drain; the thicker the SEG, the larger the spacer overlap area between gate and source or drain [23]. How much this limits the switching speed of the circuit depends upon how large this capacitance is with respect to the other parasitic capacitances, especially those in the interconnect layers. Additional parasitic capacitance is certainly a problem for applications that are optimized to achieve very high clock frequencies (for example, microprocessors).

4.5.4 *Highly Doped Drain Formation*

Ion implantation of HDDs is not so constrained by fin pitch as for the extensions (see Section 4.3.1). The larger surface area of silicon seen by vertical implants enables good dose retention over a wide range of implant conditions.

The thicker Si fins and much lower surface area to volume ratio should result in damage recovery behavior more comparable to planar bulk silicon. In practice, poor crystal quality will also degrade the series resistance of the HDD regions for the same reasons as for the extension region [24]. Epitaxy prior to HDD implant helps with damage recovery following HDD implant as there is a larger volume of unamorphized Si to provide the crystal template. However, caution must still be taken with the HDD implant conditions (see Figure 4.18). Furthermore, any implant damage during extension formation that is not recovered before epitaxy will be reflected in the crystal quality of the epitaxial regions. An example of this can be seen in Figure 4.19.

4.6 Channel Strain

Strain has been applied to great effect in planar CMOS generations ever since Intel first introduced it in their 90 nm node. The benefits for both electron and hole mobility were known for some time but the, sometimes unpredictable, effects of strain were often considered a nuisance before this. The major breakthrough of Intel was to introduce the strain late in the transistor processing and

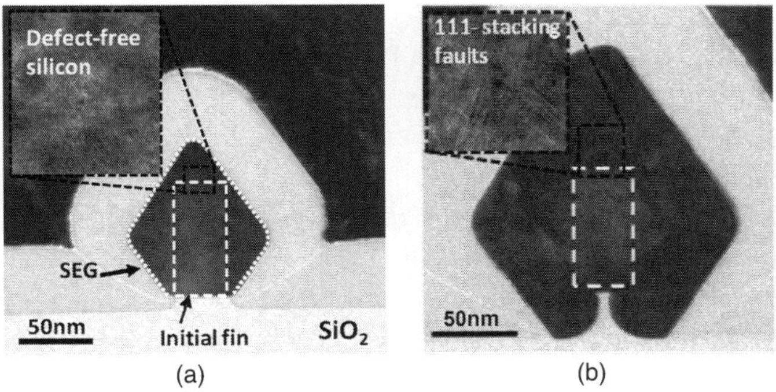

Figure 4.19. Cross-sectional TEM images of SEG region of finFET (a) grown on unimplanted Si fin and (b) grown on As-implanted Si fin. In the first case the SEG is defect-free, in the second case, 111-stacking faults are visible in the close-up image. From [24].

via compressively strained SiGe in the source drain regions. The improvements in PMOS drive current were dramatic and even improved with further device scaling. Strain in NMOS devices has been introduced via stressed SiN layers after transistor formation, where a compressive vertical channel strain, and thus, a tensile in-plane strain, is induced by the downward force on the gatestack due to the stress in the overlying layer.

These techniques do not readily transfer to a finFET geometry. First, the relative orientations of the channel confinement, current direction and strain tensors are changed with consequences that are not trivial to predict and that require careful optimization. In the case of SiGe source and drain, the device is elevated above the surrounding isolation regions so much of the compressive strain in a SiGe layer, that would normally be directed toward the channel, is relaxed away. In the case of stressed overlayers, any downward force is now distributed between the channel and the gate regions that run down the side of the fin. In both cases the desired impact on carrier mobility and current drive is reduced with respect to planar bulk CMOS.

Carrier transport is influenced by many variables; carrier type, bulk material properties, crystal orientation, strain tensor, dimensionality (e.g., fin width), electric field, the density and nature of scattering centers, etc. To the author's knowledge, no work has adequately described the impact of all of these permutations and the topic remains fertile ground for academic study. {110} surfaces seem to offer the highest hole mobility and the greatest potential for further hole mobility boost especially via uniaxial compressive strain in the channel (length) direction. Electron mobility is slightly lower on a {110} surface vs. {100} but can be boosted, particularly by uniaxial tensile strain in the channel (length) direction.

Area efficiency and modern lithography demand that the NMOS and PMOS devices have the same orientation so, without exotic hybrid substrates (see [25] for an example), a choice must be made. No study has explored exhaustively the many possible combinations of surface and channel orientation (see, for example, [16]) and most groups have focused on {110} sidewall surface orientation and a {110} channel orientation (see Figure 4.20). That this corresponds to a {100} wafer surface orientation, the industry standard for the past 30 years, is probably not coincidental. We will consider the impact of strain exclusively on this geometry in the rest of this section.

The impact of compressive and tensile strain along the three orthogonal axes (indicated in Figure 4.20) based upon two modeling approaches is shown in Figure 4.21. It is apparent from Figure 4.21 that the optimum strain configurations for NMOS and PMOS are radically different. For example, in the height direction electron mobility is boosted by compressive strain while hole mobility is only boosted by tensile strain.

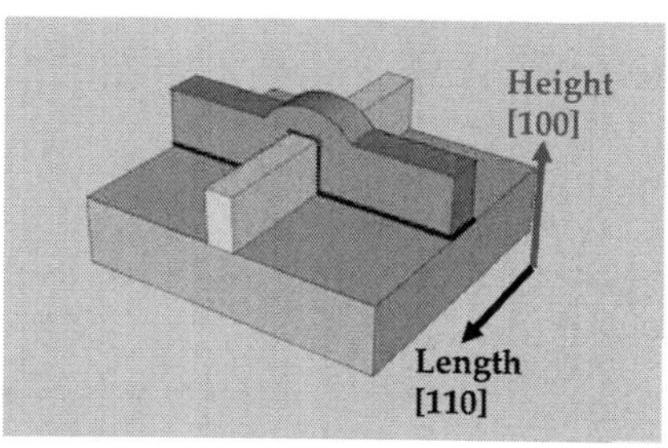

Figure 4.20. FinFET orientation (height/width/length) with respect to crystal orientation (in square brackets) considered here.

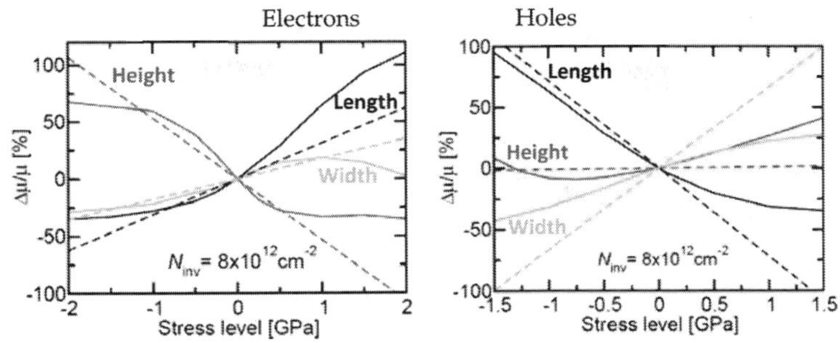

Figure 4.21. Impact upon electron and hole mobilities in the channel length direction of compressive (−ve) and tensile (+ve) stress along the three axes indicated in Figure 4.20. Results are shown for an analytical piezo-resistive model (dashed lines). Also shown are predictions for more sophisticated analyses (solid lines); for NMOS, a numerical multi-subband Monte Carlo approach and for PMOS, a **k**.**p**. band-structure calculation and mobility calculation based upon momentum relaxation time approximation. From [26]. See also Color Insert.

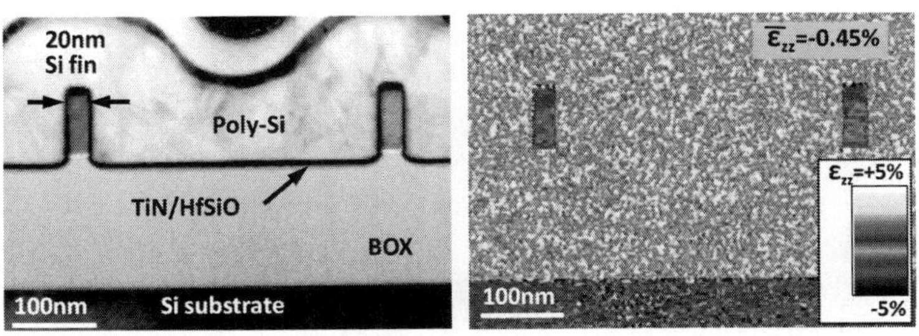

Figure 4.22. Cross-sectional TEM image through the gate-plane of FinFETs with fin width 20 nm and measurement, by holographic interferometry of the same sample, of strain in height direction, "ε_{zz}." The green shading in the fins indicates compressive strain. From [27]. See also Color Insert.

It is notable that a narrow finFET channel is especially susceptible to stress in the gate materials. This is not surprising as the gate stack is considerably wider than the fin and can readily relax its stress by compressing or extending the fin. Large vertical channel strains have been measured for narrow fins (see Figure 4.22) and it has been suggested that this may offer significant improvements in NMOS drive current [26]. How the strain due to the gate would be independently optimized for PMOS is not clear. Local relaxation of stress has been demonstrated, for example, by ion implantation into stressed SiN layers, but achieving an opposite stress type (desirable if Figure 4.21 is correct) is a much bigger challenge.

Acknowledgements

The author would especially like to thank the following: Nadine Collaert, Gilberto Curatola, Mark van Dal, Bart Degroote, Marc Demand, Gerben Doornbos, Ray Duffy, Blandine Duriez, Andriy Hikavyy, Carole Jonville, Gosia Jurczak, Anil Kottantharayil, Thomas Merelle, Axel Nackaerts, Bartek Pawlak, Rita Rooyackers, Tom Vandeweyer, Georgios Vellianitis, and Liesbeth Witters. All of these people were part of the wonderful FinFET team that provided much of the insight and understanding as well as many of the figures for this chapter.

References

1. www.itrs.net.
2. Merelle T. *et al.*, (2008). First observation of finFET specific mismatch behavior and optimization guidelines for SRAM scaling, *IEEE International Electron Devices Meeting.*
3. Pelgrom M. J. M. *et al.*, (1998). Transistor matching in analog CMOS applications, *IEEE International Electron Devices Meeting*, pp. 915.
4. www.intel.com.
5. Van Dal M. *et al.*, (2007). Highly manufacturable finFETs with sub-10nm fin width and high aspect ratio fabricated with immersion lithography, *International Symposium on VLSI Tech.*
6. Hoffmann T. *et al.*, (2005). GIDL (gate-induced drain leakage) and Parasitic Schottky barrier leakage elimination in aggressively scaled HfO_2/TiN FinFET devices, *IEEE International Electron Devices Meeting*, pp. 725–728.
7. Kawasaki H. *et al.*, (2008). Demonstration of highly scaled FinFET SRAM cells with high-κ/metal gate and investigation of characteristic variability for the 32 nm node and beyond, *IEEE International Electron Devices Meeting*, pp. 237.

8. Pelaz L. *et al.*, (2008). Atomistic modeling of impurity ion implantation in ultra-thin-body Si devices, *IEEE International Electron Devices Meeting.*
9. Lenoble D. (2002). Plasma doping as an alternative route for ultra-shallow junction integration to standard CMOS technologies, *Fabtech* 16.
10. Sasaki Y. (2008). Conformal doping for finFETs and precise controllable shallow doping for planar FET manufacturing by a novel B_2H_6/helium self-regulatory plasma doping process, *IEEE International Electron Devices Meeting.*
11. Lenoble D. (2006). Enhanced performance of PMOS MUGFET via integration of conformal plasma-doped source/drain extensions, *International Symposium on VLSI Tech.*
12. Sai-Halasz G. A. *et al.*, (1985). Antimony and arsenic segregation at Si-SiO_2 interfaces, *IEEE Electron Device Letters,* **6(6)**, pp. 285.
13. Hamilton J. J. *et al.*, (2006) Diffusion and activation of ultrashallow B implants in silicon on insulator: End-of-range defect dissolution and the buried Si/SiO_2 interface, *Applied Physics Letters,* **89**, pp. 042111.
14. Kunii Y. *et al.*, (1984). *Journal of Applied Physics,* **56**, pp. 279.
15. Pelaz L. *et al.*, (2009). Atomistic process modeling based on kinetic Monte Carlo and molecular dynamics for optimization of advanced devices, *IEEE International Electron Devices Meeting.*
16. Serra N. *et al.*, (2010). Mobility enhancement in strained finFETs: Basic insight and stress engineering, *IEEE Transactions on Electron Devices,* **57**, pp. 482.
17. Cheng K. *et al.*, (2009). Process for finFET spacer formation, *United States Patent Application* US2009/0017584.
18. Nuttinck S. *et al.*, (2006). Gate-stack analysis for 45-nm CMOS devices from an RF perspective, *IEEE Transactions on Electron Devices,* **53(4)**, pp. 925–928.
19. Kedzierski J. *et al.*, (2000). Complementary silicide source/drain thin-body MOSFETs for the 20nm gate length regime, *IEEE International Electron Devices Meeting.*
20. Wong H.-S. *et al.*, (2008). Source and drain series resistance reduction for N-channel transistors using solid antimony (Sb) segregation (SSbS) during silicidation, *IEEE Electron Device Letters,* **29(7)**, pp. 756.
21. Sinha M. *et al.*, (2009). Novel aluminum segregation at NiSi/p+-Si source/drain contact for drive current enhancement in P-channel finFETs, *IEEE Electron Device Letters,* **30(1)**, pp. 85.

22. Kaneko A. *et al.*, (2006). High-performance FinFET with dopant-segregated Schottky source/drain, *IEEE International Electron Devices Meeting.*
23. Guillorn (2008). FinFET performance advantage at 22 nm: An AC perspective, *International Symposium on VLSI Tech.*
24. Van Dal M. *et al.*, (2008). Material aspects and challenges for SOI FinFET integration, *Electrochemical Society Meeting.*
25. Yang M. *et al.*, (2006) Hybrid-orientation technology (HOT) opportunities and challenges, *IEEE Transactions on Electron Devices,* **53**, pp. 965.
26. Serra *et al.*, (2010). Mobility enhancement in strained finFETs: Basic insight and stress engineering, *IEEE Transactions on Electron Devices,* **57**, pp. 482.
27. Serra *et al.*, (2009). Experimental and physics based modeling assessment of strain induced mobility enhancement in finFETs, *IEEE International Electron Devices Meeting.*

Part II

Circuit-Related Aspects

Chapter 5

Variability and Its Implications for FinFET SRAM

Emanuele Baravelli, Luca De Marchi, and Nicolò Speciale
DEIS/ARCES — University of Bologna,
Viale Risorgimento 2, 40136 Bologna, (Italy)
ebaravelli@arces.unibo.it

While traditional scaling used to be accompanied by an improvement in device performance, this is much more challenging in sub-100 nm technology generations, causing an inefficient scaling of transistor dimensions and circuit supply voltage. Leakage and variability in devices approaching the atomic scale are major limiting factors for continued employment of conventional CMOS technology. Three-dimensional architectures ensuring a tighter electrostatic control over the channel have potential to mitigate the outlined issues. By choosing a proper combination of high-κ and metallic materials for the gate stack, it is possible to (i) resume a healthy trend of channel length scaling, (ii) limit gate leakage and (iii) set the device threshold voltage without recurring to increased channel doping. The use of undoped channels in multiple-gate structures such as FinFET significantly reduces the impact of random dopant fluctuations, which represent the major contribution to variability in planar bulk architectures. On the other hand, increased process complexity due to the intrinsic 3D

CMOS Nanoelectronics: Innovative Devices, Architectures, and Applications
Edited by Nadine Collaert

ISBN 978-981-4364-02-7 (Hardcover), 978-981-4364-03-4 (eBook)
www.panstanford.com

nature of FinFETs is reflected in a significant impact of geometry fluctuations. Line-edge roughness (LER) of the fin, top- and sidewall-gates is expected to be the dominant source of fluctuations in these devices.

Physical-level models for LER will therefore be discussed and applied to estimate the impact of the roughness on the FinFET electrical performance. An ensemble Monte Carlo (MC) approach involving both 2D and 3D simulations will be presented, which allows assessing the relative importance of different LER components at the 32 nm technology node. The dependence of gate-LER issues on doping profiles will also be addressed, thus pointing out the key role of extensions for the FinFET performance and variability. A correlation-based approach for variability estimation will be described and compared to extensive MC simulations as well as to a simplistic sensitivity analysis in order to optimize the trade-off between computational effort and statistical confidence. This analysis also allows identifying asymmetries in the device sensitivity to local geometry constrictions in different fin regions, thus further elucidating the impact of the parasitic extension resistance.

FinFET is a promising candidate for future low-voltage/low-power circuit applications. Six-transistor (6-T) SRAM will be considered as a benchmark to evaluate the impact of line-edge roughness at the circuit level. Stability of FinFET-based SRAMs in the hold, read and write operating modes will be evaluated taking into account several design options, namely cell sizing, crystal orientation and gate stack. V_{DD} scalability of these cells will be assessed, based on mixed-mode simulations and comparison with measured data. Besides demonstrating a bottom-up methodology for variability prediction, the presented analysis thus provides design guidelines at the device and circuit level for mainstream applications of FinFETs in sub-40 nm technology generations.

5.1 Introduction

Variability is inherent to the integrated circuits (IC) manufacturing process. For the purpose of circuit design, the sources of parametric variations are commonly separated into *global* and *local* components. The first group includes all parameter fluctuations occurring between different dice (*inter-die*) across a wafer or even belonging to different wafers. Instead, variations affecting two or more components within the same chip (*intra-die*) fall into the second group. While local variability used to be small with respect to the global component in the past, aggressive geometry scaling has inverted this trend in modern technologies [38]. This is because device dimensions have become so small that local fluctuations intrinsically associated with the discrete nature of charge and the atomicity of matter have gained considerable importance. Short-range variability is further enhanced by the increasing complexity of the manufacturing processes, including advanced options such as sub-wavelength lithography, junction engineering, silicide, high-κ/metal gate (HK/MG) stacks, strain and hybrid-orientation-techniques. Moreover, parameter variations produced by local sources cannot be easily compensated at the design stage because they are totally *random*.

The outlined scenario motivates the focus on short-range fluctuations in the remainder of this chapter. Most of the known sources of these unwanted phenomena are as follows:

- **Random Discrete Dopants (RDD)** refers to the variation in number and position of dopant atoms in decananometer devices.
- **Line-Edge Roughness (LER)** is the random deviation of the line edge of a printed feature from the ideal definition, mainly due to granularity of the materials, especially polysilicon and photoresist, and tolerance of optical equipments.
- **Oxide Thickness Variation (OTV)** arises from the very small thickness of gate dielectric in modern transistors, corresponding to a limited number of atomic layers, with a typical interface roughness of about 1–2 atomic layers.
- **Poly-Silicon Granularity (PSG)** inherent to the polycrystalline structure of polysilicon gates results in localized dopant penetration through the gate oxide as well as non-uniform diffusion and Fermi level pinning at grain boundaries.

- **Work-Function Variation (WFV)** is a new source of fluctuations brought about by the introduction of HK/MG stack in 45 nm generation devices: although the PSG issue is eliminated in this technology, metal gates are composed by several grains with different crystal orientations and hence different work-functions (WFs).
- **Fixed and Trapped Charge (FTC)** due to the presence of defect states near the silicon to dielectric stack interface causes electrical variability and random telegraph signals (RTS).

Fluctuations arising from these sources have been variously studied by means of Technology Computer-Aided Design (TCAD) simulations. RDD is a major threat to CMOS scalability, although it can be mitigated by using HK/MG stacks [1, 40]. Besides improving short-channel effects (SCEs) through a tighter electrostatic control over the channel, multiple-gate structures greatly enhance device robustness against RDD by leaving the channel undoped and therefore provide an effective alternative to the planar transistor architecture even from the variability standpoint. FinFET is the most promising multi-gate implementation thanks to its high compatibility with the CMOS process. However, the intrinsic 3D nature of FinFETs is expected to result in a significant impact of geometry fluctuations such as LER, because several printed features are affected, including the top- and sidewall-gates as well as the fin. A qualitative comparison of the planar and multi-gate architectures from the variability standpoint is reported in Table 5.1, where the relative importance of fluctuation sources described above is graphically represented by cell colors. The darker the color, the more critical the corresponding contribution is for threshold voltage variability of the two device structures (polysilicon is assumed as the gate material for the planar MOSFET). References in the table indicate several literature works dealing with the considered issues and taken into account to build this comparison.

Line-edge roughness clearly appears to be the most severe problem for multi-gate devices, while both RDD and OTV are much less significant. Work-function variations and the relatively high density of trapped charges associated with the introduction of high-κ

Table 5.1. Variability in planar MOSFETs and Double–Gate (DG)/FinFET devices

	Planar CMOS	FinFET/DG-FET
RDD	[2, 4, 41]	[12, 15, 52]
LER	[4, 7, 42]	[11, 15, 52, 55]
OTV	[3, 6, 41]	[22, 52, 55]
PSG	[4, 5, 16]	–
WFV	–	[9, 21, 37]
FTC	[3, 4]	[15]

Cell colors indicate the importance of each source for V_T variability, based on the reported references (dark=high impact, light=small impact).

dielectrics might have a considerable impact on FinFET variability as well, although further investigation of these phenomena is required.

Based on the reported classification, the most relevant source of fluctuations in FinFETs, i.e., LER, is analyzed in this chapter with reference to a transistor architecture designed for low-voltage/low-power applications at the 32 nm technology node, where mainstream employment of these devices might become possible. In order to provide a thorough assessment of LER-induced issues, the variability roadmap framework presented in the International Technology Roadmap for Semiconductors (ITRS) [29] is followed, which subdivides the hierarchy of design abstraction into three levels:

- *circuit/chip level*: address variability of performance figures of merit such as timing, power and/or stability;
- *device level*: address electrical variability of a single device considering relevant parameters such as threshold voltage, off- and on-current;
- *physical level*: directly address fluctuations in the manufacturing process.

Within this framework, a bottom-up analysis approach is applied. At the lowest hierarchy level, the considered source of fluctuations is physically investigated and suitable statistical models are presented, which provide a realistic TCAD representation: this is the aim of section 5.2. Based on these models, large ensembles of microscopically different devices are generated, whose simulation provides variability of FinFET electrical parameters in section 5.3. The impact of different LER contributions is compared and several characteristic options of FinFET design are considered for both n- and p-type devices, including transistor sizing, mobility dependence on crystal orientation and V_T modulation through the gate stack WF. Moreover, the role of extension profiles and junction engineering is studied in detail. To further investigate the link between geometrical and electrical variability, a correlation analysis is presented, which highlights different LER sensitivity of various device regions and provides an effective alternative to extensive Monte Carlo (MC) ensemble simulation for variability estimation. The impact of LER at the circuit level is addressed in section 5.4 with reference to SRAM cells, whose stability is evaluated in hold, read and write operating conditions. Robustness provided by the different options of FinFET design is compared at various supply voltages. Conclusions and guidelines stemming from this analysis are summarized in section 5.5.

5.2 Modeling Variation Sources at the Physical Level

At the lowest hierarchy level, the physical sources of fluctuations must be properly characterized. Line-edge roughness has multiple causes related to various steps and materials involved in the manufacturing process. These include:

- photoresist: granularity of the material, non-uniformities in the film coating, exposure issues related to the wavelength and resist smoothing/slimming, post-exposure bake, development and trim steps;
- properties of the materials and film stacks to be patterned;
- line-edge erosion produced by the etching process;
- properties of the patterned features and layout, such as stress-induced deformations in high aspect-ratio structures and proximity-related patterning errors [18, 48] (these effects introduce systematic variations that are not directly addressed in this work).

Most of the listed phenomena can hardly be mitigated by technology scaling, thus enhancing the impact of LER with shrinking device sizes.

5.2.1 *LER Metrology*

Fig. 5.1 illustrates the combined effect of all the issues mentioned above with reference to a multiple fin structure. Scanning electron microscope (SEM) images like the one in this figure are typically used for LER characterization. Highlighted in Fig. 5.1 are the top region of a fin portion and the gate area on one of the fin sidewalls. Line-edge roughness of these features is clearly visible in the three insets. Silicon fins are commonly patterned using a resist-defined process, resulting in random uncorrelated roughness on the fin edges. However, an alternative technique has been proposed [19], which is based on the use of dummy spacers and provides a significant phase correlation between the fin sidewalls, i.e., virtually zero line-width roughness (LWR). Results of the resist-defined (RDF) and spacer-defined fin patterning (SDF) techniques

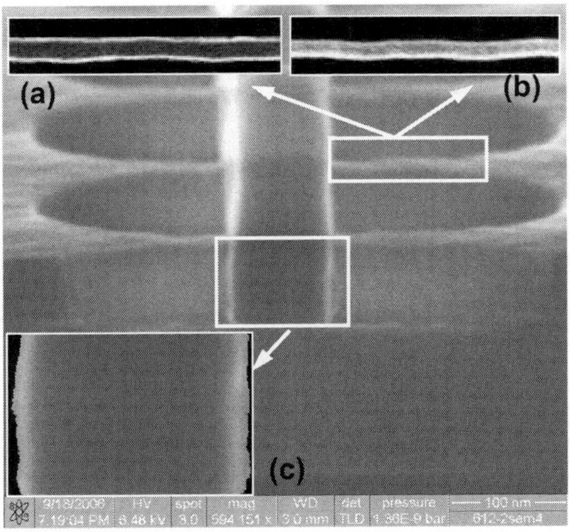

Figure 5.1. SEM image of a FinFET with multiple fins (IMEC). The insets show (a) uncorrelated and (b) correlated fin edges resulting from RDF and SDF patterning, respectively, as well as (c) LER of a sidewall gate.

are shown in Figs. 5.1(a) and (b), respectively. While top-down SEM analysis would suffice for the characterization of fin- as well as top-gate-LER, geometry fluctuations are also observed in the sidewall gates of these 3D devices, as confirmed by Fig. 5.1(c). However, sidewall (sw) metrology is still considered a difficult challenge [29], thus limiting LER measurement capabilities in FinFETs.

The characterization approach is typically based on edge detection algorithms [43] performed on SEM, or sometimes AFM (Atomic Force Microscope), images. Digitalized edge coordinates provided by this procedure are mainly used to extract two characteristic LER descriptors, i.e., rms amplitude Δ and correlation length Λ. The first parameter represents the standard deviation of line-edge fluctuations from a best straight fit, while the second one is the largest distance beyond which two points along the edge can be considered as statistically uncorrelated. Extracted values of 3Δ LWR are reported in Fig. 5.2 [22] and correspond to an rms amplitude $\Delta \simeq 1.5$ nm for the LER of individual line edges in the RDF case, while spacer-defined patterning provides a significant reduction of the LWR. Measured correlation lengths are in the 30–45 nm range. However, extraction of this parameter is difficult and should be performed on very long lines to provide reliable results; other authors report slightly smaller values [7]. Data in Fig. 5.2 were obtained through top-down SEM metrology of fin edges, while

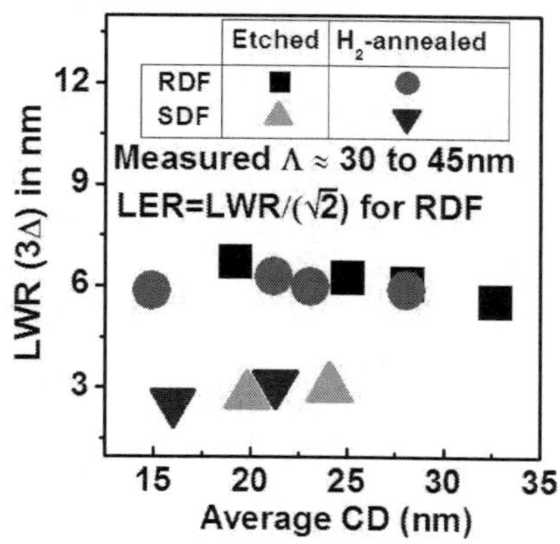

Figure 5.2. IMEC LWR measurements on resist-defined and spacer-defined fins as a function of the fin width [22].

accurate characterization of sw-gate-LER is still lacking due to difficulties in sidewall SEM as well as following edge detection and statistical analysis for the relatively short and complex shapes of sw-gate stacks [13].

5.2.2 *TCAD Representation of LER*

LER can be statistically represented by using the extracted parameters to properly model the power spectrum (PS) of digitalized fin edges. Typically, the PS of a stochastic process with Gaussian or exponential autocorrelation function (acf.) is adopted [7]. This approach can be used to synthesize LER sequences with similar statistical properties as those of the detected lines in the following way. First, realistic values of Δ and Λ are plugged into the chosen PS model and random phases are added, with the constraint that the resulting array must be symmetric with respect to its central element since it describes a real-valued process. Then, an inverse fast Fourier transform (IFFT) is applied to get the desired LER sequences. Patterns resulting from the Gaussian model are smoother than those associated with the exponential one, whose spectrum includes a wider range of spatial frequencies, as shown in Fig. 5.3(a). However, it has been shown that these two approaches provide similar estimations of LER-induced variability [11]; moreover, surface and junction profile smoothening caused by H_2 anneal and dopant diffusion, respectively, tend to suppress high frequency components of fin- and gate-LER. Therefore the Gaussian process is expected to provide a more realistic representation of line-edge roughness statistics and will be used throughout this chapter. Assuming this model, the symmetric spectra of two statistically independent lines are plotted in Fig. 5.3(b), while Fig. 5.3(c) displays the corresponding sequences obtained after IFFT.

Results of this procedure can be used to describe rough device features in a TCAD environment. For example, long LER sequences like those in Fig. 5.3(c) can be split to generate the fin edges of many FinFET instances affected by LER. Simulating the resulting ensemble of microscopically different devices provides a Monte Carlo estimation of LER impact on electrical variability, as illustrated in the following section.

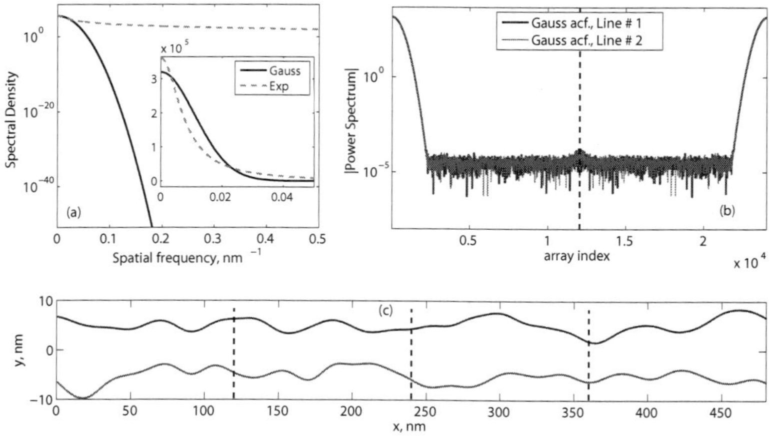

Figure 5.3. (a) Power spectral density of a stochastic process with Gaussian or exponential acf. ($\Delta = 1.5$ nm, $\Lambda = 20$ nm). A zoom on very low spatial frequencies is visible in the inset, showing a similar behavior of the two models within this range. (b) Power spectra of two statistically independent lines (Gaussian model), exhibiting symmetry w.r.t. the central element. (c) LER sequences obtained from (b) after IFFT. See also Color Insert.

5.3 Impact of Variability at the Device Level

Device simulation provides the link between microscopic variations at the physical level and fluctuations of transistor electrical performance. This will be illustrated with reference to LER in FinFETs, by exploiting an automated Matlab-TCAD flow which allows generation of large device ensembles, simulation and parameter extraction.

5.3.1 *Simulation Approach*

The devices considered throughout this chapter are LSTP-32 nm compatible FinFETs with nominal geometry and doping specifications as described in Table 5.2. In particular, N_{ch} and N_{hdd} are the channel and source/drain (S/D) doping concentrations, while $N_{ext,n}$ and $N_{ext,p}$ represent the extension concentrations for n- and p-type transistors, respectively. Resulting electrical parameters of the n-FET are also reported in the Table. A proper set of physical

Table 5.2. LSTP-32 nm FinFET specifications

Geometry	Doping	Electrical parameters
$L_{gate} = 30$ nm	$N_{ch} = 1 \times 10^{15}\text{cm}^{-3}$	$I_{ON} = 750\ \mu\text{A}/\mu\text{m}$
$W_{fin} = 10$ nm	$N_{hdd} = 1 \times 10^{20}\text{cm}^{-3}$	$I_{OFF} = 10\ \text{pA}/\mu\text{m}$
$H_{fin} = 50$ nm	$N_{ext,n} = 5 \times 10^{18}\text{cm}^{-3}$	$V_{T,sat} = 0.36$ V
$t_{ox} = 1.2$ nm	$N_{ext,p} = 2 \times 10^{19}\text{cm}^{-3}$	$SSlope = 69$ mV/dec

models must be selected to accurately predict the impact of LER on device performance. In this work, the following models have been chosen [46]:

- hydrodynamic transport, to provide a better description of the device behavior in the saturation regime, compared to the commonly used drift-diffusion approach;
- density gradient approximation (DGA), to account for quantum confinement associated with small fin widths at a reasonable computational cost;
- mobility degradation and velocity saturation in the presence of high electric fields.

As for the choice of model parameters, it must be added that standard (100) mobility conditions have been assumed in most of the simulations. However, sidewall transport in FinFETs often occurs in the (110) plane, depending on the wafer substrate orientation and fin rotation angle relative to the wafer flat [32]. Although this is expected to enhance hole mobility while depressing electron mobility [53], sidewall transport is strongly influenced by the fin patterning technique, including hard mask, corner rounding and H_2 anneal, as well as the gate stack. Different process options may even lead to opposite trends for top/sidewall mobility ratios w.r.t. theory [30]. Despite these issues, some simulations have been dedicated to estimate the impact of LER on FinFETs with (110) carrier transport: this has been done by decreasing μ_n and increasing μ_p in the low-field mobility model. Standard (100) parameters have been modified according to percentage mobility variations reported in [53]. To achieve LSTP-compatible threshold voltage values as indicated in Table 5.2, the gate WF has been set to 4.62 eV, which is consistent with TiN metal commonly used for the

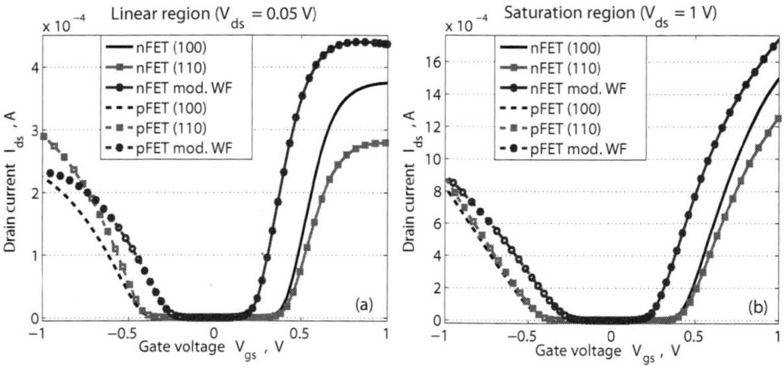

Figure 5.4. Simulated $I_{ds}-V_{gs}$ characteristics of n- and p-channel FinFETs with (100) and (110) carrier transport as well as LSTP-compatible, or LOP-compatible ("mod. WF" case), V_T. See also Color Insert.

gate stack [21]. However, work-function engineering may be applied to tune the device threshold. The impact of this design option has been investigated by adjusting the WF so as to achieve $V_T \simeq 0.2$ V, as in ITRS low operating power (LOP) specifications [29]. I_{ds}-V_{gs} FinFETs characteristics in Fig. 5.4 show the impact of the different mobility and WF settings on the nominal device performance.

Although MC is the most accurate approach to account for geometry variations, large ensembles are needed to get statistically meaningful results. Assuming representative electrical parameters, such as threshold voltage V_T and on-current I_{ON}, to be normally distributed, evaluating standard deviations with less than 5% uncertainty requires simulation of at least 200 instances [2]. Unless otherwise stated, this is the ensemble size considered to get the results shown in the following sections. Due to the high computational cost, alternatives to brute-force MC would be preferred. Many works adopt a simple sensitivity analysis: in the case of LER this consists in simulating devices with different fin widths or gate lengths but uniform features, i.e., no roughness, and estimating fluctuations from the achieved trends of electrical parameters vs. varying dimension [52]. Limitations of this approach will be discussed and an alternative methodology will be proposed, which exploits correlation between geometrical roughness and electrical performance to choose suitable corner cases for variability estimation.

5.3.2 *Assessment of LER Contributions to Electrical Fluctuations*

Impact of the three main components of line-edge roughness in FinFETs, i.e., fin-LER, top-gate LER and sw-gate LER, is discussed in this section with reference to n-channel devices with nominal features in Table 5.2. A TCAD model of FinFET affected by LER is presented in Fig. 5.5(a); however, simulating MC ensembles of similar devices is very expensive from a computational standpoint. Therefore, the three contributions have been decoupled and their effects have been separately studied considering simplified structures as shown in Figs. 5.5(b)–(d). A 2D approximation is sufficient to analyze fin- and top-gate-LER (Figs. 5.5(c) and (d), respectively), whereas a 3D approach is needed to properly account for roughness of the sidewall gate (Fig. 5.5(b)). To reduce the

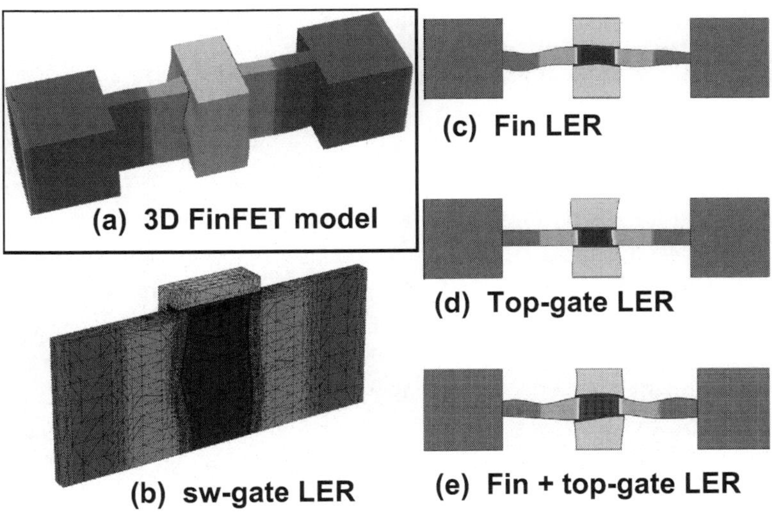

Figure 5.5. (a) 3D TCAD representation of a FinFET with fin- and gate-LER. (b)–(e) Instances of simulated structures for the investigation of sw-gate-LER, fin-LER, top-gate-LER and combined fin+top-gate LER, respectively.

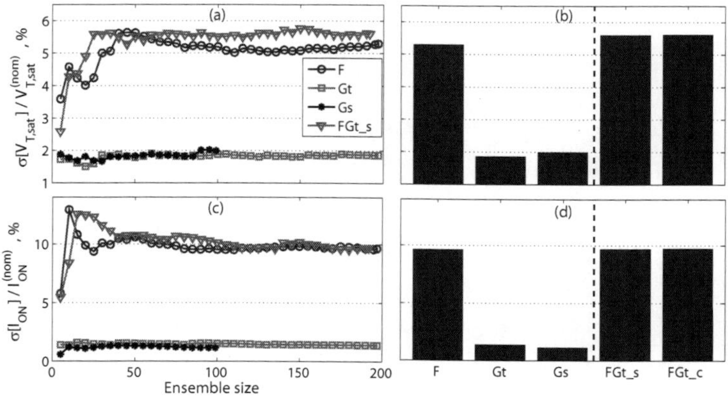

Figure 5.6. (a), (c) Normalized standard deviation of saturation threshold voltage and on-current plotted as a function of the ensemble size for simulations of fin-LER ("F"), top-gate-LER ("Gt"), sw-gate-LER ("Gs") and combined fin+top-gate LER ("FGt_s") in n-channel FinFETs (see Fig. 5.5). $V_{T,sat}$ and I_{ON} have been extracted at $V_{ds} = 1$ V and $V_{ds} = V_{gs} = 1$ V, respectively, and normalized to nominal values $V_{T,sat}^{(nom)} = 0.36$ V and $I_{ON}^{(nom)} = 750$ μA/μm (see Table 5.2). (b), (d) Statistics extracted from the full ensembles; "FGt_c" is the combined impact of fin- and top-gate-LER calculated from individual contributions through Eq. (5.1). See also Color Insert.

computational effort, the ensemble size has been limited to $N = 100$ in the latter case, while $N = 200$ devices have been considered in 2D simulations. The combined impact of fin- and top-gate-LER has also been studied through structures similar to that in Fig. 5.5(e).

For each considered case, normalized standard deviations of saturation threshold voltage and on-current extracted from $I_{ds} - V_{gs}$ simulations are plotted in Figs. 5.6(a) and (c) as a function of the ensemble size. LER parameters in this analysis are $\Delta = 1.5$ nm, $\Lambda = 20$ nm, in line with top-down SEM measurements (see Section 5.2.1). In the absence of accurate informations from sidewall metrology, the same values of Δ and Λ have been used for sw-gate-LER as well, in order to provide a fair comparison. Fin-LER ("F") is clearly seen to be the most critical issue for both V_T and I_{ON} variability, while top- ("Gt") and sw-gate-LER ("Gs") produce similar electrical fluctuations. Statistics is well stabilized when computed over the full ensembles, even in the "Gs" case with $N = 100$. Resulting values are compared in Figs. 5.6(b) and (d), confirming the predominance of fin-LER and thus motivating the prominent attention reserved to this contribution in the reminder of this chapter. Figs. 5.6(b) and (d) also indicate a good agreement between the simulated impact of combined fin- and top-gate-roughness ("FGt_s") and estimations ("FGt_c") obtained from individual components through:

$$\sigma_{FGt\_c} = \sqrt{\sigma_F^2 + \sigma_{Gt}^2} \qquad (5.1)$$

which demonstrates that these components can be considered statistically independent.

Results in Fig. 5.6 have been obtained by assuming random uncorrelated roughness of the two fin or gate edges, as in Fig. 5.5. To evaluate the impact of a spacer-defined fin patterning technique, structures with in-phase correlation between the fin edges have been simulated. Resulting electrical variability is compared to that of resist-defined devices in Figs. 5.7(a) and (c), for different rms amplitudes of the roughness. SDF patterning is found to provide more than 90% reduction of LER impact on both threshold voltage

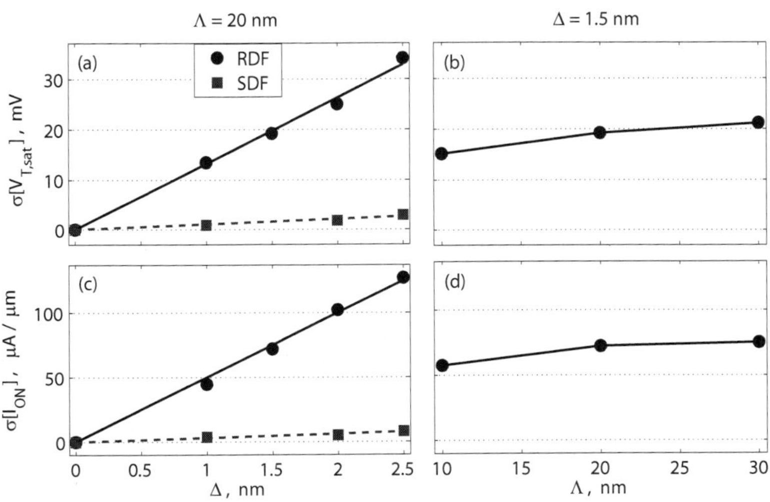

Figure 5.7. (a), (b) Threshold voltage and (c), (d) drive current variability as a function of (a), (c) LER rms amplitude and (b), (d) LER correlation length, for RDF-patterned n-channel FinFETs. Reduction of LER impact through a SDF patterning technique is also shown in (a) and (c).

and drive current fluctuations, for equal values of Δ. This technique is therefore a promising solution to alleviate line-edge roughness issues; however, SDF processes still exhibit severe instabilities, thus requiring further optimization to reach sufficient maturity [11]. On the other hand, the impact of LER on RDF-patterned devices can only be alleviated by proportionally decreasing the roughness amplitude, as demonstrated by the linear trends in Figs. 5.7(a) and (c), but this is difficult because LER causes do not scale (see Section 5.2). Smaller correlation lengths of the roughness slightly reduce electrical variability by enhancing self-averaging effects, but Figs. 5.7(b) and (d) show that this is not an effective way to suppress LER issues. Therefore, fin line-edge roughness in resist-defined devices will be further investigated in the following sections.

5.3.3 *Correlation Analysis and Comparison of LER Simulation Approaches*

Correlations between geometrical features and electrical parameters can be highlighted, which help understanding how LER affects FinFET performance and provide an alternative to both the expensive MC approach and an overly simplistic sensitivity analysis for variability estimation.

5.3.3.1 Correlation study

The considered geometrical feature is the fin width averaged either over the whole fin length ($\langle W_{fin}\rangle_{tot}$) of each device instance, or over the channel region only ($\langle W_{fin}\rangle_{ch}$), as indicated in Figs. 5.8(a) and (b), respectively [8, 12]. Threshold voltage and drive current extracted from MC simulation of several datasets with different roughness characteristics (see Fig. 5.7, RDF case) are plotted in Figs. 5.8(c)–(f) against these parameters. $V_{T,sat}$ exhibits an approximately linear dependence on $\langle W_{fin}\rangle_{ch}$ (Fig. 5.8(d)), indicating that line-edge roughness mainly impacts the device threshold by changing the average fin width in the channel, while the reduced correlation of $V_{T,sat}$ to $\langle W_{fin}\rangle_{tot}$ in Fig. 5.8(c) suggests that threshold voltage is not sensitive to LER of the S/D extensions. On the contrary, comparison of Figs. 5.8(e) and (f) demonstrates that the whole

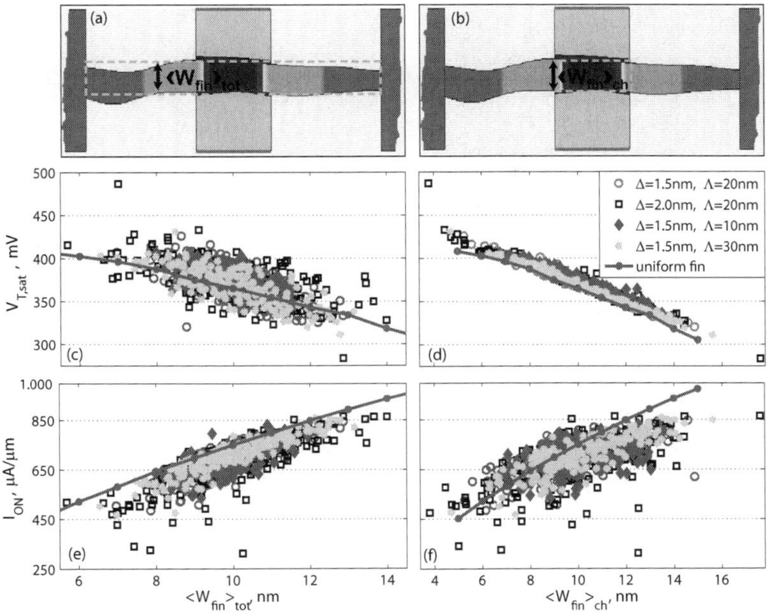

Figure 5.8. Fin width averaging (a) over the whole fin length ($\langle W_{fin}\rangle_{tot}$) and (b) over the channel region ($\langle W_{fin}\rangle_{ch}$) for correlation analysis. (c), (d) Scatter plots of saturation threshold voltage vs. $\langle W_{fin}\rangle_{tot}$ and $\langle W_{fin}\rangle_{ch}$, respectively, for RDF datasets in Fig. 5.7 (e), (f) Same for on-current.

fin region contributes to setting FinFET on-current, although the spread is quite strong for this parameter, even in Fig. 5.8(e). Solid lines in Figs. 5.8(c)–(f) were obtained by simulating straight-fin devices with different fin widths, in order to compare the MC approach with a sensitivity analysis of LER-induced fluctuations. Due to the observed correlation, such analysis may provide a fairly accurate estimation of threshold voltage spread for relatively small values of the roughness, as can be seen in the central part of Fig. 5.8(d). However, corner situations are not properly captured by this simplistic approach; moreover, Fig. 5.8(d) shows that fin-LER raises the mean value of the threshold voltage w.r.t sensitivity analysis predictions based on straight-fin devices.

This phenomenon is expected to be enhanced by scaling [55]; it is opposed to the V_T-lowering effect produced by gate-LER [7] and can be explained as follows [8]: as shown in Fig. 5.9(a), a transistor

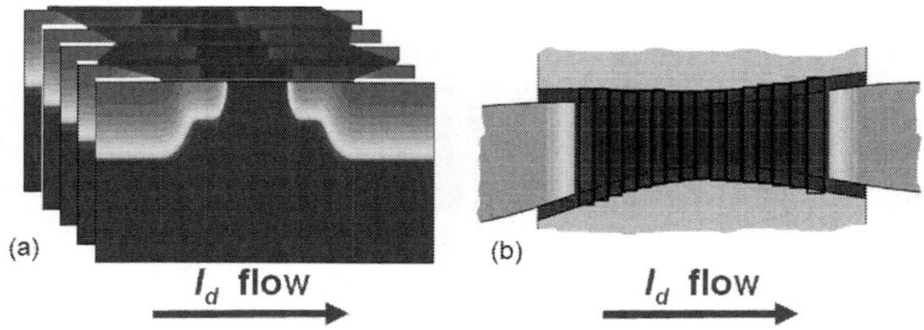

Figure 5.9. (a) Gate-LER can be modeled through a parallel combination of device slices with different L_{gate}. (b) Fin-LER is equivalent to a series composition of fin slices with different widths. See also Color Insert.

with rough gate can be thought of as a *parallel* combination of device slices with different gate lengths [42], where the early turn-on of the shorter gate-length slices lowers the overall threshold. Instead, fin-LER might be modeled through a *series* composition of fin slices with different widths (see Fig. 5.9(b)): in this case, the overall conduction is determined by the thinner slices, where higher electrostatic control and reduced SCEs contribute to raising the device V_T. Further investigation is required to check whether the opposite effects of the fin and gate roughness on FinFET threshold voltage can compensate each other.

Besides raising the device V_T, fin-LER also degrades the FinFET current drive w.r.t. the uniform fin case, as can be seen from Fig. 5.8(e). To better understand this phenomenon and reduce the scatter, I_{ON} data can be re-ordered according to an equivalent fin width W_{equiv}, which is calculated as a weighted sum of widths W_j in the M key regions of the fin [8]:

$$W_{equiv} = \sum_{j=1}^{M} c_j \cdot W_j \tag{5.2}$$

Several combinations of W_j have been explored for each device instance, including maximum, average and/or minimum fin thickness within the channel, source and drain extensions as well as the widths at the two gate ends. Corresponding weights c_j have been found by solving a least mean square problem

$$\sum_{j=1}^{M} W_{ij} c_j = I_{ON,i}, \qquad i = 1, \ldots, N \tag{5.3}$$

where i is the index of the device within the statistical ensemble ($N = 200$). The best trade-off between correlation to I_{ON} data and number M of characteristic widths has been found by considering the two end points of the gate at the source (W_s) and drain side (W_d) and the average width of the extensions $\langle W_{ex,s}\rangle$, $\langle W_{ex,d}\rangle$, as sketched in the inset of Fig. 5.10(a). Respective weights c_j assume similar values upon varying the roughness rms amplitude and correlation length: reported in Table 5.3 is the value $\overline{c}_j$ of each weight, averaged across the different datasets. This table provides information on the relative importance of LER in different fin regions: it can be seen that drive current is mainly influenced by the source side of the device, as will be better elucidated in Section 5.3.4.2. Fig. 5.10(a) shows the scatter plots of drive current vs. the equivalent width calculated by

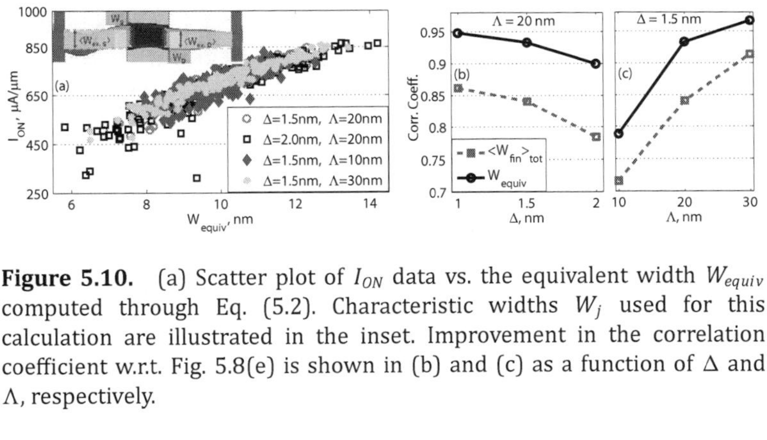

Figure 5.10. (a) Scatter plot of I_{ON} data vs. the equivalent width W_{equiv} computed through Eq. (5.2). Characteristic widths W_j used for this calculation are illustrated in the inset. Improvement in the correlation coefficient w.r.t. Fig. 5.8(e) is shown in (b) and (c) as a function of Δ and Λ, respectively.

Table 5.3. Characteristic widths W_j for W_{equiv} estimation through Eq. (5.2) and corresponding average weights $\overline{c}_j$ resulting from several datasets with different Δ and Λ values ($\sum_j \overline{c}_j = 1$)

Parameter W_j	Average weight $\overline{c}_j$
W_s	0.253
W_d	0.162
$\langle W_{ex,s}\rangle$	0.376
$\langle W_{ex,d}\rangle$	0.209

plugging into Eq. (5.2) the four characteristic widths W_j described above and respective weights c_j for each device instance. Improvement in the correlation w.r.t. Fig. 5.8(e) is plotted in Figs. 5.10(b) and (c) as a function of Δ and Λ, respectively, demonstrating the effectiveness of this approach to reduce the I_{ON} data scatter.

5.3.3.2 Exploiting correlations

Correlations highlighted so far for the FinFET threshold voltage and on-current can be exploited to achieve an approximate estimation of LER-induced variability at a low computational cost. The approach consists in calculating the statistics of a key geometrical parameter x (e.g., $\langle W_{fin}\rangle_{ch}$ or W_{equiv}) and combining this information with very few simulation data to estimate the spread of relevant electrical parameters p (e.g., V_T and I_{ON}). Standard deviation $\sigma[x]$ can be easily calculated from the considered ensemble of device structures, as depicted on Fig. 5.11(a). In contrast to the MC approach, however, only the "corner devices" corresponding to points x_L and x_R in this figure are simulated, resulting in electrical parameters p_L and p_R, respectively. An approximate estimation of electrical variability can then be calculated as:

$$\sigma[p] \simeq \left|\frac{p_R - p_L}{x_R - x_L}\right| \sigma[x] \tag{5.4}$$

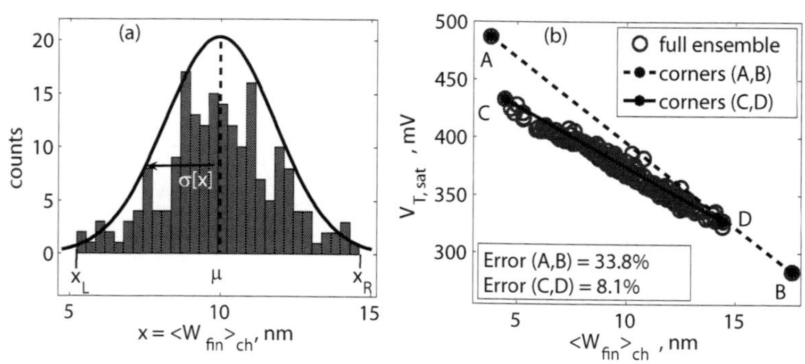

Figure 5.11. (a) Statistical analysis of geometrical parameter $x = \langle W_{fin}\rangle_{ch}$ for an ensemble of 200 FinFETs affected by fin-LER ($\Delta = 2$ nm, $\Lambda = 1.5$ nm). (b) Variability estimation of $V_{T,sat}$ exploiting correlation to $\langle W_{fin}\rangle_{ch}$. Reported errors refer to $\sigma[V_{T,sat}]$ calculated through samples (A, B) and (C, D), w.r.t. the value extracted from the full ensemble.

A modification of this technique allows handling outliers by simulating also the two devices next to the extremes, i.e., determining points C and D in addition to A and B in Fig. 5.11(b), and using these two couples to compute $\sigma_{A,B}[p]$ and $\sigma_{C,D}[p]$ through Eq. (5.4). The best estimation of electrical variability is then chosen as the maximum (i.e., the worst case) between $\sigma_{A,B}[p]$ and $\sigma_{C,D}[p]$ if their relative difference is smaller than a predefined threshold (e.g., 0.2). Instead, a large difference between the two estimates indicates the presence of outliers that normally affect the highest value: therefore, the minimum between $\sigma_{A,B}[p]$ and $\sigma_{C,D}[p]$ is retained in this case.

In Fig. 5.12, results obtained by applying the proposed technique to data of Fig. 5.8(d) are compared with those provided by the MC approach and by the sensitivity analysis. The latter procedure can only track the effect of various rms amplitudes of the roughness (Fig. 5.12(c)) on V_T spread. For the same computational expense, the "corner" method fully accounts for fin-LER impact on device threshold, including mean value and standard deviation dependence

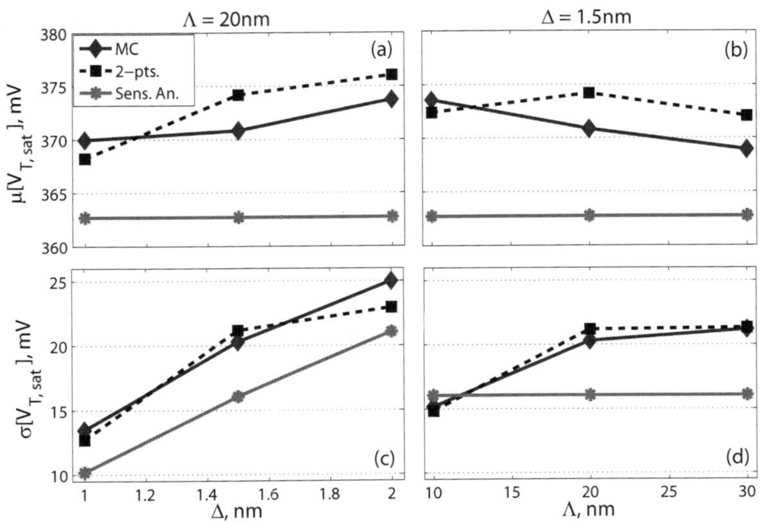

Figure 5.12. (a), (b) Mean value and (c), (d) standard deviation of saturation threshold voltage as a function of (a), (c) rms amplitude and (b), (d) correlation length of the roughness. Results of the Monte Carlo approach ("MC") are compared with estimations based on corner points ("2-pts.") and sensitivity analysis ("Sens. An.").

on LER parameters, with a fairly good accuracy (maximum error = 8% w.r.t. MC-based statistics obtained with a two orders of magnitude higher computational cost). The V_T-raising is seen to increase with increasing Δ and with decreasing Λ in Figs. 5.12(a) and (b), respectively. This is in agreement with the slice model shown in Fig. 5.9(b), since a higher rms amplitude of the roughness decreases the minimum slice thickness, while a smaller correlation length increases the probability of a thin slice occurring within the channel. Of course higher values of Δ also enhance the V_T spread, which is systematically underestimated by the sensitivity analysis, as shown in Fig. 5.12(c). Finally, Fig. 5.12(d) indicates that $\sigma[V_T]$ increases with increasing Λ as well, because of a lower self-averaging of fin thickness variations within the channel.

As for drive current fluctuations, the "corner" method has been applied both to the I_{ON} vs. $\langle W_{fin}\rangle_{tot}$ and the I_{ON} vs. W_{equiv} distributions. In the latter case, the average coefficients $\overline{c}_j$ in Table 5.3 have been used, which can be assumed as generally valid for the considered FinFET structure. Figure 5.13 shows that the W_{equiv}-based reordering improves estimation of I_{ON} statistics in most of the analyzed cases, although the "corner" method significantly deviates from the MC results at high rms amplitudes and small correlation lengths of the roughness (Figs. 5.13(c) and (d), respectively), due to a higher data spread and the presence of more outliers. Again, the sensitivity analysis can only capture the Δ-dependence of $\sigma[I_{ON}]$, while Figs. 5.13(a) and (b) indicate a significant LER-induced lowering of the mean drive current, which is approximately tracked by correlation-based estimations and will be further investigated in Section 5.3.4.2.

5.3.4 *Impact of FinFET Design on LER-Induced Variability*

Single-fin, n-channel FinFETs with nominal features specified in Table 5.2 have been considered so far. In this section, LER-induced variability of both n- and p-type devices with various design options will be investigated, including transistor sizing, crystal orientation, gate stack and extension engineering. The impact of line-edge roughness on both channel and extension parasitic resistance will be studied in detail.

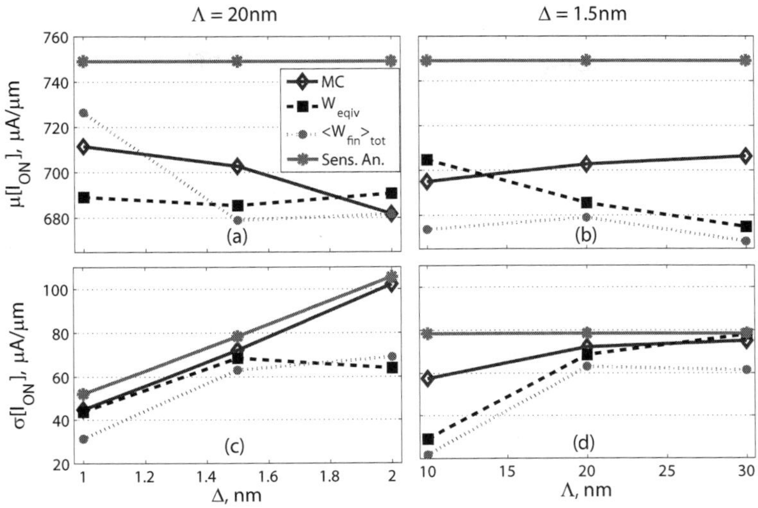

Figure 5.13. (a), (b) Mean value and (c), (d) standard deviation of drive current as a function of (a), (c) rms amplitude and (b), (d) correlation length of the roughness. Results of the Monte Carlo approach ("MC") are compared with estimations based on sensitivity analysis ("Sens. An.") and on corner points selected from the I_{ON} vs. W_{equiv} and I_{ON} vs. $\langle W_{fin}\rangle_{tot}$ distributions.

5.3.4.1 Number of fins, crystal orientation and WF engineering

FinFETs with (100) and (110) carrier transport have been compared; moreover, the effect of a lower threshold voltage ($V_T \simeq 0.2$ V, compatible with LOP applications) obtained by WF tuning has been considered to evaluate the influence of gate stack engineering on LER-induced variability. Transfer characteristics of the nominal n-FETs and p-FETs are shown in Fig. 5.4. As the channel width in these devices is quantized in multiples of the fin height, multi-finger structures have also been simulated to check how LER-robustness is improved by increasing transistor area. Results of this analysis are summarized in Fig. 5.14, where the standard deviation of both $V_{T,sat}$ and I_{ON} is normalized to the mean value of these quantities and plotted versus the inverse square root of the number of fins in each device. Linear trends in this figure are in agreement with Pelgrom's law on variability being inversely proportional to the transistor area [44]. Devices with (100) and (110) conduction but relatively

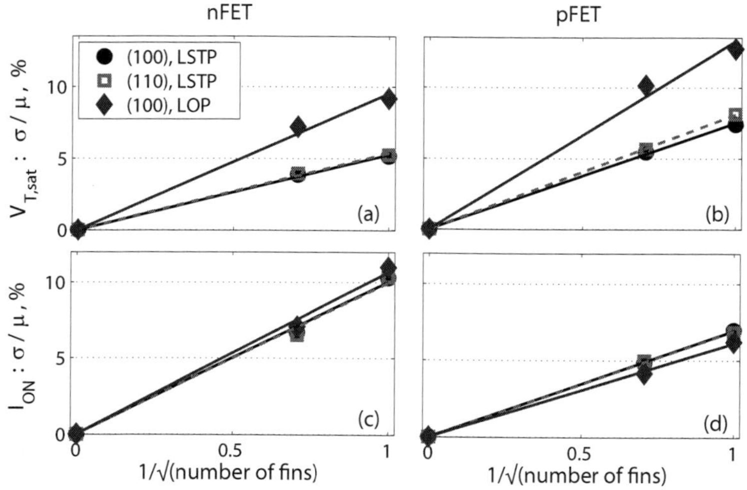

Figure 5.14. LER-induced variability of (a), (c) n-type and (b), (d) p-type FinFETs with (100) and (110) conduction as well as WF modulation for LOP compatibility. Variability is expressed as the ratio between standard deviation σ and mean value μ of (a), (b) saturation threshold voltage $V_{T,sat}$ and (c), (d) on-state current I_{ON}. Statistics is based on ensembles ranging from 200 up to 300 devices.

high nominal V_T for LSTP compatibility are equally affected by LER. Instead, decreasing the threshold voltage by WF tuning is seen to enhance sensitivity of this parameter to LER (Figs. 5.14(a) and (b), "LOP" case), while drive current fluctuations in Figs. 5.14(c) and (d) are not significantly worsened. In all considered cases, line-edge roughness appears to be slightly more critical for threshold voltage variability in p-channel than in n-channel FETs, while opposite trends are observed for I_{ON}; however, differences between the fluctuations of n- and p-type FinFETs are small.

5.3.4.2 Doping profiles and role of the extensions

While the FinFET channel is typically left undoped and very high concentrations are used in the S/D pads (see Table 5.2), extension doping is a critical process step. In particular, low-energy, high-dose implants are desired at high tilt angles and dopant penetration underneath the gate should be avoided to effectively suppress

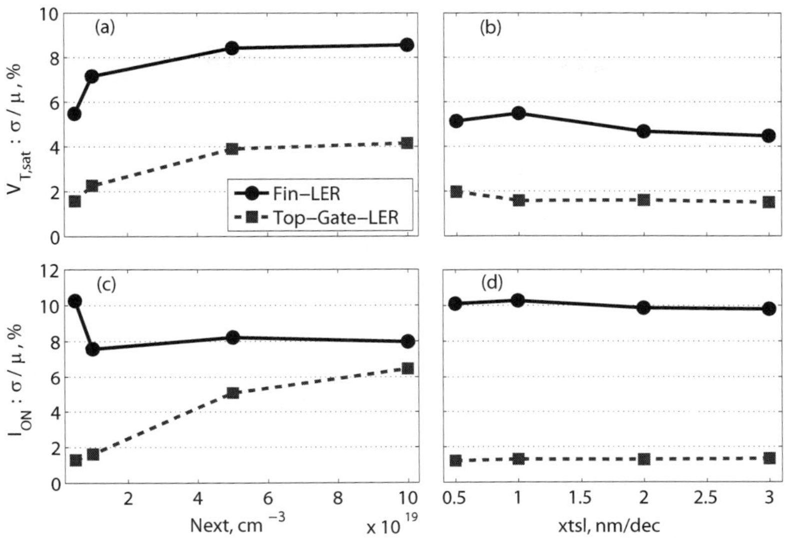

Figure 5.15. Impact of fin and top-gate roughness as a function of extension profiles. (a), (c): impact of different extension concentrations N_{ext}. (b), (d): impact of extension slope $xtsl$.

short channel effects [27]. Advanced techniques as Solid-Phase Epitaxial Regrowth (SPER) are being explored to achieve abrupt junctions [34] and improve device performance [23]. The two basic parameters which characterize resulting profiles, i.e., extension levels N_{ext} and decay rates $xtsl$, have been varied in order to estimate the LER dependence on extension doping.

Simulation results in Fig. 5.15(a) indicate that the impact of both fin- and gate-LER on the threshold voltage is enhanced with higher N_{ext}, but the trends are approximately parallel to each other. On the other hand, increasing the peak doping concentration in the extensions is seen to considerably enhance I_{ON} sensitivity to gate-LER in Fig. 5.15(c), while the fin roughness contribution is not significantly changed. This can be explained in terms of parasitic resistances, as sketched in Fig. 5.16. The more ideal extension profiles with high concentration may be required to boost the saturation drain current through reduction in S/D resistance [23]. Such reduction is probably responsible for the decreasing or roughly constant impact of fin-LER in Fig. 5.15(c). However, this causes

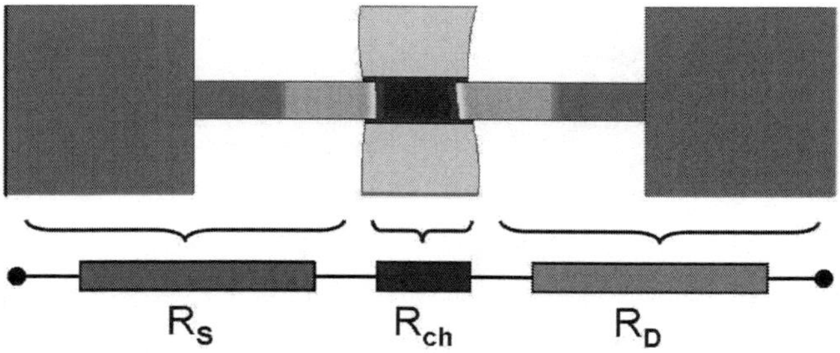

Figure 5.16. Parasitic resistance model of a FinFET. Fluctuations in physical channel length due to gate-LER change the channel resistance R_{ch}. Increasing extension profile concentration and slope (junction engineering) reduces S/D resistances (R_S, R_D), thus enhancing the relative importance of R_{ch}.

the drive current to be more sensitive to the effective channel resistance, which in turn is particularly affected by gate-LER: hence, importance of this contribution increases in Fig. 5.15(c) and becomes comparable to that of the fin-LER for very high N_{ext} values.

The effect of different profile decay rates on V_T and I_{ON} sensitivity to LER is shown in Figs. 5.15(b) and (d), respectively. It can be seen that steeper junctions correspond to slightly higher fluctuations, but the impact of $xtsl$ is clearly negligible w.r.t. that of the extension concentration. Moreover, increasing N_{ext} is also expected to enhance dopant fluctuation issues [12], thus posing critical difficulties to junction engineering.

Even at moderate extension levels like those in Table 5.2, for which fin-LER is the dominant source of variability, it was shown in Section 5.3.3.1 that the impact of thickness fluctuations on drive current is dependent on the affected fin region. In particular, the S end of the channel and the S extension have a stronger impact on I_{ON} w.r.t. the D side of the device, as indicated by the dominant weights of W_s and $\langle W_{ex,s} \rangle$ in Table 5.3. To further investigate local effects of fin-LER on parasitic resistances, W_{fin} has been varied linearly over the whole fin length (Fig. 5.17(a)) or just in the channel (Fig. 5.17(b)) or extensions (Fig. 5.17(c)), while keeping the overall average fin width fixed to 10 nm. The tapering has been applied either from S to D or vice versa, in order to highlight asymmetries.

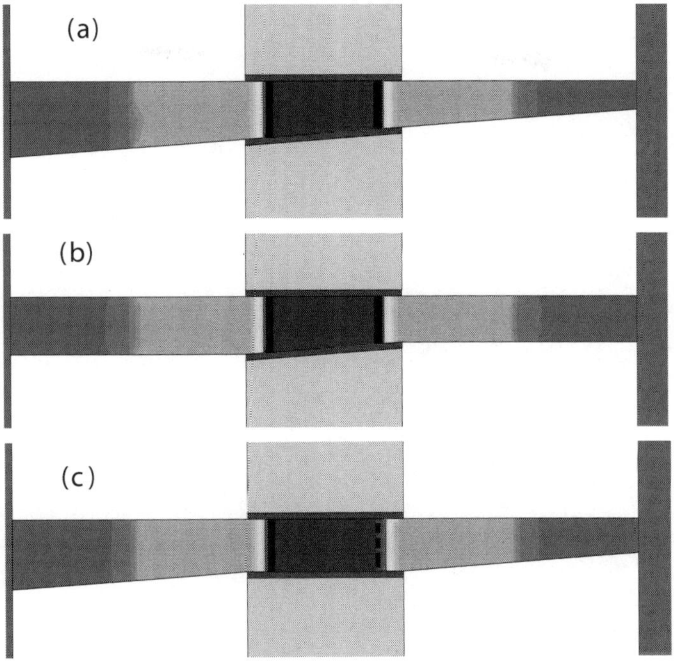

Figure 5.17. Simplified device structures with tapering of (a) the whole fin, (b) just the channel region, and (c) just the extensions, considered to evaluate the impact of local thinning in different fin regions on device performance.

Electrical parameters resulting from this analysis are reported in Fig. 5.18, where "W_{fin} change rate" indicates the fin thickness change per unit fin length associated with different slopes of the inclined edge in Fig. 5.17. A local thinning of one fin end always degrades the FinFET current with respect to the nominal case, although it is compensated by an equal thickening at the other end: this is in agreement with the LER-induced I_{ON}-lowering discussed in Section 5.3.3. A similar impact of the thinning regardless of the taper direction is seen in Figs. 5.18(a)–(c), due to the small asymmetry of S/D bias conditions (V_{ds} = 50 mV). However, remarkable asymmetries appear in the saturated regime (Figs. 5.18(d)–(f)), where geometry constrictions towards the source cause a strong reduction of I_{ON}, while the "Drain thinning" case is not critically

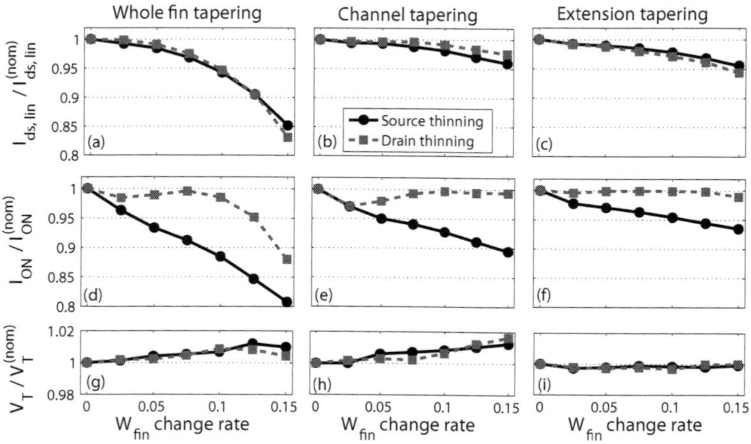

Figure 5.18. Relative variation of linear ($I_{d,lin}$) and saturated drain current (I_{ON}) as well as threshold voltage (V_T) as a consequence of different fin tapering, as described in Fig. 5.17. Fin width variation per unit fin length "W_{fin} change rate" represents the taper magnitude, while "source thinning" and "drain thinning" indicate the taper direction. $I_{d,lin}$ and I_{ON} were extracted at $V_{DS} = 50$ mV and $V_{ds} = 1$ V, respectively, and $V_{gs} = 1$ V.

degraded, except for extremely small values of the minimum thickness close to the D pad (see Fig. 5.18(d)). Since $V_{T,sat}$ is basically set by the average fin width in the channel ($\langle W_{fin}\rangle_{ch}$, see Section 5.3.3), it is not sensitive to the tapering, as shown in Fig. 5.18(g)–(i), and thus cannot be responsible for the observed I_{ON} variability. The I_{ON}-lowering must therefore be attributed to increased parasitic resistance in both the channel (R_{ch}) and S/D extension regions ($R_{S/D}$). Although the former contribution seems to be dominant when comparing Figs. 5.18(e) and (f), the dependence of $R_{S/D}$ on the taper direction in the former plot is not completely eliminated (see the simulated structure in Fig. 5.17(b)).

A tapered device with very short extensions of length $L_{ext} =$ 12 nm has been considered to better decouple the role of channel and extension regions. I_{ON} degradation for the structures with channel tapering and long/short extensions is compared in Figs. 5.19(a) and (b), highlighting opposite effects of the taper direction. The more pronounced on-current reduction in the "Drain

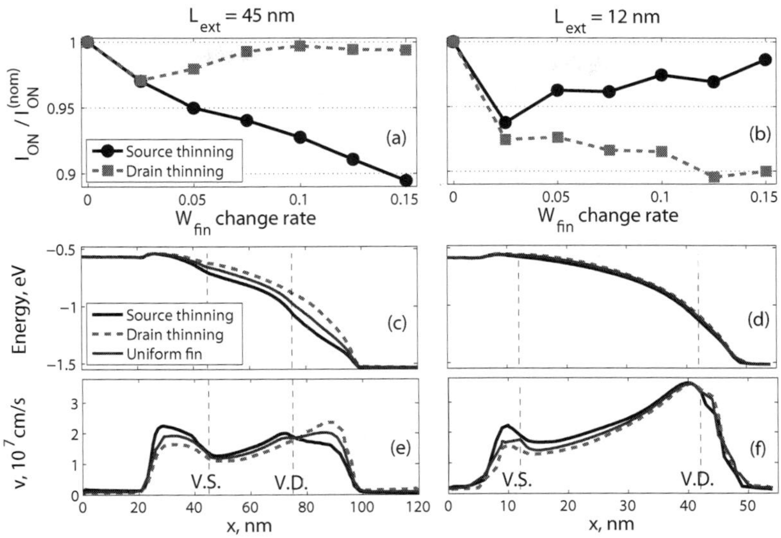

Figure 5.19. Relative variation of I_{ON} w.r.t. the uniform fin case due to channel tapering, for a device with (a) long and (b) short extensions (L_{ext} = 45 nm and L_{ext} = 12 nm, respectively). (c), (d) Potential energy and (e), (f) electron velocity for the two FinFET structures. x indicates the position along the fin (V.S = virtual source, V.D. = virtual drain). These cuts were taken inside the fin, 5 nm away from the axis-aligned edge (see Fig. 5.17), but similar trends were observed at different y positions. See also Color Insert.

thinning" case for the FinFET with L_{ext} = 12 nm can be interpreted according to Lundstrom's model for quasi-ballistic transport [36]. Geometrical constriction toward the D locally increases the subband energy, thus producing a wider kT-layer, i.e., a less steep decay of the potential energy along the channel compared to the device with uniform fin. This results in a larger backscattering coefficient and therefore in a smaller injection velocity at the virtual source (V.S.). Swapping the thinning direction is expected to produce an opposite effect and ideally improves drive current of the *intrinsic* (i.e., no extensions) device with respect to the straight-fin case [47]. Figs. 5.19(c) and (d) show a wider kT-layer in the "drain thinning" case for both devices with long and short extensions: therefore, injection velocity at the V.S. is lower in these structures than in those with uniform fin, as can be seen from Figs. 5.19(e) and (f). Opposite trends are observed for the "source thinning" case, confirming that conduction of the *intrinsic* transistor is degraded by a fin thinning towards the virtual drain (V.D.) and enhanced if the tapering direction is swapped. However, the asymmetric impact of parasitic resistances in the S and D extensions suppresses I_{ON} enhancement even with $L_{ext} = 12$ nm and produces an opposite effect of the thinning direction w.r.t. the intrinsic case for longer L_{ext}. Since the sheet resistance R_{sh} is inversely proportional to W_{fin} [23], decreasing the fin width in the S extension results in a higher R_{sh} in this region, thus reducing the effective V_{gs} and hence drive current [50]:

$$V_{gs,eff} = V_{gs} - R_S I_d \tag{5.5}$$

The impact of R_D is much lower because $V_{gs,\,eff}$ is not affected by this parameter.

The critical importance of extension resistances for FinFET variability is confirmed by measurements [39] and the asymmetric role of R_S and R_D, in agreement with results of the correlation analysis in Section 5.3.3, makes electrical fluctuations especially sensitive to LER in the source side of the device. This may provide design guidelines for an improved LER robustness through optimized extension engineering.

5.4 Impact of Variability at the Circuit Level

Electrical variability of individual devices is reflected in performance fluctuations and potential yield losses at the circuit level. Static random access memory (SRAM) is especially susceptible to process variations because minimum-size transistors are typically employed to comply with area requirements and each cell within large memory arrays must be functional. SRAM is one of the most likely candidates for circuit application of FinFETs [25, 31, 51]. Therefore, the investigation of line-edge roughness impact on this circuit block is particularly interesting and will be carried on in this section.

5.4.1 *Simulation Approach and SRAM Stability Metrics*

Circuit-level variability is commonly studied through SPICE simulations featuring sensitivity analysis [26, 33]. However, it has been shown in Section 5.3.3 that this approach cannot fully capture the impact of LER even on the single device; when applied to circuit blocks, this worst-case analysis is often highly inaccurate and can lead to overly pessimistic design constraints. A more reliable technique is based on Monte Carlo circuit simulation where variability is incorporated into compact model parameters of each transistor according to electrical data obtained at the device level [17]. Since compact modeling of the FinFET device is a relatively recent topic and is still in progress, the approaches described above are hardly applicable to FinFET-based circuits. Therefore, statistical mixed-mode simulations have been used. These combine the device and circuit level of the variability framework (Section 5.1), directly computing the impact of microscopic fluctuations on circuit performance. However, large statistical ensembles of circuits with different device realizations need to be simulated, thus requiring a trade off between the circuit and ensemble size.

When applied to SRAM arrays, these simulations aim to predict yield losses caused by cell instability. In the hold and read mode of SRAM operation, the considered metric is the static noise margin (SNM) [45], i.e., the minimum noise voltage needed to flip the cell state, which can be extracted from transfer characteristics f_1 and f_2 as illustrated in Fig. 5.20. Conversely, the write noise margin (WNM) is the minimum DC noise that prevents the cell state from being flipped during a write access and is measured as described in the same figure. Transfer curves in Fig. 5.20(b) are simulated by setting $V_{BL} = V_{BLB} = V_{DD}$ in the read mode, $V_{BL} = V_{DD}$ and $V_{BLB} = 0$ V or vice-versa during write operation, while the word-line WL is kept low in the hold state.

Given an SRAM matrix of size dim and a target yield Y_T, the maximum tolerated failure probability caused by insufficient SNM or WNM is

$$P_{FAIL} = (1 - Y_T)/dim \tag{5.6}$$

To evaluate modern SoC applications, a large SRAM size dim = 10 Mbit and a tight target Y_T = 99.9% are considered in this

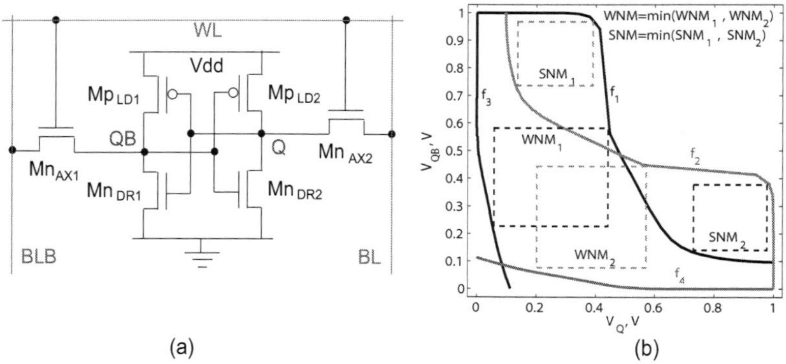

Figure 5.20. (a) Schematic of a 6-T SRAM cell. (b) Voltage transfer curves for storage nodes Q and QB during read and write operation. SNM is computed as the minimum between edges of the largest squares that can be inscribed into the eyes of f_1 and f_2. Similarly, WNM is calculated considering the largest squares between the bottom-right parts of f_1 and f_3 or the top-left portions of f_2 and f_4.

section [24, 39], resulting in a very strict failure specification $P_{FAIL} = 10^{-10}$. Assuming a Gaussian distribution with mean μ_{SNM} and standard deviation σ_{SNM} for the static noise margin, such probability corresponds to a critical value SNM_{crit} which is $6.4\sigma_{\text{SNM}}$ away from the average. Following [49], here it is assumed $\text{SNM}_{crit} > 4\% V_{DD}$ for safe operation, while $0\text{ V} < \text{SNM} < 4\% V_{DD}$ represents a critical zone below which the cell is certainly unstable. The sample size N allowed by our computational resources varies between 200 and 300 cells, which is larger than commonly reported for mixed-mode simulations [54], but still quite small for MC extrapolation down to 6.4σ. Therefore, statistical noise has been accounted for by providing 95% confidence intervals CI for SNM mean and variance [10]. The former is computed as:

$$CI_{1-\alpha}[\mu_{\text{SNM}}] = \mu_{\text{SNM}} \pm t_{\alpha/2}\sigma_{\mu} \tag{5.7}$$

where $t_{\alpha/2}$ is the critical two-tailed value of Student's t distribution with $N-1$ degrees of freedom, the standard deviation of μ_{SNM} is estimated as $\sigma_{\mu} = \sigma_{\text{SNM}}/\sqrt{N}$ and the accepted tolerance is $\alpha = 0.05$. To improve robustness against moderate deviations from normality observed in SNM distributions [24, 35], the CI for σ_{SNM} has been calculated through a more sophisticated approach provided by Eq. (4) in [14]. The same methodology has been applied to WNM when analyzing the write operation of SRAM cells.

5.4.2 *FinFET-Based SRAM Design*

The design of six-transistor (6-T) SRAM cells is commonly carried on by choosing the cell ratio CR and pull-up ratio PR, which are defined as suitable ratios between current factors β of access, driver and load devices (respectively $Mn_{AX,i}$, $Mn_{DR,i}$ and $Mp_{LD,i}$, $i = 1, 2$, in Fig. 5.20(a)). Specifications for robust read and write operations are

$$CR = \frac{\beta_{DR}}{\beta_{AX}} > 1 \quad , \qquad PR = \frac{\beta_{LD}}{\beta_{AX}} < 1 \tag{5.8}$$

i.e., stronger driver and weaker load w.r.t. the access FET. In SRAMs based on narrow-fin FinFETs, the cell ratio is quantized in multiples of the fin height and the corresponding requirement in Eq. (5.8) can be met by designing driver FETs with two fins [33]. Since this leads to area penalty in RDF processes, however, single fins are often used for all six transistors [20], thus penalizing read stability. The PR specification in Eq. (5.8) is fulfilled with (100) conduction due to the lower mobility of p-channel w.r.t. n-channel devices, but cannot be guaranteed in FinFETs with (110) sidewall transport, where mobility is influenced by several factors (see Section 5.3.1). N-channel FETs (especially $Mn_{AX,i}$) are sometimes designed with 45°-rotated fins to recover (100) conduction and avoid WNM degradation, at the expense of a larger cell area and possibly enhanced process variations due to additional lithography difficulties [28]. Moreover, accurate V_T control through the high-κ/metal gate stack is challenging.

The five scenarios in Table 5.4 will be considered to illustrate the impact of LER on low-voltage/low-power compatible FinFET SRAMs with different design options [10]. Cell $S1$ has driver transistors with two fins and (100) conduction, thus ensuring stability criteria to be met. The considered mobility conditions may be the result of fin rotation and/or the fin and gate formation process. The second SRAM ($S2$) is a minimum-area version of the former, with all single-fin devices, while the impact of sidewall transport in the (110) plane is addressed in cell $S3$. The last two scenarios explore the impact of

Table 5.4. Considered SRAM designs

Design	Driver FET sizing	Conduction	Nominal V_T
$S1$	2 fins	(100)	0.36 V (LSTP-32 nm)
$S2$	1 fin	(100)	0.36 V (LSTP-32 nm)
$S3$	1 fin	(110)	0.36 V (LSTP-32 nm)
$S4$	1 fin	(100)	0.2 V (LOP-32 nm)
$S5$	2 fins	(100)	0.2 V (LOP-32 nm)

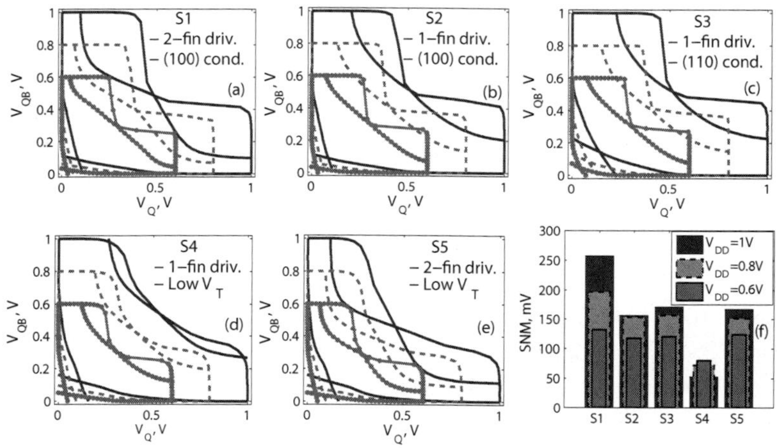

Figure 5.21. (a)–(e): nominal butterfly curves of cells $S1$ to $S5$ (Table 5.4), at V_{DD} = 1 V, 0.8 V and 0.6 V. (f): comparison of resulting static noise margins. See also Color Insert.

a lower, LOP-compatible, threshold voltage on the cells with 1-and 2-fin driver FETs ($S4$ and $S5$, respectively), which might be the result of a different gate stack and WF engineering. The basic building blocks of these circuits are FinFETs with nominal I–V curves shown in Fig. 5.4. Device dimensions are reported in Table 5.2 and are analogous to those of fabricated cells in ref. [20], which will be used for comparison. Figs. 5.21(a)–(e) display simulated butterfly curves of the nominal cells $S1$ to $S5$, respectively. The comparison of resulting SNMs in Fig. 5.21(f) indicates $S1$ as the most robust design, as expected, while $S2$, $S3$ and $S5$ exhibit a similar behavior; poor read stability is observed in cell $S4$. The following sections discuss

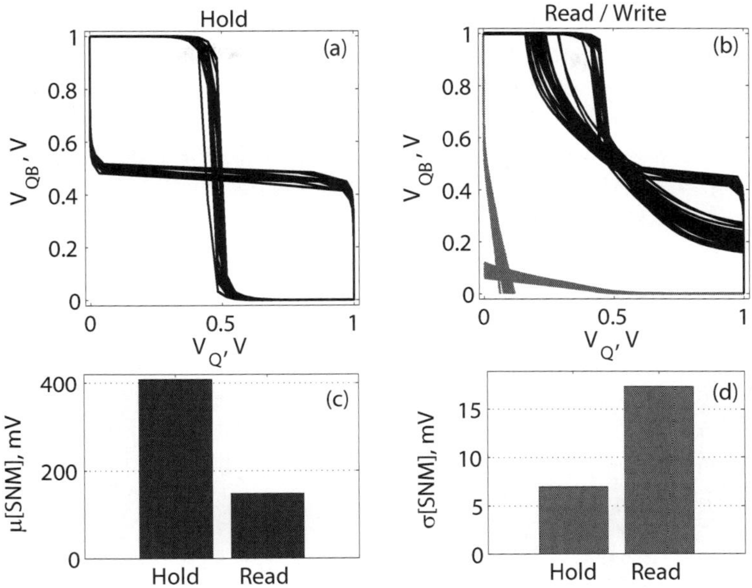

Figure 5.22. Voltage transfer curves in the hold (a) and read/write operating mode (b) for cells *S*2 (Table 5.4) with fin-LER (Δ = 1.5 nm, Λ = 20 nm). (c) Mean value and (d) standard deviation of SNM extracted from (a) and (b).

robustness of each design case to fin-LER, considering different operating conditions and supply voltage scaling.

5.4.3 *Hold, Read and Write Operating Conditions*

The impact of LER on SRAM stability in the hold, read and write operating modes has been studied with reference to the minimum-area cell *S*2 in Table 5.4, in order to determine the most critical situations to be monitored in further investigations. Respective butterfly curves obtained by statistical mixed-mode simulations are shown in Figs. 5.22(a) and (b). Only driver and load transistors are active in the hold state, resulting in a relatively high SNM and limited fluctuations, as can be seen from Fig. 5.22(a). In ref. [13] it was shown that these fluctuations are mainly determined by pull-down FETs and significant correlations were found between the SNM of each cell and the average fin width in the channel of these devices. The activity of the access transistors during read raises the minimum voltage at the storage nodes, thus reducing the average static noise margin, but these devices also enhance the spread of butterfly curves in in Fig. 5.22(b) considerably. The degradation of both mean value and dispersion of SNM in the read w.r.t. hold operating mode is quantitatively assessed in Figs. 5.22(c) and (d), respectively. Moreover, the additional contribution from variability of the access transistors makes noise margin statistics more complicated, so that correlations cannot be exploited to simplify the analysis. These observations justify the adoption of a MC approach and the choice of the read mode as the most critical operating condition for evaluating static noise margin variability. Although write operation seems to be relatively robust from Fig. 5.22(b), WNM statistics will be monitored as well in the following sections.

5.4.4 *SRAM Stability vs. Cell Sizing*

Comparison of design options $S1$ and $S2$ in Table 5.4 allows predicting the stability-area trade off for LSTP-32 nm compatible FinFET SRAMs. SNM and WNM histograms for these cells are reported in Fig. 5.23, revealing an enhanced read variability for the cells with single-fin driver FETs. This is mainly caused by the smaller area, and hence larger electrical fluctuations, of these devices w.r.t. their 2-fin counterparts (see Pelgrom plots in Fig. 5.14), thus further degrading the inherently poorer stability of $S2$ cells due to a smaller CR w.r.t. $S1$ design. As a result, SRAM arrays with all single-fin devices may not comply with yield requirements when operated at 1 V supply voltage. This can be seen from Fig. 5.24, where mean value, standard deviation and $\mu - 6.4\sigma$ statistics of both SNM and WNM are plotted as a function of V_{DD} for the considered design cases. Error bars represent 95% confidence intervals calculated as described in Section 5.4.1. As expected, $\mu - 6.4\sigma$ statistics of SNM for minimum-area cells $S2$ is found to lay in the highlighted critical zone at $V_{DD} = 1$ V (see Fig. 5.24(c)). However, supply voltage scaling allows $S2$ SRAMs to recover sufficient read stability. Figs. 5.24(d)–(f) indicate that the write operation of these cells is not significantly affected by LER issues. On the other hand, design

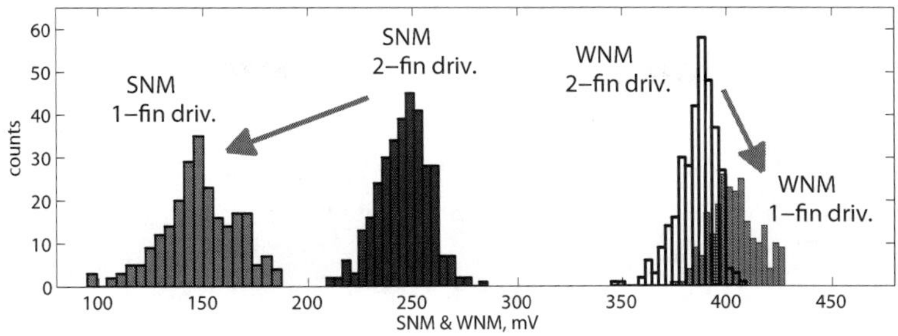

Figure 5.23. SNM and WNM histograms for SRAMs $S1$ and $S2$ with 2-fin and 1-fin drivers, respectively. All cell FinFETs have fin-LER with $\Delta = 1.5$ nm, $\Lambda = 20$ nm.

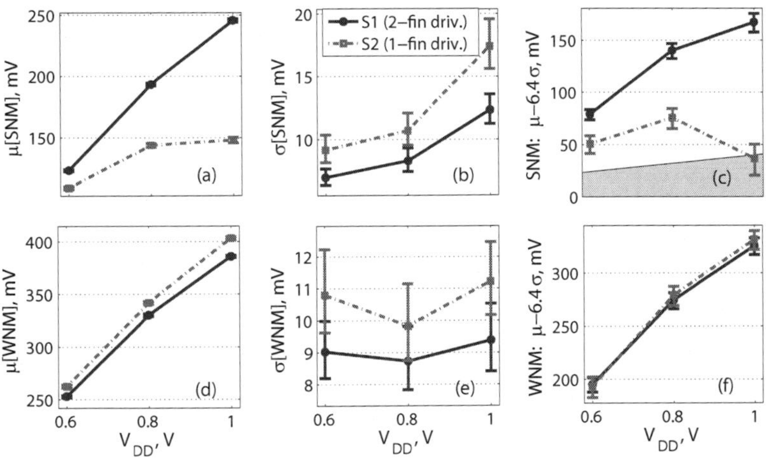

Figure 5.24. Mean value and standard deviation of (a), (b) SNM as well as (d), (e) WNM as a function of V_{DD}, for cases $S1$ and $S2$. (c), (f): corresponding $\mu - 6.4\sigma$ statistics. Error bars represent 95% confidence intervals, while the highlighted region in (c) is the critical zone bounded by $4\% V_{DD}$.

$S1$ exhibits a satisfactory behavior in both read and write mode. Therefore, FinFET SRAMs with 2-fin drivers represent a safe design option; nevertheless, single-fin drivers can also be used to improve the cell area in low-voltage applications.

5.4.5 *SRAM Stability vs. Crystal Orientation*

Top and sidewall carrier mobility in FinFETs is influenced by many factors, as discussed in Section 5.3.1. Moreover, the effective change in (110) current drive w.r.t. (100) transport is much weaker than theoretical mobility modifications, especially at high V_{ds}, as shown in Fig. 5.4.

To evaluate the effect of different fin orientations and other causes of mobility changes, (100) and (110) carrier transport in minimum-size SRAMs $S2$ and $S3$ (Table 5.4) with fin-LER has been simulated as described in Section 5.3.1. Resulting statistics in Figs. 5.25(a) and (b) indicate that the enhanced strength of p-type FETs in (110) conduction slightly increases the mean SNM, without significantly affecting its standard deviation. Therefore, $\mu - 6.4\sigma$ metrics in Fig. 5.25(c) is improved for cell $S3$, providing better read stability even at $V_{DD} = 1$ V, although the lower bound of the corresponding confidence interval still crosses the critical zone. As a trade-off, WNM statistics is degraded by the stronger pull-up vs. access devices, but overall the write operation is not severely affected (see Fig. 5.25(d)–(f)).

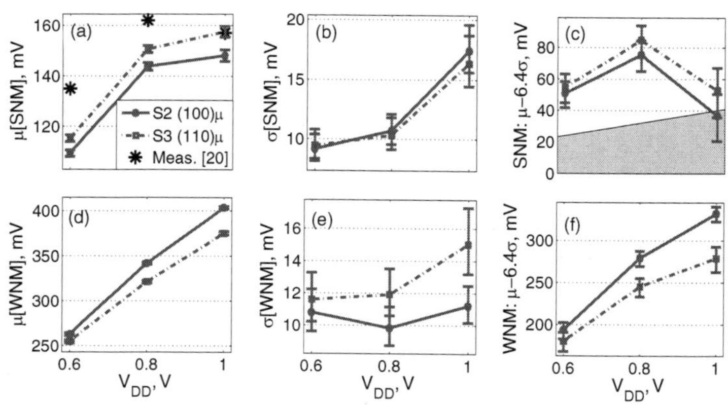

Figure 5.25. Mean value and standard deviation of (a), (b) SNM as well as (d), (e) WNM as a function of V_{DD}, for cases $S2$ and $S3$. (c), (f): corresponding $\mu - 6.4\sigma$ statistics. 95% confidence intervals are indicated. The critical zone bounded by $4\% V_{DD}$ is highlighted in (c). Measurement data reported in (a) refer to fabricated SRAMs with analogous features [20].

This analysis shows that sidewall transport on the (110) plane has potential to improve, rather than compromise, SRAM stability, since the measured change in $I_{d,n}/I_{d,p}$ ratio w.r.t. (100) conduction is typically smaller than the theoretical μ_n/μ_p modifications. This helps relaxing the supply voltage constraints. In Fig. 5.25(a), simulation results for $\mu[\mathrm{SNM}]$ are also compared to measurements performed on fabricated SRAMs featuring single-fin devices with $L_g = 30$ nm, $W_{fin} = 10$ nm [20]. The good agreement observed in this figure supports the validity of the presented TCAD study.

5.4.6 *SRAM Stability vs. Gate Stack*

Low standby power applications require relatively high threshold voltages like those of cell devices in SRAMs $S1$ to $S3$ (nominal $V_T \simeq 0.36$ V). In this section, the impact of gate stack WF tuning to achieve a lower V_T, compatible with ITRS-LOP specifications [29], is investigated considering cells $S4$ and $S5$ with 1-fin and 2-fin drivers, respectively. The same mobility conditions as in cases $S1$ and $S2$ are assumed for comparison.

Butterfly curves reported in Fig. 5.26(a) for SRAMs $S4$ indicate read failures at $V_{DD} = 1$ V, due to LER. It is further clarified by Figs. 5.27(a)–(c) that these cells cannot achieve sufficient yield, even though V_{DD} scaling rapidly improves the SNM statistics.

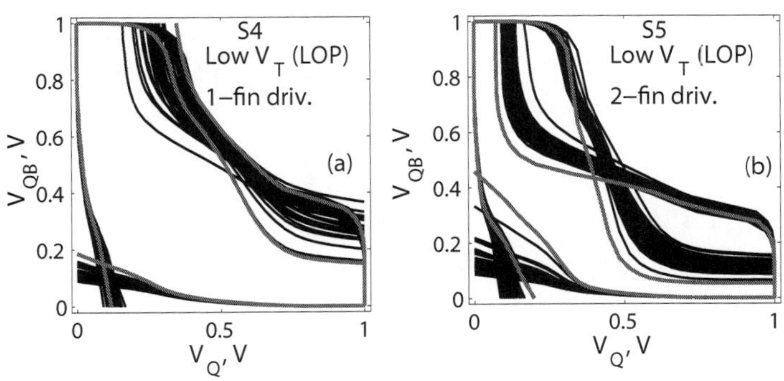

Figure 5.26. Transfer curves of LOP-compatible cells $S4$ (a) and $S5$ (b) with 1-fin and 2-fin drivers, respectively, in the presence of fin-LER ($\Delta = 1.5$ nm, $\Lambda = 20$ nm). Read failure and degraded write characteristics are highlighted in (a) and (b), respectively.

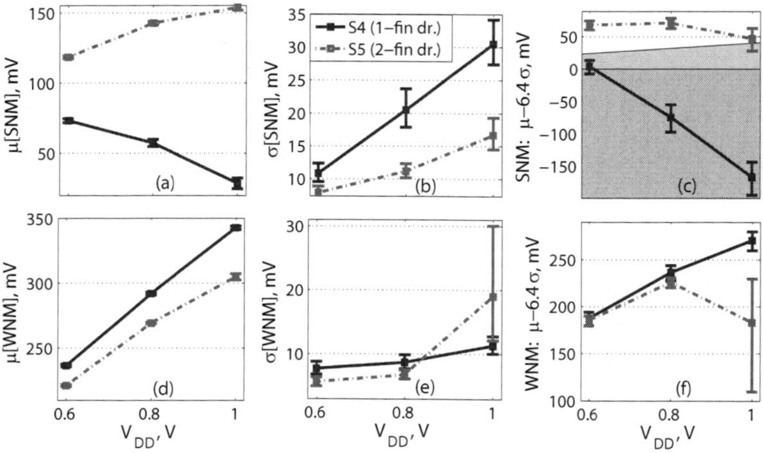

Figure 5.27. Mean value and standard deviation of (a), (b) SNM as well as (d), (e) WNM as a function of V_{DD}, for cases $S4$ and $S5$. (c), (f): corresponding $\mu - 6.4\sigma$ statistics. 95% confidence intervals are indicated. Highlighted in (c) are the critical zone bounded by $4\% V_{DD}$ and the failure region $\mu - 6.4\sigma < 0$ V. See also Color Insert.

Further supply voltage reduction might provide acceptable read margins for design $S4$, although the write operation tends to become more difficult, as suggested by Fig. 5.27(f). The increased cell ratio of LOP-compatible SRAMs with 2-fin drivers ($S5$ design) effectively improves read performance, as shown by butterfly curves in Fig. 5.26(b). SNM distribution is thus shifted to considerably higher values for these SRAMs, as shown in Fig. 5.27(a). Although confidence intervals in Fig. 5.27(c) still cross the critical zone at $V_{DD} = 1$ V, supply voltage scaling is found to provide sufficient SNM and the read performance of these cells becomes similar to that of their high-V_T counterparts $S1$ at $V_{DD} = 0.6$ V (compare SNM statistics in Figs. 5.27 and Fig. 5.24)

The write operation is negatively influenced by the stronger pull-down devices in SRAMs $S5$, but it should not be compromised, as suggested by Fig. 5.27(f). Nevertheless, the WNM sensitivity to LER is considerably enhanced for these cells and degraded transfer curves like the ones highlighted in Fig. 5.26(b) can be generated by anomalous access devices with extremely pronounced fin thinning.

This is the reason for the large error bars of $S5$ WNM statistics in Fig. 5.27(e)–(f). The impact of anomalous cells on the write operation is, however, reduced when V_{DD} is lowered.

Scaling down the device threshold is thus seen to dangerously affect read stability of SRAM cells due to fin-LER. However, sufficient SNM can be achieved at the expense of a larger cell area with 2-fin drivers. Although requiring a careful trade-off between read and write margins, this allows successful application of FinFETs in LOP SRAM technologies.

5.5 Conclusions

An extensive TCAD investigation of the variability issues in multiple-gate architectures was presented. Combining our analysis with several literature works, line-edge roughness was indicated as the major source of fluctuations in these devices. The impact of LER on FinFET structures suitable for low-voltage/low-power applications at the 32 nm technology node was studied at the physical, device and circuit level.

Starting from SEM metrology and edge detection, suitable stochastic models were described, which capture the basic statistical properties of rough printed features and can be exploited for a realistic representation of LER in a TCAD environment. A Fourier synthesis technique can thus be used to generate large ensembles of microscopically different device realizations, whose simulation provides distributions of meaningful electrical parameters, such as threshold voltage and drive current. Combining 2D and 3D analysis, it was shown that roughness of the fin edges is the most critical source of variability in aggressively scaled FinFETs, more so than top- and sidewall-gate-LER, although it could be mitigated through an optimized spacer-defined patterning process. Comparison of our Monte Carlo approach with a naïve sensitivity analysis indicated that fin-LER raises the average V_T in threshold voltage distributions and degrades the on-current w.r.t. the uniform fin case. The causes of these phenomena were clarified and correlation of the considered electrical parameters to suitable geometrical features (average fin thickness in the channel or a weighted sum of widths in some key regions of the fin) was highlighted, which provides approximate variability estimation at the same computational cost as sensitivity analysis, but with improved accuracy.

Comparing several design options it was found that the impact of LER is similar in n- and p-channel devices and does not change with fin rotation, which results in (100) or (110) carrier transport on the fin sidewalls. Electrical variability is reduced by increasing the number of fins, in agreement with Pelgrom's law, while work-function tuning through the gate stack can sensibly enhance the impact of LER when it lowers the device threshold. This makes FinFETs designed for low operating power (LOP) applications more sensitive to LER than their LSTP-compatible counterparts. Moreover, WF variability due to the granular structure of the metal gates might be another significant cause of electrical fluctuations: the combined impact of this issue and geometrical roughness needs to be further investigated. Extension doping was found to be a critical design step: increasing the peak concentration in these regions enhances the relative importance of gate-LER, which can become comparable to the fin-related contribution, and increases random dopant fluctuation issues. Any local thinning of the fin has a negative impact on I_{ON}, but the degradation is stronger when the source side of the device is affected, due to the asymmetric role of parasitic S/D extension resistances: engineering these regions therefore requires special attention.

LER-induced variability at the circuit level was investigated through mixed mode simulations of LSTP/LOP-32 nm compatible SRAMs. Several design options were compared by employing a restrictive $\mu - 6.4\sigma$ criterion for 99.9% yield in 10 Mbit arrays. Statistics was computed over relatively large MC ensembles ranging from 200 to 300 cells and 95% confidence intervals were provided to improve robustness of the performed analysis. It was found that designing driver transistors with two fins provides sufficient stability in all operating conditions, i.e., hold, read and write, for both LSTP and LOP SRAM applications. In a low standby power framework, minimum-area cells with all single-fin devices exhibit significant static noise margin variability during read at 1 V supply voltage. However, safe read operation is rapidly recovered as V_{DD} is scaled down. (110) sidewall transport does not compromise write ability of these cells and can slightly improve SNM statistics. Instead, LOP-compatible SRAMs with smaller device threshold voltages are subject to read failure when designed with single-fin drivers, although this issue might be alleviated at very low operating voltages. Our simulation results compare favorably with measurements performed on fabricated cells with similar features. The presented analysis thus provides variability-aware design guidelines at both the device and circuit level for mainstream employment of FinFETs at and beyond the 32 nm technology node.

References

1. Arnaud, F., Liu, J., Lee, Y. M., K. Y. Lim, S., Chen, J., Moon, B. K., Lai, C. W., Lipinski, M., Sang, L., Guarin, F., Hobbs, C., Ferreira, P., Ohuchi, K., Li, J., Zhuang, H., Mora, P., Zhang, Q., Nair, D. R., Lee, D. H., Chan, K. K., Satadru, S., Yang, S., Koshy, J., Hayter, W., Zaleski, M., Coolbaugh, D. V., Kim, H. W., Ee, Y. C., Sudijono, J., Thean, A., Sherony, M., Samavedam, S., Khare, M., Goldberg, C. and A.Steegen (2008). 32nm general purpose bulk CMOS technology for high performance applications at low voltage, in *IEDM Tech. Dig.*
2. Asenov, A. (1998). Random dopant induced threshold voltage lowering and fluctuations in sub 0.1 micron MOSFETs: a 3D 'atomistic' simulation study, *IEEE Trans. Electron Devices*, **45**, pp. 2505–2513.
3. Asenov, A., Brown, A. R., Davies, J. H., Kaya, S. and Slavcheva, G. (2003). Simulation of intrinsic parameter fluctuations in decananometer and nanometer-scale MOSFETs, *IEEE Trans. Electron Devices*, **50**, 9, pp. 1837–1852.
4. Asenov, A., Brown, A. R., Roy, G., Cheng, B., Alexander, C., Riddet, C., Kovac, U., Martinez, A., Seoane, N. and Roy, S. (2009). Simulation of statistical variability in nano-CMOS transistors using drift-diffusion, Monte Carlo and non-equilibrium Green's function techniques, *Journal of Computational Electronics*, **8**, pp. 349–373.
5. Asenov, A., Cathignol, A., Cheng, B., McKenna, K. P., Brown, A. R., Shluger, A. L., Chanemougame, D., Rochereau, K. and Ghibaudo, G. (2008). Origin of the asymmetry in the magnitude of the statistical variability of n- and p-channel Poly-Si gate bulk MOSFETs, *IEEE Electron Dev. Lett.* **29**, 8, pp. 913–915.

6. Asenov, A. and Kaya, S. (2000). Effect of oxide interface roughness on the threshold voltage fluctuations in decanano MOSFETs with ultrathin gate oxides, in *Proc. SISPAD*, pp. 135–138.
7. Asenov, A., Kaya, S. and Brown, A. R. (2003). Intrinsic parameter fluctuations in decananometer MOSFETs induced by gate line edge roughness, *IEEE Trans. Electron Devices*, **50**, 5, pp. 1254–1260.
8. Baravelli, E., De Marchi, L. and Speciale, N. (2009). Fin shape fluctuations in FinFET: correlation to electrical variability and impact on 6-T SRAM noise margins, *Solid-State Electronics*, **53**, 12, pp. 1303–1312.
9. Baravelli, E., De Marchi, L. and Speciale, N. (2010). Physical insight and Monte Carlo statistical analysis of Work-Function variability in FinFETs based on 2D slice composition, in *Proc. ULIS*, pp. 49–52.
10. Baravelli, E., De Marchi, L. and Speciale, N. (2010). V_{DD} scalability of FinFET SRAMs: robustness of different design options against LER-induced variations, *Solid-State Electronics*, **54**, 9, pp. 909–918.
11. Baravelli, E., Dixit, A., Rooyackers, R., Jurczak, M., Speciale, N. and De Meyer, K. (2007). Impact of line-edge roughness on FinFET matching performance, *IEEE Trans. Electron Devices*, **54**, 9, pp. 2466–2474.
12. Baravelli, E., Jurczak, M., Speciale, N., De Meyer, K. and Dixit, A. (2008). Impact of LER and random dopant fluctuations on FinFET matching performance, *IEEE Trans. Nanotechnology*, **7**, 3, pp. 291–298.
13. Baravelli, E., Speciale, N., Dixit, A. and Jurczak, M. (2008). TCAD modeling and characterization of short-range variations in multiple-gate devices and circuit blocks, in *15th Int. Conf. on Mixed Design (MIXDES)*, pp. 85–90.
14. Bonett, D. G. (2006). Approximate confidence interval for standard deviation of nonnormal distributions, *Computational Statistics & Data Analysis*, **50**, 3, pp. 775–782.
15. Brown, A. R., Asenov, A. and Watling, J. R. (2002). Intrinsic fluctuations in sub 10-nm double-gate MOSFETs introduced by discreteness of charge and matter, *IEEE Trans. Nanotechnology*, **1**, 4, pp. 195–200.
16. Brown, A. R., Roy, G. and Asenov, A. (2007). Poly-Si-gate-related variability in decananometer MOSFETs with conventional architecture, *IEEE Trans. Electron Devices*, **54**, 11, pp. 3056–3063.
17. Cheng, B., Roy, S., Roy, G., Adamu-Lema, F. and Asenv, A. (2005). Impact of intrinsic parameter fluctuations in decanano MOSFETs on yield and functionality of SRAM cells, *Solid-State Electronics*, **49**, 5, pp. 740–746.
18. Chiang, C. C. and Kawa, J. (2007). *Design for Manufacturability and Yield for Nano-Scale CMOS*, chap. Variability & Parametric Yield (Springer Netherlands), pp. 151–168.

19. Choi, Y. K., Lindert, N., Xuan, P., Tang, S., Ha, D., Anderson, E., King, T. J., Bokor, J. and Hu, C. (2001). Sub-20nm CMOS FinFET technologies, in *IEDM Tech. Dig.*, pp. 421–424.
20. Collaert, N., von Arnim, K., Rooyackers, R., Vandeweyer, T., Mercha, A., Parvais, B., Witters, L., Nackaerts, A., Sanchez, E. A., Demand, M., Hikavyy, A., Demuynck, S., Devriendt, K., Bauer, F., Ferain, I., Veloso, A., De Meyer, K., Biesemans, S. and Jurczak, M. (2008). Low-voltage 6T FinFET SRAM cell with high SNM using HfSiON/TiN gate stack, fin widths down to 10nm and 30nm gate length, in *Proc. ICICDT*, pp. 59–62.
21. Dadgour, H., Endo, K., De, V. and Banerjee, K. (2008). Modeling and analysis of grain-orientation effects in emerging Metal-Gate devices and implications for SRAM reliability, in *IEDM Tech. Dig.*
22. Dixit, A., Anil, K. G., Baravelli, E., Roussel, P., Mercha, A., Gustin, C., Bamal, M., Grossar, E., Rooyackers, R., Augendre, E., Jurczak, M., Biesemans, S. and De Meyer, K. (2006). Impact of stochastic mismatch on measured SRAM performance of FinFETs with resist/spacer-defined fins: Role of line-edge-roughness, in *IEDM Tech. Dig.*
23. Dixit, A., Anil, K. G., Collaert, N., Goodwin, M., Jurczak, M. and De Meyer, K. (2005). Analysis of the parasitic S/D resistance in multiple-gate FETs, *IEEE Trans. Electron Devices*, **52**, 6, pp. 1132–1140.
24. Doorn, T. S., ter Maten, E. J. W., Croon, J. A., Bucchianico, A. D. and Wittich, O. (2008). Importance Sampling Monte Carlo simulations for accurate estimation of SRAM yield, in *Proc. ESSCIRC*, pp. 230–233.
25. Endo, K., O'uchi, S., Ishikawa, Y., Liu, Y., Matsukawa, T., Sakamoto, K., Masahara, M., Tsukada, J., Ishii, K., Yamauchi, H. and Suzuki, E. (2008). Independent-gate four-terminal FinFET SRAM for drastic leakage current reduction, in *Proc. ICICDT*, pp. 63–66.
26. Gangwal, S., Mukhopadhyay, S. and Roy, K. (2006). Optimization of surface orientation for high-performance, low-power and robust FinFET SRAM, in *Proc. CICC*, pp. 433–436.
27. Gossmann, H.-J. L., Agarwal, A., Parrill, T., Rubin, L. M. and Poate, J. M. (2003). On the FinFET extension implant energy, *IEEE Trans. Nanotechnology*, **2**, 4, pp. 285–290.
28. Guo, Z., Balasubramanian, S., Zlatanovici, R., King, T.-J. and Nikolic, B. (2005). FinFET-based SRAM design, in *Proc. ISLPED*, pp. 2–7.
29. ITRS (2007 Edition). http://public.itrs.net.
30. Iyengar, V. V., Kottantharayil, A., Tranjan, F. M., Jurczak, M. and De Meyer, K. (2007). Extraction of the top and sidewall mobility in FinFETs and the impact of fin-patterning processes and gate dielectrics on mobility, *IEEE Trans. Electron Devices*, **54**, 5, pp. 1177–1184.

31. Kawasaki, H., Khater, M., Guillorn, M., Fuller, N., Chang, J., Kanakasabapathy, S., Chang, L., Muralidhar, R., Babich, K., Yang, Q., Ott, J., Klaus, D., Kratschmer, E., Sikorski, E., Miller, R., Viswanathan, R., Zhang, Y., Silverman, J., Ouyang, Q., Yagishita, A., Takayanagi, M., Haensch, W. and Ishimaru, K. (2008). Demonstration of highly scaled FinFET SRAM cells with High-κ/Metal Gate and investigation of characteristic variability for the 32 nm node and beyond, in *IEDM Tech. Dig.*

32. Kretz, J., Dreeskornfeld, L., Schröter, R., Landgraf, E., Hofmann, F. and Rösner, W. (2004). Realization and characterization of nano-scale FinFET devices, *Microelectronic Engineering*, **73–74**, pp. 803–808.

33. Lekshmanan, D., Bansal, A. and Roy, K. (2007). FinFET SRAM: optimizing silicon fin thickness and fin ratio to improve stability at iso area, in *Proc. CICC*, pp. 623–626.

34. Lindsay, R., Pawlak, B., Kittl, J., Henson, K., Torregiani, C., Giangrandi, S., Surdeanu, R., Vandervorst, W., Mayur, A., Ross, J., McCoy, S., Gelpey, J., Elliott, K., Pages, X., Satta, A., Lauwers, A., Stolk, P. and Maex1, K. (2003). A comparison of spike, flash, SPER and laser annealing for 45nm CMOS, in *2003 MRS Spring Meeting*.

35. Lu, D. D., Lin, C.-H., Yao, S., Xiong, W., Bauer, F., Cleavelin, C. R., Niknejad, A. M. and Hu, C. (2009). Design of FinFET SRAM cells using a statistical compact model, in *Proc. SISPAD*.

36. Lundstrom, M. and Ren, Z. (2002). Essential physics of carrier transport in nanoscale MOSFETs, *IEEE Trans. Electron Devices*, **49**, 1, pp. 133–141.

37. Matsukawa, T., O'uchi, S., Endo, K., Ishikawa, Y., Yamauchi, H., Liu, Y. X., Tsukada, J., Sakamoto, K. and Masahara, M. (2009). Comprehensive analysis of variability sources of FinFET characteristics, in *Sympos. on VLSI Tech.*, pp. 118–119.

38. McAndrew, C. C. (2003). Statistical modeling for circuit simulation, in *Proc. ISQED*, pp. 357–362.

39. Mérelle, T., Curatola, G., Nackaert, A., Collaert, N., van Dal, M., Doornbos, G., Doorn, T., Christie, P., Vellianitis, G., Duriez, B., Duffy, R., Pawlak, B., Voogt, F., Rooyackers, R., Witters, L., Jurczak, M. and Lander, R. (2008). First observation of FinFET specific mismatch behavior and optimization guidelines for SRAM scaling, in *IEDM Tech. Dig.*

40. Mistry, K., Allen, C., Auth, C., Beattie, B., D. Bergstrom and, M. B., Brazier, M., Buehler, M., Cappellani, A., Chau, R., Choi, C.-H., Ding, G., Fischer, K., Ghani, T., Grover, R., Han, W., Hanken, D., Hattendorf, M., He, J., Hicks, J., Huessner, R., Ingerly, D., Jain, P., James, R., Jong, L., Joshi, S., Kenyon, C., Kuhn, K., Lee, K., Liu, H., Maiz, J., McIntyre, B., Moon, P., Neirynck, J.,

Pae, S., Parker, C., Parsons, D., Prasad, C., Pipes, L., Prince, M., Ranade, P., Reynolds, T., Sandford, J., Shifren, L., Sebastian, J., Seiple, J., Simon, D., Sivakumar, S., Smith, P., Thomas, C., Troeger, T., Vandervoorn, P., Williams, S. and Zawadzki, K. (2007). A 45nm logic technology with High-k+Metal Gate transistors, strained silicon, 9 Cu interconnect layers, 193nm dry patterning, and 100% Pb-free packaging, in *IEDM Tech. Dig.*, pp. 247–50.

41. Mizuno, T., Okamura, J. and Toriumi, A. (1994). Experimental study of threshold voltage fluctuation due to statistical variation of channel dopant number in MOSFET's, *IEEE Trans. Electron Devices*, **41**, 11, p. 2216–2221.
42. Oldiges, P., Lint, Q., Petrillot, K., Sanchez, M., Ieong, M. and Hargrove, M. (2000). Modeling line edge roughness effects in sub 100 nanometer gate length devices, in *Proc. SISPAD*, pp. 131–134.
43. Patsis, G. P., Tsikrikas, N., Constantoudis, V. and Gogolides, E. (2005). Combined metrology and simulation of imprinted photopolymer lines/spaces. Extraction of line-edge roughness descriptors, in *Proc. International Symposium on Nanomanufacturing*.
44. Pelgrom, A. J. M., Duinmaijer, A. C. J. and Welbers, A. P. G. (1989). Matching properties of MOS transistors, *IEEE Journal of Solid-State Circuits*, **24**, 5, pp. 1433–1440.
45. Seevinck, E., List, F. J. and Lohstorn, J. (1987). Static-noise margin analysis of MOS SRAM cells, *IEEE Journal of Solid-State Circuits*, **SC-22**, 5, pp. 748–754.
46. Sentaurus Device MANUAL (Version Z-2007.3). Synopsys, Inc.
47. Serra, N., Palestri, P., Smit, G. and Selmi, L. (2009). Multi-subband Monte Carlo simulations of I_{ON} degradation due to fin thickness fluctuations in FinFETs, *Solid-State Electronics*, **53**, 4, pp. 424–432.
48. Sponton, L., Bomholt, L., Pramanik, D. and Fichtner, W. (2006). A full 3D TCAD simulation study of line-width roughness effects in 65 nm technology, in *Proc. SISPAD*, pp. 377–380.
49. Stolk, P. A., Tuinhout, H. P., Duffy, R., Augendre, E., Bellefroid, L. P., Bolt, M. J. B., Croon, J., Dachs, C. J. J., Huisman, F. R. J., Moonen, A. J., Ponomarev, Y. V., Roes, R. F. M., Rold, M. D., Seevinck, E., Sreerambhatla, K. N., Surdeanu, R., Velghe, R. M. D. A., Vertregt, M., Webster, M. N., van Winkelhoff, N. and Duijnhoven, A. T. A. Z.-V. (2001). CMOS device optimization for mixed-signal technologies, in *IEDM Tech. Dig.*, pp. 10.2.1–4.

50. Subramanian, V., Mercha, A., Parvais, B., Loo, J., Gustin, C., Dehan, M., Collaert, N., Jurczak, M., Groeseneken, G., Sansen, W. and Decoutere, S. (2007). Impact of fin width on digital and analog performances of n-FinFETs, *Solid-State Electronics*, **51**, 4, pp. 551–559.

51. Veloso, A., Demuynck, S., Ercke, M., Goethals, A. M., Demand, M., de Marneffe, J.-F., Altamirano, E., Keersgieter, A. D., Delvaux, C., Backer, J. D., Brus, S., Hermans, J., Baudemprez, B., Roey, F. V., Lorusso, G. F., Baerts, C., Goossens, D., Vrancken, C., Mertens, S., Versluijs, J. J., Truffert, V., Huffman, C., Laidler, D., Heylen, N., Ong, P., Parvais, B., Rakowski, M., Verhaegen, S., Hikavyy, A., Meiling, H., Hultermans, B., Romijn, L., Pigneret, C., Lok, S., Dijk, A. V., Shah, K., Noori, A., Gelatos, J., Arghavani, R., Schreutelkamp, R., Boelen, P., Richard, O., Bender, H., Witters, L., Collaert, N., Rooyackers, R., Absil, P., Lauwers, A., Jurczak, M., Hoffmann, T., Vanhaelemeersch, S., Cartuyvels, R., Ronse, K. and Biesemans, S. (2008). Full-field EUV and immersion lithography integration in 0.186μm^2 FinFET 6T-SRAM cell, in *IEDM Tech. Dig.*

52. Xiong, S. and Bokor, J. (2003). Sensitivity of double-gate and FinFET devices to process variations, *IEEE Trans. Electron Devices*, **50**, 11, pp. 2255–61.

53. Yang, M., Gusev, E. P., Ieong, M., Gluschenkov, O., Boyd, D. C., Chan, K. K., Kozlowski, P. M., D'Emic, C. P., Sicina, R. M., Jamison, P. C. and Chou, A. I. (2003). Performance dependence of CMOS on silicon substrate orientation for ultrathin oxynitride and HfO_2 gate dielectrics, *IEEE Electron Dev. Lett.* **24**, 5, pp. 339–341.

54. Yu, S., Zhao, Y., Du, G., Kang, J., Han, R. and Liu, X. (2009). The impact of line edge roughness on the stability of a FinFET SRAM, *Semiconductor Science and Tech.* **24**, 2.

55. Yu, S., Zhao, Y., Song, Y., Du, G., Kang, J., Han, R. and Liu, X. (2008). 3-D simulation of geometrical variations impact on nanoscale FinFETs, in *Proc. ICSICT*, pp. 408–411.

Chapter 6

Specific Features of MuGFETs at High Temperatures over a Wide Frequency Range

Valeriya Kilchytska, Jean-Pierre Raskin, and Denis Flandre
ICTEAM Institute, Université catholique de Louvain, 3 Place du Levant, Louvain-la-Neuve, B-1348, Belgium
valeriya.kilchytska@uclouvain.be

6.1 Introduction

The high-temperature electronics market is widely considered one of the main areas for silicon-on-insulator (SOI) device applications. In the last decade, integrated circuit technology advanced towards the deep submicron era to improve device performance, lower power consumption, reduce die area, etc. This unavoidably resulted in the appearance of new physical phenomena and/or significant changes to existing ones. Indeed, progress in technology does not mean simply device shortening, which is directly related to gate oxide thinning, doping level change or introduction of high-k/metal gate stacks, but at the same time requests the introduction of new architectural solutions for the control of short-channel effects (SCE), such as various multiple-gates devices.

CMOS Nanoelectronics: Innovative Devices, Architectures, and Applications
Edited by Nadine Collaert

ISBN 978-981-4364-02-7 (Hardcover), 978-981-4364-03-4 (eBook)
www.panstanford.com

Furthermore, the shrinkage of the device dimensions results in higher current drive through the device and therefore higher device temperature (or stronger device heat) under normal (or room temperature) operation condition. This "intrinsic heating" has a particular importance for the SOI-like devices featuring a buried oxide (BOX) with poor thermal conductivity and hence known to be suffering from self-heating effects (SHE). Increased "intrinsic temperature" of advanced devices (which can attain more than a hundred degree Celsius) thus requests for a deep understanding of the device behavior at high operation temperatures.

Nowadays multiple-gates FETs (MuGFETs), and particularly FinFETs, are widely considered promising candidates to satisfy the semiconductor roadmap requirements for the devices downscaling to the deca-nanometer range thanks to the improved control of the channel from multiple gates [1]. Therefore, their high-temperature behavior attracted large attention during last years [2–11]. With this regard, the questions to be addressed are "what are their specific features in high-temperature behavior?" and "do they maintain their performance advantages at high temperatures?"

In this chapter we try to answer these two questions by summarizing experimental and simulation results on MuGFETs obtained mostly in our laboratory during these last years [4–6]. We will first focus on specific features of the MuGFET threshold voltage, V_T, and subthreshold slope, S, high-temperature behavior. Particular attention will be paid to the influence of the fin width on the temperature evolution of these parameters. Next we will describe the DC to RF FinFET performance in a temperature range up to 200°C, assessing temperature variation of such important parameters as: on-to-off current ratio, I_{on}/I_{off}, transconductance maximum, $G_{m\,max}$, early voltage, V_{EA}, transconductance to drain current ratio, G_m/I_d, intrinsic gain, A_v, current gain and maximum oscillation gain cut-off frequencies, f_T and f_{max}. The influence of device geometry will be also analyzed.

6.2 Devices, Measurements and Simulation Details

The experimental results presented in this chapter were obtained on FinFETs processed at Imec, Leuven, Belgium. Triple-gate FinFETs with Ω-configuration and mid-gap metal gate electrodes were fabricated on SOI wafers with 60 nm film and 145 nm buried oxide. The active area fins were patterned using 193 nm optical lithography with resist and oxide hard mask trimming. Hydrogen anneal and sidewall oxidation were used for surface smoothening and corner rounding. Details of the fabrication process can be found in [12]. A nitrided oxide (SiON) with effective oxide thickness (EOT) of 1.6 nm, or atomic layer deposited (ALD) HfO_2 deposited on a chemical oxide with total EOT of about 1.4 nm were used as gate dielectrics. A mid-gap MOCVD (metal-organic chemical vapor deposition) TiN was used as the gate electrode. The metal was capped with 100 nm polySi. As and BF_2 extensions were implanted with high angle and 45 nm PECVD nitride spacers were formed. No selective epitaxial growth was used to reduce the source/drain resistance. After spacer etch, HDD (highly doped drain) implantations were done, followed by a spike anneal and a standard NiSi process and Cu BEOL (Back-End-Of-Line) metallization.

The experimental DC devices had a gate length, L, from 10 μm down to 40 nm, a fin height, H_{Fin}, of 60 nm and a fin width, W_{Fin}, varying from 10 nm to 3 μm. The silicon body in these devices was left undoped (i.e., with expected residual doping on the level of $10^{15}-10^{16}$ cm^{-3}) and hence the very wide 1–3 μm-wide fin FinFETs can be considered a single-gate (SG) quasi-planar fully depleted (FD) SOI MOSFETs with 60 nm-thick Si film, whereas the devices with 10–40 nm fin width can be considered double-gate (DG) devices.

Multi-finger devices were used and embedded in coplanar waveguide access pads for performing RF characterization. They are composed of 50 gate fingers 3 μm long, each finger controlling 9 fins. The fin length was varied from 40 nm to 0.5 μm, the fin width from 20 nm to 40 nm and a quasi-planar single gate with fin width of 1 μm was available and used for the sake of comparison.

I_D–V_G in linear and saturation regimes as well as I_D–V_D curves were measured on devices with different geometries in a temperature range from room temperature up to 250°C.

2D Atlas simulations [13] used simplified long-channel symmetrical planar double-gate MOSFET structures with various silicon film thicknesses (to emulate different fin widths) [4, 5]. The use of long-channel devices allowed for avoiding the inclusion of parasitic short channel and self-heating effects. Quantum effects were excluded in the simulations since their influence on the MOSFET current-voltage characteristics can be neglected for the device parameters and operation regimes under consideration. The thickness of the Si film, t_{Si}, was varied from 5 nm to 60 nm. The thickness of the gate oxide, t_{gox}, of 2 nm and the Si film doping level of 10^{15} cm^{-3} used in simulations correspond in a first approximation to the experimental devices. Simulations were performed in the temperature range up to 300°C.

6.3 Threshold Voltage

We will first describe the temperature variation of the threshold voltage, the parameter of prime importance for any transistor. Threshold voltage was extracted from linear I_D–V_G curves (V_D = 20 mV) using the second derivative of the drain current method, which was considered one of the most appropriate for the multiple-gate devices [14]. Figure 6.1 presents the threshold voltage evolution with temperature in 10 μm-long FinFETs with different

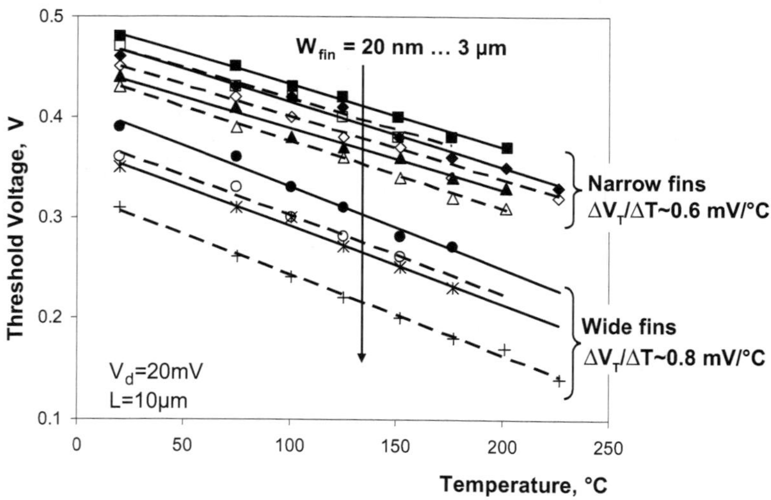

Figure 6.1. Threshold voltage variation as a function of temperature experimentally obtained on undoped 10 μm-long FinFETs with different fin widths. H_{fin} = 60 nm.

fin widths. First important observation which should be pointed out is that the threshold voltage shift with temperature is very small, on the level of 0.6 mV/°C. Similar numbers have also been reported for the shorter devices [6, 7, 9, 10]. It has also been demonstrated that thanks to the undoped body and multiple-gate control of the channel, transition from fully depleted to partially depleted (PD) operation often observed with temperature increases, due to depletion width reduction, does not occur in FinFETs [7], which was predictable according to the fin height and doping level.

Two-dimensional, 2D, Atlas simulations have been performed in [4, 5] to ensure the generality of obtained experimental results. Simulation results confirm the general trends of the threshold voltage behavior with temperature increase which have been obtained experimentally. Similar to the experiments, the threshold voltage shifts are as low as about 0.6 mV/°C for thin-film planar DG devices.

Such experimental and simulation results are rather surprising, because these values of V_T shift are much smaller than those expected from planar FD SOI MOSFETs theory. It is well known that in the case of FD SOI MOSFETs, the variation of the threshold voltage with temperature is defined by the temperature variation of the Fermi potential only and can be expressed as [15]:

$$\partial V_T/\partial T = \partial \phi_F/\partial T \tag{6.1}$$

where ϕ_F is the Fermi potential, given as $\phi_F = kT/q \cdot \ln(N_A/n_i)$ with N_A the doping level, n_i the intrinsic doping concentration and other symbols having their usual meaning. Therefore, the temperature variation of the Fermi potential, and hence threshold voltage in FD SOI MOSFETs, is independent on the gate dielectric and Si film thickness, depending only on the doping level. As can be seen in Fig. 6.2, the lower the doping level, the stronger the decrease of the Fermi potential with temperature. This classical approach gives us values of the threshold voltage shift for undoped devices (i.e., with $N_A \sim 10^{15} - 10^{16}$ cm^{-3}) of about 1–1.2 mV/°C, which is much higher than those obtained from both the experimental data on FinFETs and the simulations on planar DG devices [5].

A second conclusion that can be derived from the experimental curves (Fig. 6.1), and also confirmed by 2D Atlas simulations results

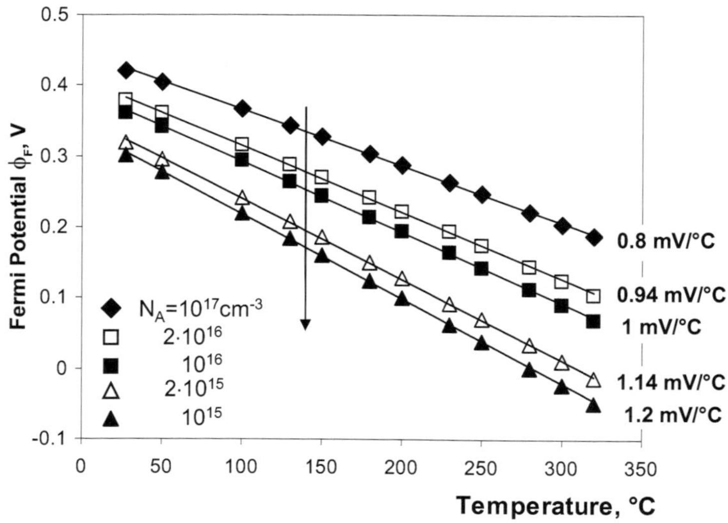

Figure 6.2. Fermi potential variation with temperature for different doping levels.

[4, 5] is that the V_T temperature shift depends on the fin width (or Si body thickness in the case of planar DG FETs). This can be clearly seen from Fig. 6.3, which plots the variation of the V_T shift with temperature as a function of fin width (in the case of measurements) or Si film thickness (in the case of simulations) [5], evidencing the decrease of V_T temperature shift with Si film thinning (or fin narrowing). Moreover, simulations and experimental results agree surprisingly well, keeping in mind the difference between planar DG and FinFETs structures. This is especially true for wider fin devices, which should be considered more as triple-gate devices and cannot simply be approximated as DG. This suggests one more time the generality of such MuGFET high-temperature behavior for devices operated under volume inversion conditions around the V_T regime.

Nevertheless, such clearly apparent Si film thickness dependence is surprising and intriguing. This is different from common considerations for FD SOI MOSFETs, which according to Eq. 6.1, supposes the V_T temperature variation to be independent of Si film thickness. The reason of this disagreement lies in the inadequateness of

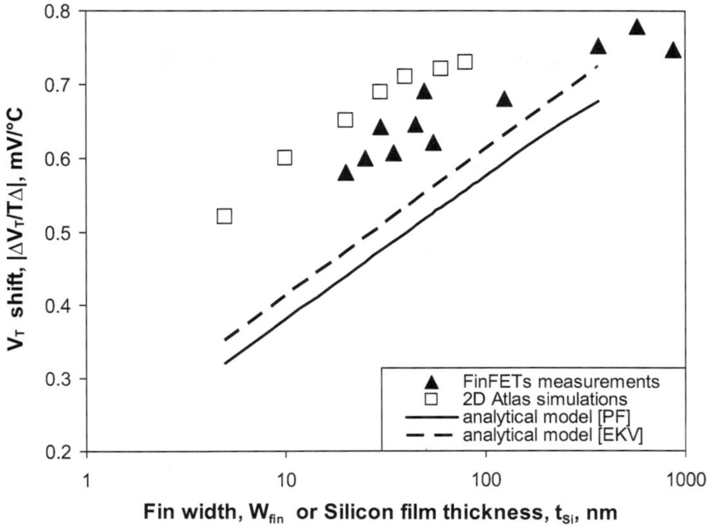

Figure 6.3. Comparison of the absolute value of the threshold voltage temperature shift as a function of the Si film thickness (or W_{fin}) obtained from experiments on FinFETs (L = 1 or 10 μm), from 2D Atlas simulations, and predicted by the analytical models (Eqs. 6.2, 6.3).

the classical V_T definition, fixing the surface potential at $2\phi_F$ independently of film thickness, in the case of multiple-gate devices.

There exist, indeed, several analytical models for DG MOSFETs, which include the temperature and Si film thickness-dependent terms and hence can predict the dependence of the V_T shift with temperature on the Si film thickness [16, 17]. The model proposed in 1994 by Pascal Francis *et al.* [16] provides an explicit expression for both the V_T and surface potential, ϕ_S^*, at V_T, as follows:

$$V_T = \phi_S^* + V_{FB} + \frac{Q_{depl}}{2C_{ox}}\sqrt{1 + \frac{2kTC_{ox}}{qQ_{depl}}} \tag{6.2a}$$

$$\phi_S^* = 2\phi_F + \frac{kT}{q}\ln\left(\frac{C_{ox}}{4C_{Si}}\frac{1}{1-\exp\left(-\frac{q}{kT}\frac{Q_{depl}}{8C_{Si}}\right)}\right) \tag{6.2b}$$

where $Q_{depl} = qN_A t_{Si}$ and other notations have their usual meaning. The advantage of this model is that it can be used for doped devices as well.

Another model formulated in 2005 by the EKV group for undoped devices [17] is design oriented, giving a very simple expression for V_T in the following way:

$$V_T = \phi_{MS} - \frac{kT}{q}\ln\left(\frac{q^2 n_i t_{Si} t_{ox}}{4\varepsilon_{ox} kT}\right) \tag{6.3}$$

Both models give the same trends as the experimental and simulation data for the V_T temperature shift with fin width (and Si film thickness) (Fig. 6.3) and even the quantitative values are rather fairly reproduced. We may now explain why the V_T shift physically becomes Si film thickness dependent in MuGFETs. A detailed analysis of Eq. 6.2 (which can be found in [5]) shows that its 3rd term is nearly T-independent, while its second term (V_{FB} or finally ϕ_{MS}) does not depend on the t_{Si}, so that the variation of $\Delta V_T/\Delta T$ with Si film thickness lies in the 1st term, i.e., surface potential (detailed in Eq. 6.2b). Reference [5] demonstrates rather good correspondence between analytical (using Eq. 6.2b) and simulated dependences of ϕ_s^* on both temperature and Si film thickness as well as between simulated, measured and analytical dependences of $\Delta V_T/\Delta T$ on Si film thickness. Nevertheless, there remains a small discrepancy especially at very high temperatures, and therefore, a further upgrade of the existing analytical models is still needed for better understanding of the surface potential behavior and hence more correct prediction of the MuGFET temperature behavior. Moreover, when applied to FinFETs with intermediate fin widths, the existing models have to be further modified to account for the charge sharing between the three gate electrodes.

6.4 Subthreshold Slope

The MOSFETs subthreshold slope, S, is classically determined as the inverse slope of semi-logarithmic I_D–V_G curve:

$$S = \frac{dV_G}{d(\log(I_D))} = \frac{\ln 10}{\frac{d(\ln I_D)}{dV_G}} = \frac{\ln 10 \cdot I_D}{\frac{dI_D}{d\phi_s}\frac{d\phi_s}{dV_G}} \tag{6.4a}$$

Then, using the charge-sheet model, which yields $I_D/(dI_D/d\phi_s) = kT/q$ and the gate-to-surface potential coupling through the differential surface capacitance $C_s = dQ_s/d\phi_s$, this equation is usually rewritten as [15]:

$$S = \frac{\ln 10 dV_G}{d(\ln I_D)} = \frac{kT}{q} \cdot \ln(10) \cdot \left(1 + \frac{C_s}{C_{ox}}\right) \quad (6.4b)$$

It is usually assumed that C_s can be obtained by the depletion approximation, $C_s = \varepsilon_{Si}/x_{d\,max}$, (with $x_{d\,max}$ the maximum depletion width) which is temperature independent for FD devices and varies for PD devices due to the decrease of $x_{d\,max}$ with temperature. As a result, classical theory predicts a linear dependence of S on temperature for FD devices and a superlinear dependence for PD devices [15]. However, it was also shown that the classical theory fails at $T > 150$–$200°$C, as both the charge-sheet model and the depletion approximation become invalid [18]. In fact, with temperature increase, we cannot neglect anymore the contribution from the free carriers in C_s: this capacitance increases both in PD and FD devices, resulting in the increase of S. Another factor is the lowering of the surface electric field in weak inversion due to the decrease of ϕ_F with temperature, resulting in broadening of inversion layer [18]. As a consequence the charge-sheet model becomes inaccurate. Consequently, the increase of S with temperature is non-linear even in FD devices, and the non-linear dependence in PD devices is stronger than predicted by classical theory [18].

Subsequently, for the multiple-gate devices, assuming perfect gate-to-channel coupling, i.e., $d\phi_s/dV_G = 1$, the classical theory predicts ideal "$kT/q \cdot \ln(10)$" values of the subthreshold slope and a linear temperature dependence is expected. Experimental and simulation results deviate, however, from these expectations. Figure 6.4 shows the experimental and simulated variations of the subthreshold slope with temperature in FinFETs with different fin widths (and different Si film thicknesses in the simulations) [4, 5]. Similarly to the threshold voltage, the high-temperature behavior of the subthreshold slope depends on the fin width (Si film thickness). Very wide-fin devices (which, taking into account the undoped film and 60 nm of fin height, can be considered quasi-planar FD SOI devices) exhibit the typical behavior of FD SOI MOSFETs with superlinear dependence for temperatures higher than 150°C, as

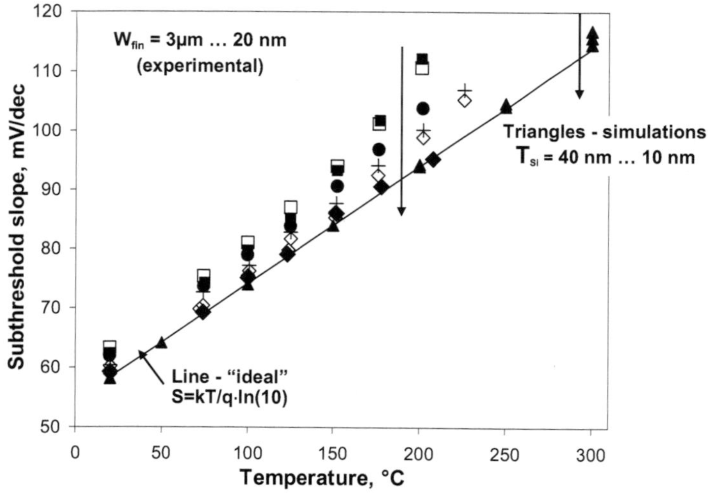

Figure 6.4. Variation of the subthreshold slope with temperature obtained from the experiments on 10 μm-long FinFETs with different fin widths and simulations on DG MOSFETs with different Si film thicknesses. The solid line indicates the ideal linear subthreshold slope vs. temperature dependence.

observed previously [18] and briefly described above. Narrow-fin devices reveal improved high-temperature stability, keeping almost an ideal linear subthreshold slope variation up to 200–225°C. 2D Atlas simulations confirm the experimentally observed tendencies [5]. Furthermore, simulations reveal a deviation of the subthreshold slope from the ideal "$kT/q \cdot \ln(10)$" values in DG MOSFETs at temperatures higher than 250°C. Moreover, this deviation from the ideal behavior increases for thicker Si films (from 10 to 40 nm).

Therefore the question we have to answer is "can we still rely on the two assumptions used above to derive the ideal subthreshold slope in MuGFETs, i.e., the "perfect" gate-to-channel coupling and the charge-sheet approximation for a temperature increase higher than 225–250°C?"

An interpretation used in single gate SOI MOSFET, showing degradation of the capacitive coupling to the substrate with temperature, even in FD devices, cannot be directly applied to the MuGFET high-temperature subthreshold slope variation. Nevertheless, 2D

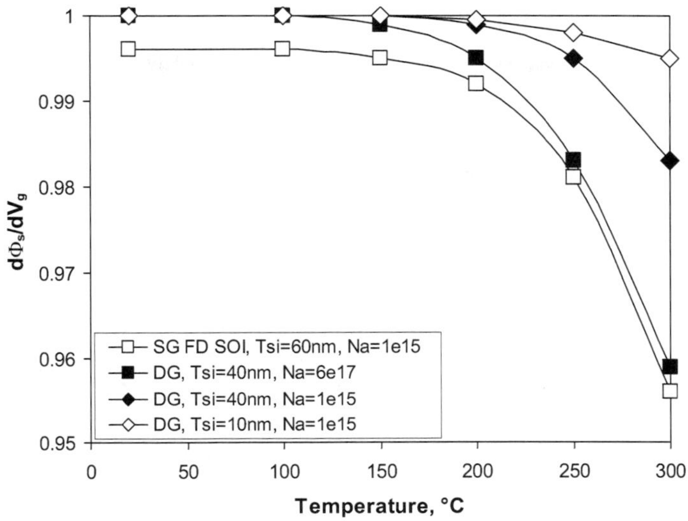

Figure 6.5. Simulated temperature variation of $d\phi_s/dV_G$ in the subthreshold region of undoped DG MOSFETs with 10 nm- (open diamonds) and 40 nm- (full diamonds) thick Si film, doped 40 nm-thick Si film (full squares) and undoped SG MOSFETs with 60 nm-thick Si film (open squares), which can be considered the analog of very wide fin devices with $H_{fin} = 60$ nm. $L = 3\,\mu$m. $t_{gox} = 2$ nm.

Atlas simulations shown in Fig. 6.5 reveal that for undoped DG MOSFETs, $d\phi_s/dV_G$ is no longer equal to one at temperatures higher than 200–250°C. Furthermore, the deviation from ideal becomes stronger in the case of doped devices and starts at lower temperatures, thus assuming stronger degradation of the subthreshold slope with temperature in such devices. Contrarily, the deviation decreases with Si film thinning, and this suggests a weaker degradation of the subthreshold slope with temperature in narrower/thinner devices. This agrees with both simulations and measurement results. Anyway, the deviation from the ideality in DG MOSFETs is smaller than in undoped SG MOSFETs and starts only at very high temperatures in undoped DG MOSFETs.

The reason for this non-ideal high-temperature dependence was questioned in [5] by analyzing the analytical model. Starting from the model of Taur [19] for undoped DG devices (i.e., considering only minority carriers), one can obtain:

$$\frac{d\phi_s}{dV_g} = 1 - \frac{1}{C_{ox}}\sqrt{2\varepsilon_{Si}kT\frac{n_i^2}{N_A}\frac{d}{d\phi_s}\left(e^{q\phi_s/kT} - e^{q\phi_0/kT}\right)} \quad (6.5)$$

and hence $d\phi_s/dV_g = 1$ only when $\phi_s = \phi_0$, i.e., mid-film and surface potentials are equal, which corresponds to volume inversion conditions. Then, [5] shows that when the temperature becomes higher than ~250°C, ϕ_s is no longer equal to ϕ_0, According to Eq. 6.5 this results in a $d\phi_s/dV_g$ deviation from 1 and corresponds well to the values obtained by 2D Atlas simulations. Moreover, at high temperatures Eq. 6.5 has to be modified to take into consideration majority carriers. More details can be further found in [5].

Next, can we still assume an exponential inversion charge, Q_n, versus surface potential dependence in MuGFETs at high temperatures, especially since this was already shown to be invalid at $T > 150$°C in FD SOI MOSFETs [18]? Indeed, we have shown that this assumption also fails at high temperatures [5]. In order to assess the non-exponential behavior of the inversion charge versus ϕ_s we used the coefficient introduced in [18] as:

$$n = \left[\frac{kT}{q}\frac{d\ln Q_n}{d\phi_s}\right]^{-1} \quad (6.6)$$

Figure 6.6 demonstrates that similarly to the FD SOI case, the dependence of the inversion charge on ϕ_s becomes non-exponential with temperature increase. However, the deviation from the exponential dependence in DG MOSFETs starts at higher temperatures and is much smaller than in FD SOI devices (at 300°C the coefficient n equals 1.04 for 40 nm-thick DG undoped devices versus 1.17 for 60 nm-thick undoped FD SOI) and decreases further with Si film thinning down to 1.001 (i.e., negligible) in 10 nm-thick undoped DG device. Here again, similarly to the coupling factor, the use of a doped body degrades the n-coefficient compared with the undoped one with the same Si film thickness, while the effect is not as strong as in the case of the coupling factor (Fig. 6.5).

Therefore, summarizing the discussion above, two modifications need to be introduced in the ideal equation for the subthreshold slope to take into account these deviations from ideality:

$$S = \frac{kT}{q}\cdot\ln(10)\cdot\frac{n}{d\phi_s/dV_G} \quad (6.7)$$

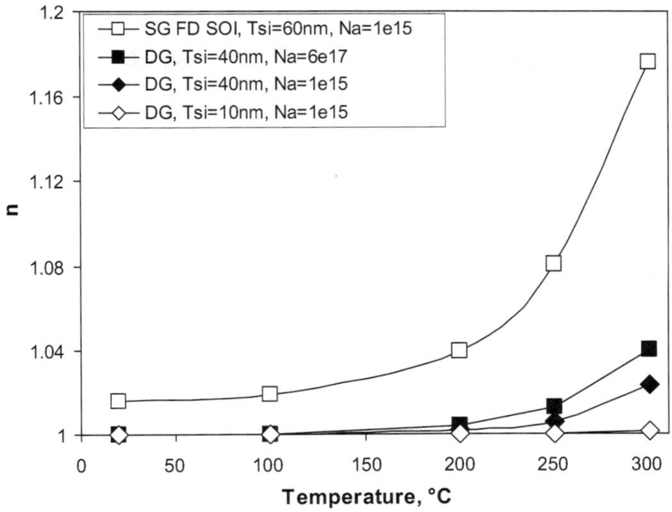

Figure 6.6. Simulated temperature variation of n, coefficient of the non-exponential behavior of the inversion charge on ϕ_s, in the subthreshold region of undoped DG MOSFETs with 10 nm-(open diamonds) and 40 nm-(full diamonds) thick Si film, doped 40 nm-thick Si film (full squares) and undoped SG FD SOI MOSFETs with 60 nm-thick Si film (open squares), which can be considered the analog of very wide fin devices with $H_{fin} = 60$ nm. $L = 3$ μm. $t_{gox} = 2$ nm.

A good correspondence between the subthreshold slope temperature evolution obtained by 2D Atlas simulations and using Eq. 6.7 was demonstrated in [5], proving that nothing but the two above-mentioned reasons are responsible for the high-temperature subthreshold slope deviation from the ideal linear temperature dependence.

Table 6.1 summarizes the subthreshold slope values at 300°C for different devices. Keeping in mind that the ideal subthreshold slope value at 300°C would be ~114 mV/dec, we can see that the deviation from this ideal behavior is quite small for 40 nm-thick undoped DG MOSFETs and can be further improved by the thinning of the Si film body. Indeed, DG MOSFETs with a 10 nm Si film thickness can provide S = 115 mV/dec at 300°C, that is almost the ideal value. It is worthwhile to emphasize that the "non-ideality" in the high-temperature subthreshold slope is much stronger in doped DG

Table 6.1. $d\phi_s/dV_G$ and the n-coefficient obtained by 2D Atlas simulations and the subthreshold slope calculated using Eq. 6.7 for different device types at $T = 300°$C

Device type	$d\phi_s/dV_G$	n	S
Ideal	1	1	114
DG, $T_{Si} = 40$ nm, $N_A \sim 10^{15}$ cm^{-3}	0.983	1.02	118
DG, $T_{Si} = 10$ nm, $N_A \sim 10^{15}$ cm^{-3}	0.995	1.001	115
SG, $T_{Si} = 60$ nm, $N_A \sim 10^{15}$ cm^{-3}	0.956	1.17	143
DG, $T_{Si} = 40$ nm, $N_A \sim 6{\cdot}10^{17}$ cm^{-3}	0.959	1.04	124

MOSFETs, while even that value is still smaller than in the undoped SG counterpart.

It is worth to mention that an analytical model to describe the high-temperature behavior of the subthreshold slope of undoped DG MOSFETs, which accounts for both the non-ideality factors discussed above, was recently proposed [8]. It points out that the deviation of the subthreshold slope from the "ideal" trends observed at high temperatures occurs when the intrinsic Debye length becomes comparable to the fin width/Si film thickness [8]. This again suggests that narrower/thinner body devices and undoped devices are more robust to high-temperature operations, being in agreement with the above discussed simulations/measurements results.

6.5 On-to-Off Current Ratio, I_{on}/I_{off}

In this performance-related part of this chapter we mostly used multi-fins multi-fingers devices, which are closer to the devices to be used in real applications. One needs to note that these devices were not optimized for high temperature applications. Figure 6.7 gives an example of the high-temperature I_D–V_G curves of 60 nm- and 120 nm-long FinFETs in the saturation regime. The I_{off} (i.e., drain current taken at $V_G = 0$ V) normalized to the total device width reaches 200 nA/μm and 20 nA/μm for 60 nm and 120 nm-long devices, respectively, at 200°C. At the same time, the minimum leakage current (achievable at slightly negative V_G) is 2–3 orders of magnitude lower, thus leaving space for optimization. Moreover,

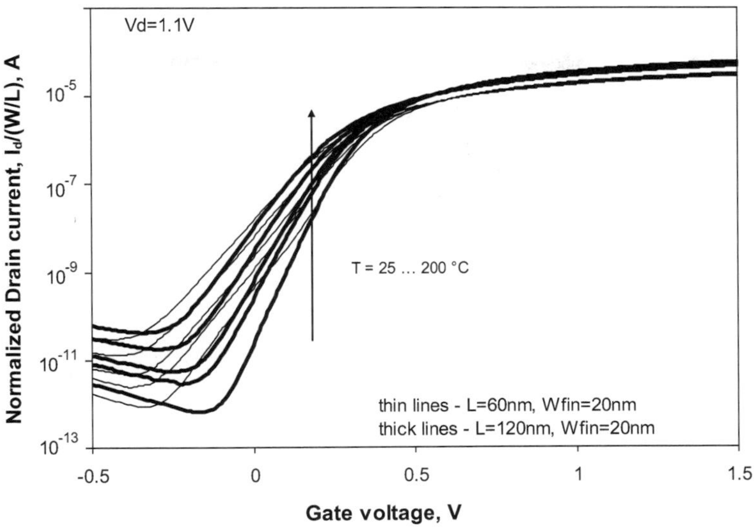

Figure 6.7. I_D–V_G curves 60 nm- and 120 nm-long narrow-fin FinFETs in saturation at different temperatures up to 200°C. $W_{tot} = 50 \times 9 \times (2 \times 0.06 + W_{Fin})$. $V_D = 1.1$ V.

the device maintains rather high values of on-to-off current ratio, I_{on}/I_{off}, up to 200°C.

In order to compare FinFETs with quasi-planar SG FD SOI as well as to demonstrate the influence of W_{Fin} on the I_{on}/I_{off} ratio, we introduce the "maximum operating temperature" figure of merit [20]. This parameter is arbitrarily defined as the temperature at which I_{on}/I_{off} ratio becomes lower than 10^4. We consider this value the lowest limit, after which the device cannot be used for digital applications, but this device can still be used for analog applications where a high I_{on}/I_{off} is not necessary. This chosen value of 10^4 can be too low for some application requirements, but in any case it reflects the fin-width influence and serves as a tool for the FinFET versus SG FD SOI comparison. It would be worthwhile to point out that not all wide-fin and SG quasi-planar FD SOI devices, depending on the device length, are able to satisfy this requirement even at room temperature.

Figure 6.8 shows that FinFETs are advantageous compared with the SG FD SOI 60-nm-thick film counterpart, allowing sub-100 nm

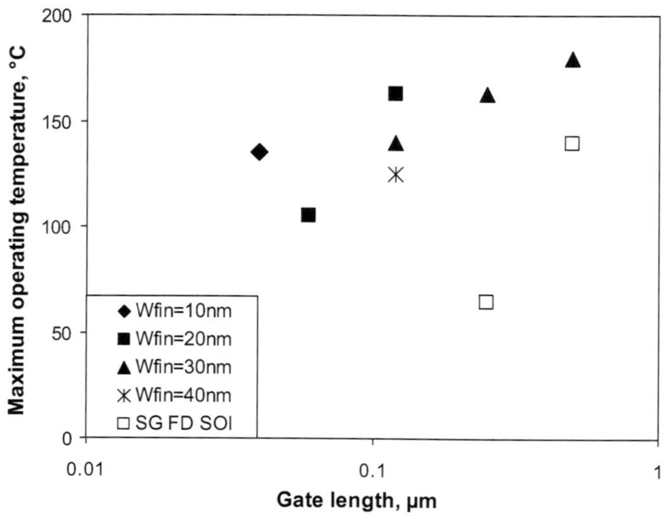

Figure 6.8. Gate length dependence of the "maximum operating temperature", taken at $I_{on}/I_{off} = 10^4$ for FinFETs with different W_{Fin} and SG FD SOI 60 nm-thick film counterpart. $V_D = 1.1$ V.

devices operation up to 150°C and even higher (depending on the fin width and length). Moreover, fin width narrowing clearly improves the achieved figures of merit.

6.6 Analog and RF Applications

6.6.1 *Maximum Transconductance-to-Drain Current Ratio, $G_m/I_{d\,max}$*

The attenuated subthreshold slope degradation in FinFETs compared with its SG FD SOI counterpart, is directly translated into an attenuated decrease of the transconductance-to-drain current ratio maximum, $(G_m/I_d)_{max} = \ln(10)/S$, which is further reduced in the narrowest fins (Fig. 6.9). Moreover, fin width narrowing allows a larger drive current range with about maximal G_m/I_d values as well as higher drive currents at the same fixed G_m/I_d. This can be related to the improved gate control and hence lower body factor as well as the improved mobility (volume inversion and lower electric field

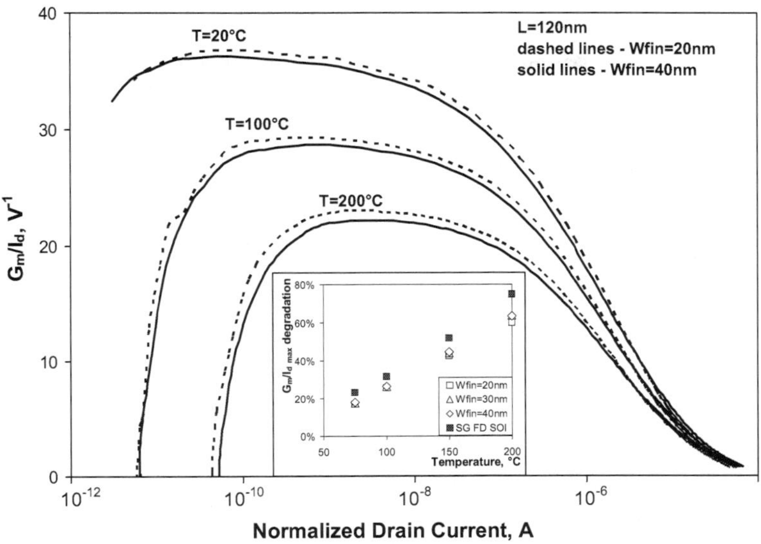

Figure 6.9. G_m/I_d as a function of the normalized drain current $(I_d/(W/L))$ at different temperatures for FinFETs with 20 and 40 nm fin width. $L = 0.12$ μm. $V_D = 1.1$ V. The insert gives the percentage of the $G_m/I_{d\,max}$ degradation as a function of temperature for different devices.

degradation). Such trends have been also confirmed and even better evidenced by 2D Atlas simulations of long-channel DG MOSFETs with different Si film thicknesses (Fig. 6.10).

6.6.2 G_m/I_d, Early Voltage and Intrinsic Gain

First, using room-temperature measurements the bias range for the comparative analysis of the analog performance was chosen. We have found that it is most advantageous for FinFETs to work at gate voltages, V_G, close to V_T in order to have a benefit of the volume inversion regime both on V_{EA} and G_m/I_d (through mobility enhancement), while applying a nominal drain voltage, V_D, equal to 1.1 V. It is worth to note that this bias point is furthermore closer to the zero temperature coefficient (ZTC) point, which corresponds to the gate voltage at which drain current remains constant with temperature. The ZTC point was clearly observed in all studied devices (see Fig. 6.7).

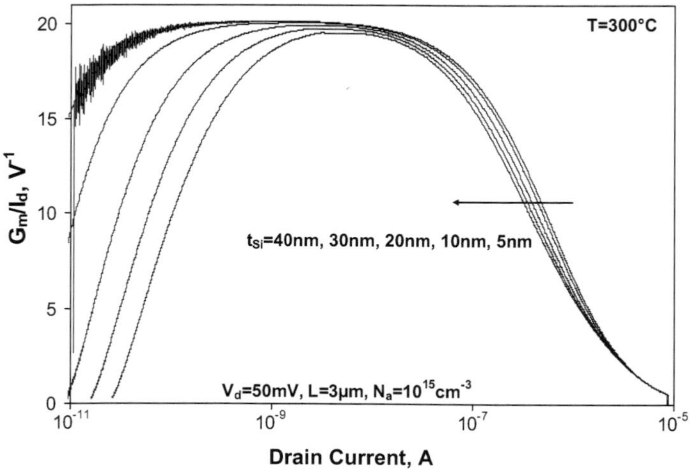

Figure 6.10. Simulated G_m/I_d vs. the drain current at $T = 300°C$ for undoped DG MOSFETs with different Si film thicknesses from 5 nm to and 40 nm. $L = 3$ μm. $V_D = 50$ mV.

Figure 6.11 shows the temperature evolution of G_m/I_d at fixed biases in FinFETs and quasi-planar SG FD SOI with different gate lengths. The observed G_m/I_d degradation with temperature is related to the mobility and body factor degradation with temperature as well as the threshold voltage shift and hence higher gate-voltage overdrive at constant V_G. A slightly smaller degradation can be seen in FinFETs compared with the SG counterparts, which is further improved with fin narrowing.

The early voltage was calculated from I_D–V_D characteristics as $V_{EA} = g_D/I_D$, where g_D is the output conductance. Figure 6.12 compares V_{EA} in FinFETs and SG FD SOI MOSFETs with different gate lengths. FinFETs clearly show more than twice improved V_{EA} values compared with the 60 nm-thick SG FD SOI counterparts over the whole temperature range. However, it is noticeable that the V_{EA} of FinFETs degrades slightly more with temperature than for the SG FD SOI ones, which could be related to the reduction of the channel control from the gates at high temperature as well as possibly the reduced advantage of volume inversion.

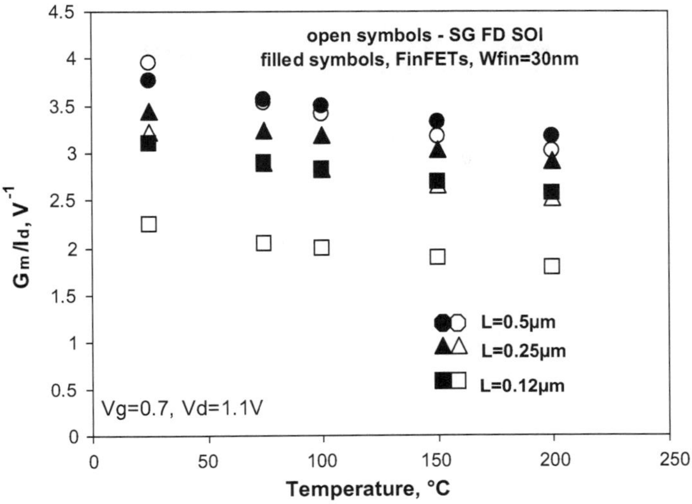

Figure 6.11. Temperature dependence of G_m/I_d at fixed biases $V_G = 0.7$ V, $V_D = 1.1$ V, in FinFETs with $W_{Fin} = 30$ nm (filled symbols) and 60 nm-thick film SG FD SOI MOSFETs (open symbols) with different gate lengths.

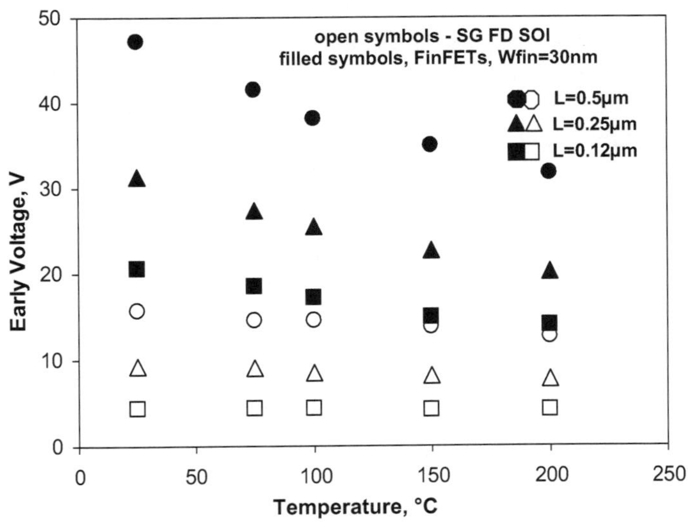

Figure 6.12. Temperature dependence of the Early voltage in FinFETs with $W_{Fin} = 30$ nm (filled symbols) and 60 nm-thick film SG FD SOI MOSFETs (open symbols) with different gate lengths. $V_G = 0.7$ V, $V_D = 1.1$ V.

Intrinsic gain, A_v, was then estimated as $A_v = V_{EA} \cdot G_m/I_D$. Figure 6.13 compares the intrinsic gain in FinFETs and SG FD SOI MOSFETs and shows also the influence of fin width narrowing. Here again the advantages of FinFETs are clear:

(1) More than 10 dB higher values for all FinFET devices are observed in the whole temperature range compared with the SG devices.
(2) The gain degradation in FinFETs does not exceed 5 dB over 200°C.

Moreover, the achieved values are higher than those we previously obtained on FD [21] and PD [20] SOI MOSFETs with similar gate lengths (about twice for $L = 0.12$ to 0.15 μm [20, 21]).

Figure 6.13b shows that a further 5–10 dB increase of the intrinsic gain can be achieved in the whole temperature range when the fin is thinned down, giving values as high as 27–30 dB at 200°C even for 60 nm-long devices.

6.6.3 *Transconductance Maximum, $G_{m\,max}$*

The device transconductance appears as a very important parameter since it determines the frequency limit of the device operation. It is commonly believed that the maximum transconductance degradation with temperature is directly related to the degradation of the low-field mobility with temperature. This can be related to the phonon scattering in this temperature range and therefore follows the same power law [22]:

$$\mu(T) = \mu(T_0) \cdot \left(\frac{T}{T_0}\right)^{\alpha} \tag{6.8}$$

where α is a constant in the range of $-1.5 \ldots -1.8$.

However, another parameter affecting the transconductance variation with temperature, namely the series resistance, has to be taken into account. The series resistance normally slightly increases with temperature, which in turn, similarly to the mobility effect, also results in a degradation of the transconductance maximum, but its temperature dependence is weaker than that of the mobility [6].

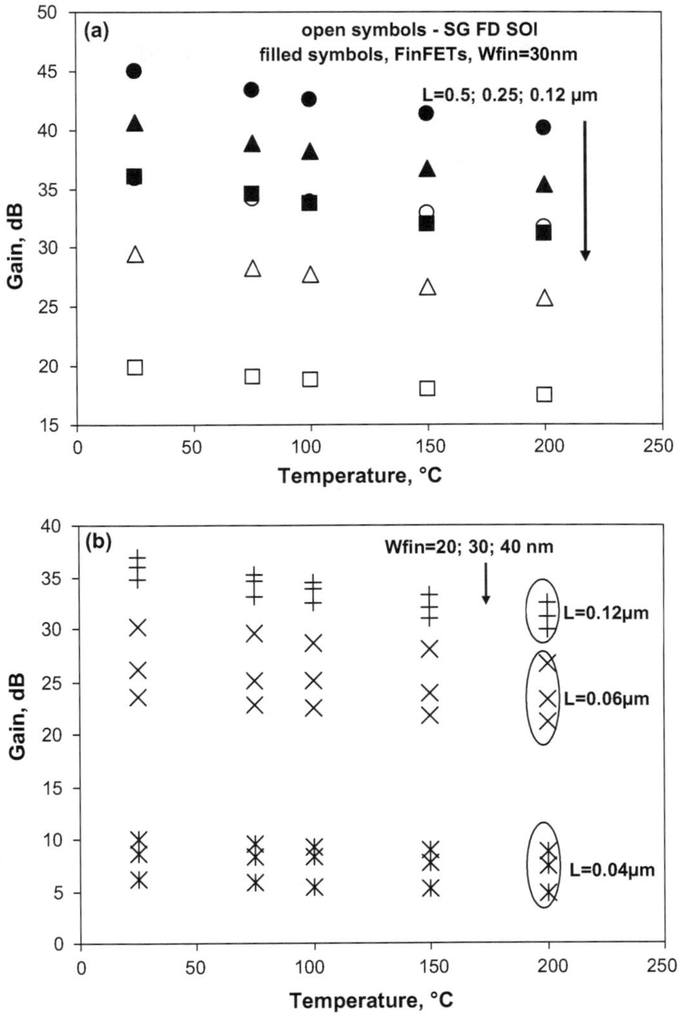

Figure 6.13. (a) Temperature dependence of the intrinsic gain in FinFETs with $W_{Fin} = 30$ nm (filled symbols) and 60 nm-thick film SG FD SOI MOSFETs devices (open symbols) with different gate lengths. $V_G = 0.7$ V, $V_D = 1.1$ V. (b) Influence of the fin width on the temperature dependence of the intrinsic gain for FinFETs with different gate lengths.

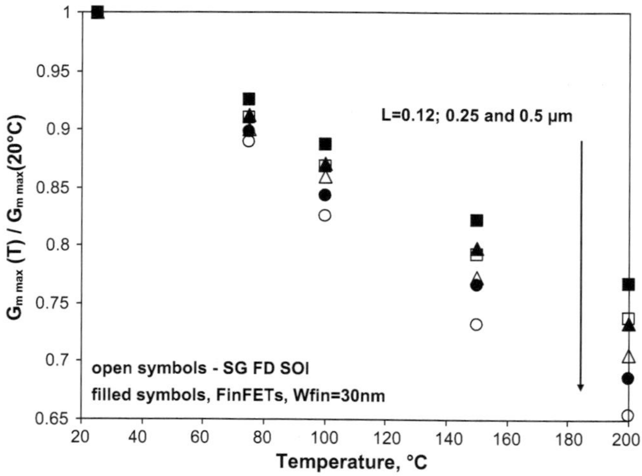

Figure 6.14. Degradation of the transconductance maximum with temperature for FinFETs with $W_{Fin} = 30$ nm (filled symbols) and 60 nm-thick film SG FD SOI MOSFETs devices (open symbols) with different gate lengths. $V_D = 1.1$ V.

The effect of the series resistance on the $G_{m\,max}$ temperature degradation is naturally of particular importance for devices with high series resistance such as FinFETs. Therefore, we may expect to have different trends in the $G_{m\,max}$ vs. T behavior in narrow-fin FinFETs (known to suffer from high series resistance, which moreover increases with fin narrowing [23]) and in short-channel devices (more strongly affected by series resistance).

This expectation is confirmed experimentally [6, 7]. Figure 6.14 compares the degradation rate of the transconductance maximum for the FinFETs and SG FD SOI MOSFETs with different gate lengths. Two important features are demonstrated by this comparison:

(1) The $G_{m\,max}$ degradation is weaker in FinFETs compared with the quasi-planar SG FD SOI counterpart;
(2) The $G_{m\,max}$ degradation decreases with gate length reduction. Moreover, based on our experience with different PD/FD/FinFETs devices, it is worthwhile to point out that such behavior is a general one and independent on technology or supplier.

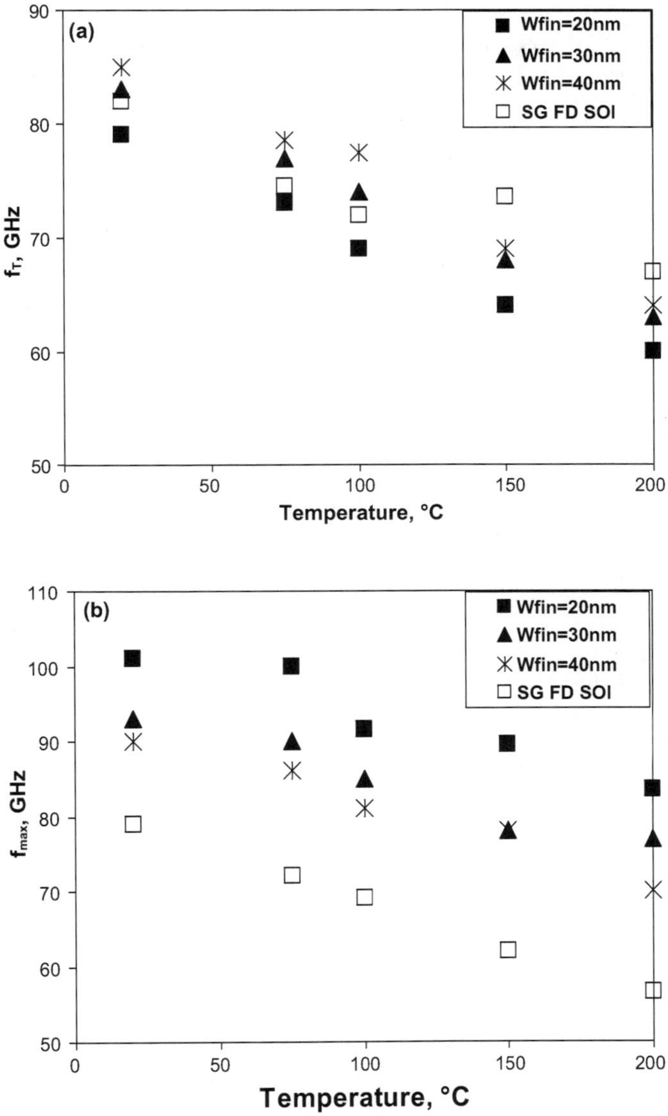

Figure 6.15. (a) f_t and (b) f_{max} evolution with temperature for FinFETs with different fin widths of 20 to 40 nm and the 60 nm-thick film SG FD SOI MOSFETs devices. $L = 60$ nm.

Therefore, we can assume that the enhanced role of the series resistance in FinFETs and short-length devices is indeed a possible explanation for their attenuated $G_{m\,max}$ degradation with temperature.

6.6.4 f_T, f_{max}

Figures 6.15a and 6.15b compare the temperature degradation of f_T and f_{max}, respectively, in FinFETs with different fin widths and quasi-planar SG FD SOI devices with a fixed gate length of 60 nm [6]. It is seen that the f_T and f_{max} degradations are slightly smaller in FinFETs compared with SG FD SOI devices, which correlates with the obtained results on the $G_{m\,max}$ degradation. It is worth pointing that [9] shows that the intrinsic capacitances (C_{gs} and C_{gd}) are almost constant over the whole temperature range. Furthermore, fin width narrowing allows further attenuation. Over a 200°C temperature range, we can obtain about 17–22% of f_{max} degradation for FinFETs with W_{Fin} = 20–40 nm, respectively, contrarily to about 27% in SG FD SOI devices. The f_T degradation in FinFETs is about 23–25%, almost independent on fin width and comparable to the 25% f_T degradation in the SG FD SOI counterparts. Nevertheless, in FinFETs both the f_T and f_{max} degradations with temperature do not exceed 15–20 GHz over the 200°C, which is slightly smaller than in SG FD SOI devices with the same gate length.

6.7 Conclusions

This chapter discusses some particular features of the high-temperature behavior of advanced MuGFETs and assesses their perspectives for high-temperature applications through detailed wide-band measurements and simulations in a temperature range up to 300°C. It has been demonstrated that narrow-fin FinFETs outperform their quasi-planar 60 nm-thick film SG FD SOI counterparts, showing better threshold voltage and subthreshold slope temperature stabilities, higher values of the on-to-off current ratio, Early voltage, intrinsic gain over the whole considered temperature range and a slightly attenuated degradation of the $G_{m\,max}$, f_T and f_{max}.

Summarizing the analysis presented above, it can be concluded that advanced MuGFETs appear to have a great potential for future high-temperature applications and are worth of further detailed investigation of their high-temperature stability and reliability.

Acknowledgements

The authors thank Imec (Belgium) for providing experimental devices. We also thank our colleagues both from UCL and the Imec teams, particularly Mr. Pascal Simon, Dr. Julio Tinoco, Dr. Nadine Collaert, Dr. Malgorzata Jurczak, Dr. Rita Rooyakers, Dr. Bertrand Parvais, Dr. Morin Dehan for their direct or indirect participation in this work and fruitful discussions.

This work was partially funded by the European Commission through the NoE "SINANO" (IST-506844).

References

1. www.itrs.net.
2. Lemme, M., Mollenhauer, T., Henschel, W. (2003). Subthreshold characteristics of p-type Triple-gate MOSFETs, *Proceedings of ESSDERC 2003*, pp. 123–127.
3. Colinge, J.-P., Floyd, L., Quinn, A. J., *et al.* (2006). Temperature effects on trigate SOI MOSFETs, *IEEE Electron Device Letters*, **27**, pp. 172–175.
4. Kilchytska, V., Collaert, N., Jurczak, M., Flandre, D. (2007) Multi-gate MOSFET behavior at high temperatures, *Proceedings of EuroSOI 2007*, 25–26 January 2007, Leuven, Belgium, pp. 30–31.
5. Kilchytska, V., Collaert, N., Jurczak, M., Flandre, D. (2007). Specific features of multiple-gate MOSFET threshold voltage and subthreshold slope behavior at high temperatures, *Solid State Electronics*, **51**, pp. 1185–1193.
6. Kilchytska, V., Flandre, D., Simon, P., Raskin, J.-P., Parvais, B., Collaert, N., Jurczak, M. (2007). FinFETs perspectives for high-temperature applications, *Proceedings of HITEN 2007*, available online at http://science24.com/paper/12252.
7. Akarvardar, K., Mercha, A., Simoen, E., Subramanian, V., Claeys, C., Gentil, P., Cristoloveanu, S. (2007). High-temperature performance of state-of-

the-art triple-gate transistors, *Microelectronics Reliability*, **47**, pp. 2065–2069.

8. Lee, C.-W., Lederer, D., Afzalian, A., Yan, R., Akhavan, N. D., Colinge, J.-P. (2009). Analytical model for the high-temperature behaviour of the subthreshold slope in MuGFETs, *Microelectronic Engineering*, **86**, pp. 2067–2071.
9. Tinoco, J. C., Parvais, B., Mercha, A., Decoutere, S., Raskin, J.-P. (2008). DC and RF characteristics of FinFET over a wide temperature range, *Proceedings of EuroSOI 2008*, pp. 57–58.
10. Talmat, R., Put, S., Collaert, N., *et al.* (2010). High-temperature characterization of advanced strained nMuGFETs, *Proceedings of EuroSOI 2010*, pp. 75–76.
11. Doria, R., Pavanello, M. (2010). Threshold voltage dependence on the temperature in strained and standard nFinFETs, *Proceedings of EuroSOI 2010*, pp. 87–88.
12. Collaert, N., *et al.* (2005). Tall triple-gate device with TiN/HfO_2 gate stack, *Proceedings of Symposium on VLSI Technology*, pp. 108–109.
13. Atlas Manual 2005.
14. Colinge, J.-P., Park, J. W., Xiong, W. (2003). Threshold voltage and subthreshold slope of multiple-gate SOI MOSFETs, *IEEE Electron Device Letters*, **24**, pp. 515–517.
15. Colinge, J.-P. (1997) *Silicon-on-Insulator Technology: Materials to VLSI*. 2nd Ed. (Dordrecht: Kluwer Academic Publishers).
16. Francis, P., Terao, A., Flandre, D., Van de Wiele, F. (1995). Moderate inversion model of ultrathin double-gate nMOS/SOI transistors, *Solid State Electronics*, **38**, pp. 171–176.
17. Sallese, J. M., Krummenacher, F., Pregaldiny, F., Lallement, C., Roy, A., Enz, C. (2005) A design oriented charge-based current model for symmetric DG MOSFET and its correlation with the EKV formalism, *Solid State Electronics*, **49**, pp. 485–489.
18. Rudenko, T., Kilchytska, V., Colinge, J.-P., Dessard, V., Flandre, D. (2002). On the high-temperature subthreshold slope of thin-film SOI MOSFETs, *IEEE Electron Device Letters*, **23**, pp. 148–151.
19. Taur, Y. (2001). Analytic solutions of charge and capacitance in symmetric and asymmetric double-gate MOSFETs, *IEEE Transactions on Electron Devices*, **48**, pp. 2861–2869.
20. Kilchytska, V., de Meyer, K., Flandre, D. (2004). In-depth investigation of 0.13 μm SOI MOSFETs for high-temperature applications, *Proceedings of ULIS 2004*, pp. 163–166.

21. Vancaillie, L., Kilchytska, V., Delatte, P., Matsuhashi, H., Ichikawa, F., Flandre, D. (2003). 0.15μm Fully Depleted SOI for Mixed-Signal Applications up to 250°C: Are We Approaching the Limits of Device Scaling for High-Temperature Electronics?, *Proceedings of HITEN 2003*, pp. 127–132.

22. Reichert, G., Ouisse, T., Pelloie, J. L., Cristoloveanu, S. (1996). Mobility modeling of SOI MOSFETs in the high temperature range, *Solid-State Electronics*, **39**, pp. 1347–1352.

23. Subramanian, V., Mercha, A., Parvais, B. *et al.* (2007). Impact of fin width on digital and analog performances of n-FinFETs, *Solid-State Electronics*, **51**, pp. 551–559.

Chapter 7

ESD Protection in FinFET Technology

Steven Thijs
IMEC, Kapeldreef 75, 3001 Heverlee, Belgium
steven.thijs@imec.be

Despite a small silicon volume to dissipate the heat from ESD discharges, it is demonstrated that FinFET devices can have reasonably good ESD robustness, depending strongly on layout and process parameters. Different normalization techniques are required for correct data interpretation.

7.1 Introduction

The reliability of sub-micrometer devices and circuits is a major issue that determines both their manufacturability and application lifetime. Design for reliability should be implemented during technology, device and circuit development to avoid undesirable product development cycles and costly yield loss and field failures. As CMOS keeps scaling down, new technology options arise and their ElectroStatic Discharge (ESD) robustness should be preferably considered in the early technology development phase as these technology evolutions might lead to a 'drastic' reduction in ESD robustness as it has been the case in the past when new technology

CMOS Nanoelectronics: Innovative Devices, Architectures, and Applications
Edited by Nadine Collaert

ISBN 978-981-4364-02-7 (Hardcover), 978-981-4364-03-4 (eBook)
www.panstanford.com

features, such as silicides and Lightly Doped Drain (LDD), were introduced [Amerasekara and Duvvury (2002)].

In [Russ *et al.* (2005)] and [Russ *et al.* (2007)], it was shown that early FinFET structures displayed an extremely low ESD robustness. In the succeeding work [Gossner *et al.* (2006)], localized heating was demonstrated to be the cause for the high sensitivity and consequently FinFET optimization requires understanding of the thermal effects.

First, a brief general introduction to ESD is given in Section 7.2. After discussing the normalization methodology in Section 7.3, Section 7.4 describes the impact of all FinFET geometrical parameters, such as fin width, gate length, fin spacing, fin height, number of fins and BOX thickness for MOS devices and gated diodes. Section 7.5 discusses the impact of different process options, such as extension implants, fin doping, selective epitaxial growth (SEG), silicide blocking (SB) and strain.

7.2 Brief Introduction to ESD

The most famous type of ESD is lightning. In fact, lightning is nothing else but ESD on a large scale, with voltages up to 10^7 V and currents up to 30 kiloamperes. The world's tallest and most expensive ESD protection structure is the Burj Dubai skyscraper located in Downtown Dubai, United Arab Emirates. It has a giant lightning-rod on its top to safely discharge the lightning events as shown in Fig. 7.1.

Triboelectric charging of objects results from electron transfer during friction of two objects. For example, a person can acquire charges by simply walking across a room. ESD is the transfer of an electrostatic charge which occurs when two objects of different electrostatic potential are brought close together.

The amount of charge induced depends on various parameters, such as the position of the relevant materials in the triboelectric series, the relative humidity, the texture of the material surfaces, speed of separation, area of contact, etc. When such a charged person or object then approaches a grounded conductor, for example a pin of a packaged integrated circuit (IC), an electrostatic discharge (ESD)

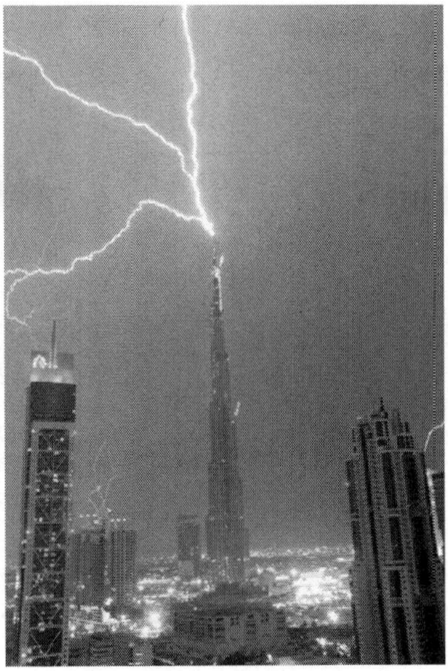

Figure 7.1. The Burj Dubai is world's tallest ESD protection structure [Courtesy of HALEX].

event occurs, characterized by a high current (~A) during a few nanoseconds. An ESD event of amplitude of 3000 V or below (corresponding to a current level of typically 2 A) will not be detected by humans by sensory perception. However, such ESD event can cause various types of damage in an IC, resulting in catastrophic failure.

To avoid circuit damage during ESD stress, ESD protection elements need to be placed around the integrated circuit (IC), which can safely remove the ESD current, similar as the lightning-rod in Fig. 7.1. The ideal ESD protection element is basically a switch that is open during normal operation and closed during ESD.

The ESD design window can be defined as the region in which the ESD protection elements need to operate, as shown in Fig. 7.2. On one hand, the window is limited by the normal operation regime, with which the ESD protection should not infere. On the other hand, the window is limited by the IC reliability, caused by gate oxide breakdown, turn-on of parasitics, etc. A typical snapback device IV characteristic is shown in the ESD design window in Fig. 7.2. In such

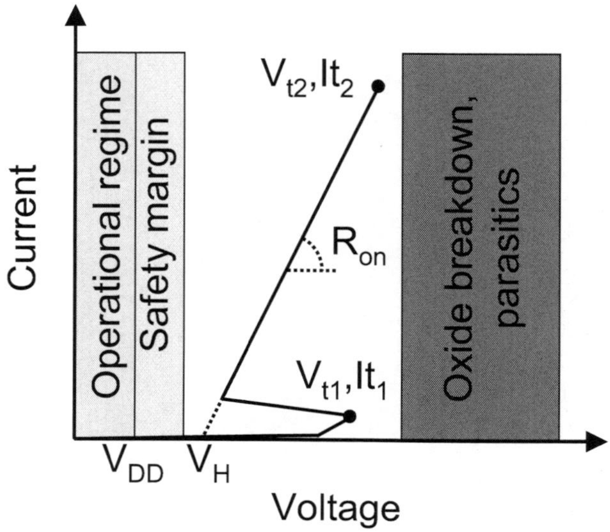

Figure 7.2. ESD design window.

devices, at a certain moment a parasitic device inside will turn on which allows efficient dissipation of the ESD current. These devices need to turn on at their trigger point (V_{t1}, I_{t1}) before core damage occurs. The holding voltage (V_h) denotes the minimum voltage to maintain the parasitic device action and should be at a safe level above V_{DD} to avoid latchup issues. After snapback, the parasitic device dissipates the ESD current with a certain on-resistance (R_{on}) until its failure point (V_{t2}, I_{t2}) is reached. I_{t2} should be above the minimum required ESD current level.

7.2.1 *Basic ESD Protection Devices*

In this section, two basic ESD protection devices, diode and grounded-gate NMOS, are summarized.

Diode

Diodes are excellent ESD protection devices when operated under forward bias. A cross section is shown in Fig. 7.3. The anode is formed by the P+ terminal and the cathode by the N+ terminal.

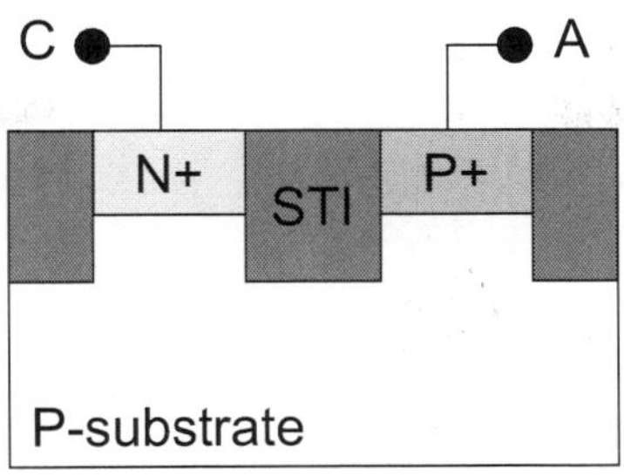

Figure 7.3. Cross section of a diode.

Anode and cathode can be separated by either STI isolation or by a poly gate. The diode can be created either in an nwell or pwell. When placing diodes in series, nwell diodes are required to avoid shortening of the P+ anodes via the P-substrate resistance.

Diodes have a low turn-on voltage around 0.7 V and exhibit a low on-resistance. They have a high ESD current capability, up to 50 mA/um. Under reverse bias however, they have a high turn-on voltage and high on-resistance, leading to a low ESD current capability. Therefore, diodes can only conduct current efficiently in a single direction, namely in forward bias mode.

Grounded-gate NMOS

The cross section of a grounded-gate nMOS (ggNMOS) is shown in Fig. 7.4. In a ggNMOS, the N+ drain forms the anode, while the source, gate and bulk are shorted together and form the cathode. Under normal V_{DD} bias conditions, the ggNMOS is not conducting as the gate terminal is grounded. However, when the voltage at the drain rises high enough, avalanche breakdown of the drain to substrate junction will occur generating electron–hole pairs. As the generated holes flow to the P+ substrate terminal, the substrate voltage under the source rises until the substrate source diode gets forward biased. At this moment, the source will start to emit electrons that are collected at the drain. Avalanche multiplication occurs at the drain side creating a positive feedback mechanism, which allows the drain voltage to collapse (i.e., snapback). As such, a parasitic bipolar npn device is triggered which has an ESD current capability of typically 8–14 mA/um. For negative ESD

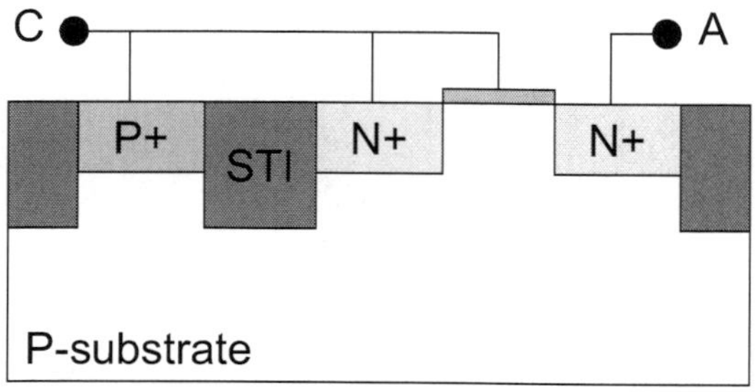

Figure 7.4. Cross section of a grounded-gate NMOS (ggNMOS).

stress, the substrate-drain diode gets forward biased, making the ggNMOS a bidirectional ESD protection device. Despite its rather high ESD robustness, the ggNMOS has some important drawbacks. The parasitic snapback effect is difficult to model and simulate. Its behavior is also difficult to predict as it depends heavily on the process parameters. Uniformity problems can occur for large devices. However, even with these drawbacks, the ggNMOS remains a widely used ESD protection device.

7.2.2 *Transmission Line Pulsing (TLP) Measurements*

An engineering tool called transmission line pulse (TLP) measurements has been developed, which gives information on how the device reacts during ESD stress. TLP was first introduced by Intel in 1985 [Maloney and Khurana (1985)]. Standard TLP has a typical pulse duration of 100 ns and a rise time between 2 and 10 ns.

If one would try to measure a device with DC up to ESD current levels, which are in the order of Amps, the device would fail early due to self-heating caused by the high instantaneous power dissipation. Therefore, very short rectangular pulses are created, using transmission lines, with a pulse duration in the same order as the ESD-timeframe. This prevents self-heating and allows device qualification in the ESD time-, voltage- and current-domain. TLP is not designed to give accurate measurement results in the low-current region (below a few mA), where DC remains preferred.

A full TLP test consists of applying TLP pulses for increasing voltage levels, yielding each time an averaged voltage-current point,

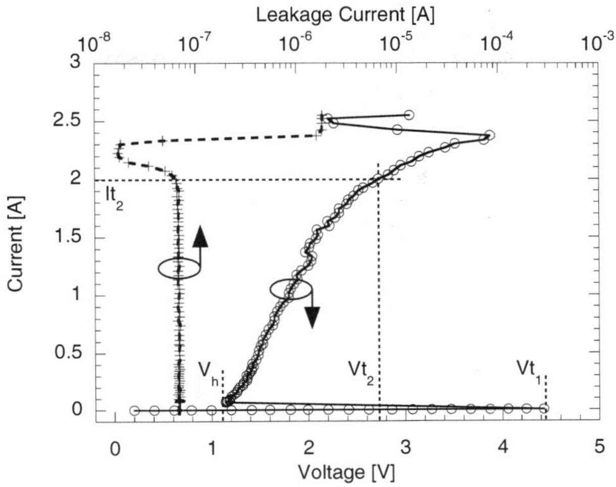

Figure 7.5. Example TLP-IV curve of an ESD protection device.

which is plotted in the TLP-IV graph. After each stress pulse, a leakage current measurement is performed to see whether any change has occured comparing to the initial leakage current of the DUT before the TLP test, which would indicate device failure. This leakage current is typically plotted versus the TLP current in the same TLP-IV graph on a double X-axis on top. Figure 7.5 shows such a TLP-IV graph for an ESD protection device. The typical quasi-static TLP parameters for ESD snapback devices, such as the SCR, are also shown in Fig. 7.5: trigger voltage V_{t1}, holding voltage V_h, failure voltage V_{t2} and second (thermal) breakdown current I_{t2}. I_{t2} is defined as the TLP current level at which any change in leakage current is measured.

7.3 Normalization Methodology

For interpretation of the results, different device width normalization techniques are possible for FinFETs due to the larger number of geometrical dimensions compared to planar devices. It should always be indicated which normalization was used.

First, there is normalization possible toward intrinsic silicon width W_{intr} (7.1).

$$W_{intr} = N W_{fin} \tag{7.1}$$

This normalization is preferred when current is flowing through the full cross section ($W_{fin}{}^{*}H_{fin}$) of the fins, e.g., as will be shown for MOS devices operating in parasitic bipolar mode and for gated diodes. This is a measure for the intrinsic ESD performance of the device, which relates to the current density in the silicon volume.

Second, a normalization can be used to investigate the layout efficiency of the device, considering the total layout width W_{layout} (7.2).

$$W_{layout} = N W_{fin} + (N-1)S \tag{7.2}$$

W_{layout} includes the overhead due to the fin-to-fin spacing S. The gate overlap on fins W_{ext} and the size of the poly contacts are neglected. An additional layout optimization could be performed by folding the transistor and sharing different source and drain regions, reducing the overall layout area. The total layout width normalization is most important for an I/O layout engineer since it is related to the total space occupied by the devices on chip.

Third, the normalization can take into account the fact that FinFET devices have a total channel width W_{chan} (7.3), defined by the top and sidewalls of the fin, per silicon footprint area. This normalization relates to the total drive current of a MOS transistor. For a given amount of drive current of an output driver, the ESD robustness of the standalone driver is then known.

$$W_{chan} = N(W_{fin} + 2H_{fin}). \tag{7.3}$$

Finally, a synthetic view of all normalization can be made giving a rough number to compare different technologies. To exploit the FinFET 3D channel benefit, an effective width W_{eff} (7.4) is proposed, which corrects the intrinsic width W_{intr} by the ratio of W_{layout} and W_{chan}.

$$W_{eff} = W_{intr}\frac{W_{layout}}{W_{chan}} \tag{7.4}$$

As such, the effective width normalization relates to intrinsic performance, the total drive current and the layout efficiency of the device. This method is more applicable when MOS current is flowing, and therefore is used for MOS devices operating in active MOS mode. For this normalization, the device was considered to behave as a triple-gate transistor. For W_{fin} of 10 nm and below, the contribution of the top channel can be neglected and the device acts like a double-gate transistor. This is also the preferred normalization when comparing FinFET ESD performance with other technologies. Note that for wide fin devices, all three normalizations yield almost identical results.

7.4 Geometrical Dependencies

The influence of the geometrical parameters, L_g, W_{fin}, N, H_{fin}, S and T_{BOX}, on the different ESD performance parameters is investigated in this section. Section 7.4.1 discusses the parasitic bipolar operation mode where ESD stress is applied to the drain, while source and gate are grounded. Gated diodes are discussed in Section 7.4.2.

7.4.1 *MOS Devices — Parasitic Bipolar Mode*

ESD stress is applied to the drain, while source and gate are grounded. The MOS devices are thus first in off-mode and later operated in parasitic bipolar mode, which means that each fin forms its own parasitic bipolar transistor. The analysis done in this section applies to both dedicated MOS ESD protection devices operating in bipolar mode and to MOS output drivers which could be made self-protecting based on these results.

TLP measurements of narrow and wide fin NMOS and PMOS FinFET devices are shown in Fig. 7.6 and Fig. 7.7 respectively, for different gate lengths. The last point indicated in each IV-curve corresponds to the maximum failure current I_{t2}. After the next TLP stress level, an increase in leakage current was noticed, indicating device failure. Extraction of I_{t2}, V_{t1}, V_h and R_{on} is indicated in Fig. 7.6. The narrow fin devices have a W_{fin} of 30 nm and N is 400, resulting in W_{intr} of 12 um and W_{layout} of 80 um, according to Section 7.3. The wide fin devices consist of a single 'fin' of 40 um wide resembling a planar SOI device. Since the parasitic

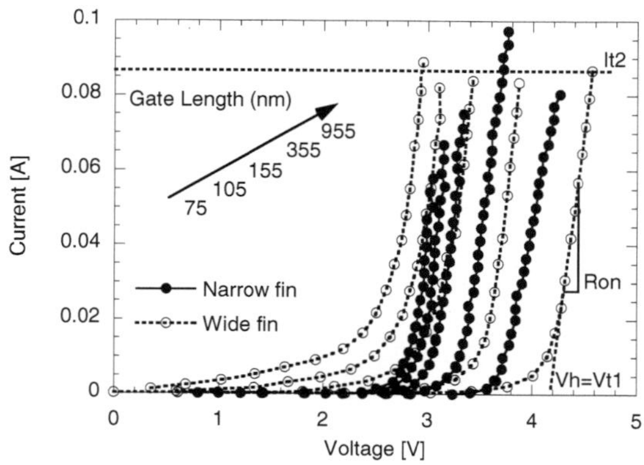

Figure 7.6. TLP-IV curves for different gate lengths of N-type FinFET in bipolar mode for both narrow (400 fins of 30 nm W_{fin}) and wide (single 40 um) fin devices.

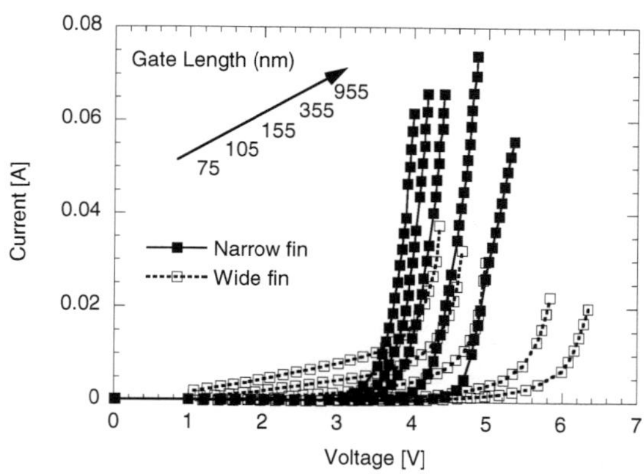

Figure 7.7. TLP-IV curves for different gate lengths of P-type FinFET in bipolar mode for both narrow (400 fins of 30 nm W_{fin}) and wide (single 40 um) fin devices.

bipolars have their bases floating, no snapback is seen in the TLP I-V curves. This floating body effect is typical for any SOI process [Amerasekara and Duvvury (2002)], even though for planar SOI a body contact could be provided from the device side. The trigger voltage is not BV_{CBO}, for example, for bulk technologies, but the device starts to conduct current immediately at the lower BV_{CEO}. This means that the trigger voltage, V_{t1}, and holding voltage, V_h, are equal [Amerasekara and Duvvury (2002)], which helps for uniform turn-on of all fingers. Both Fig. 7.6 and Fig. 7.7 show that small gate lengths cannot control SCE for wide fin devices, leading to a significant amount of current flow, even at voltages of 2 V and below. Based on the TLP measurements in Fig. 7.6 and Fig. 7.7, the different ESD performance parameters can be investigated.

7.4.1.1 Gate length dependence

The impact of L_g is investigated on the different ESD performance parameters I_{t2}, V_h and R_{on}.

Failure current I_{t2}

I_{t2} as a function of L_g for both NMOS and PMOS is shown in Fig. 7.8 and Fig. 7.9 respectively, using the different normalizations as discussed in Section 7.3. For narrow fin NMOS and PMOS devices, I_{t2} increases with increasing gate length and slightly drops down for the largest gate length. At high current levels, the current tends to localize in a few fins near the onset of failure, as described in [Gossner *et al.* (2006)]. This "non-uniform failure" is not a matter of "non-uniform turn-on" in multifinger devices. Remember that the floating base and thus absence of snapback ensures all fingers to turn-on. In [Gossner *et al.* (2006)], failure analysis was used to show that fusing of single fins was the cause of failure. Increasing

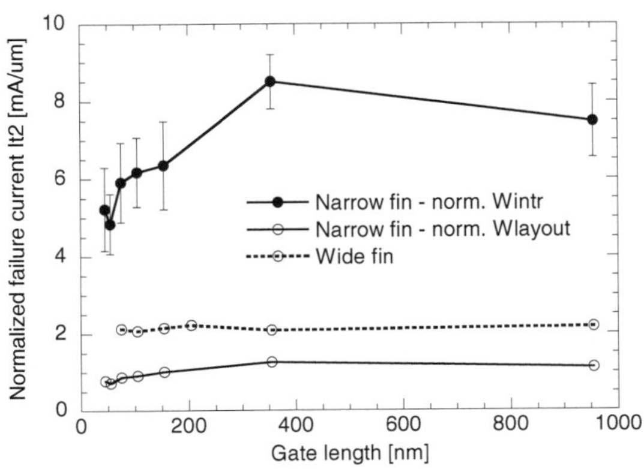

Figure 7.8. Normalized I_{t2} as a function of gate length for narrow and wide fin N-type FinFET devices in bipolar mode.

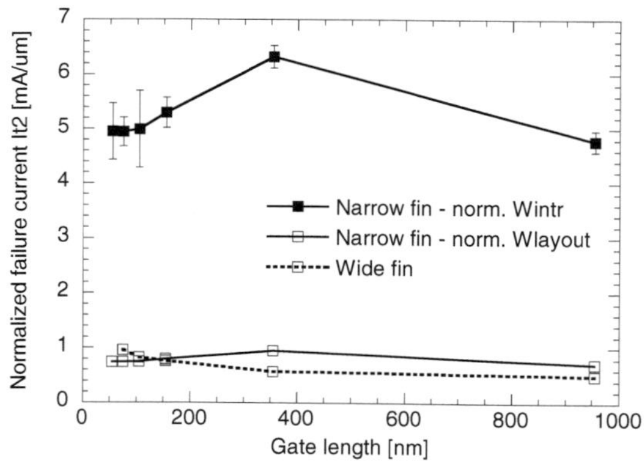

Figure 7.9. Normalized I_{t2} as a function of gate length for narrow and wide fin P-type FinFET devices in bipolar mode.

L_g for narrow fin devices does not only increase the silicon volume below the gate and hence its heat capacity, but it also seems to have the same effect as a ballast resistance which improves the current uniformity at high current levels. This explains the increase of I_{t2} with increasing L_g. When further increasing L_g also the voltage drop increases (increased V_h and R_{on}, Fig. 7.10 and Fig. 7.12 respectively, explained in the next subsections). As a consequence, the dissipated energy is increased, which leads to a maximum I_{t2} at medium L_g, Fig. 7.8 and Fig. 7.9. For 45 nm L_g for narrow fin NMOS devices, the very small increase of I_{t2} compared to 75 nm, is due to incorrect normalization because of a fin-widening due to the Optical Proximity Correction (OPC) of the active etch mask. The shortest L_g leads to the shortest fin length and thus the fins are inevitably processed at slightly larger fin width.

For wide fin NMOS devices, I_{t2} is independent of L_g. For a single fin of 40 um, much less problems exist with current uniformity at high current levels, since now the current is located within one single wide fin, and not among different narrow fins. However, it is important to notice that the failure is located at a constant current level, rather than a constant power level. This can be attributed to isothermal current instability, which is initiated by impact ionization under high field conditions [Vas (2008)]. Locally a high Joule power level is generated, which results in a filament formation and finally

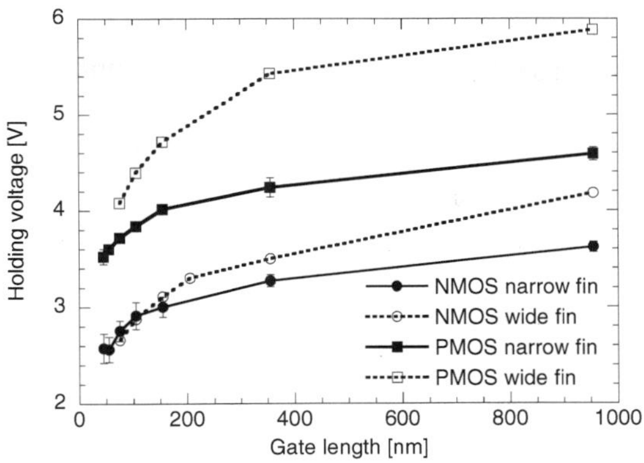

Figure 7.10. Holding voltage as a function of gate length for narrow and wide fin FinFET devices in bipolar mode.

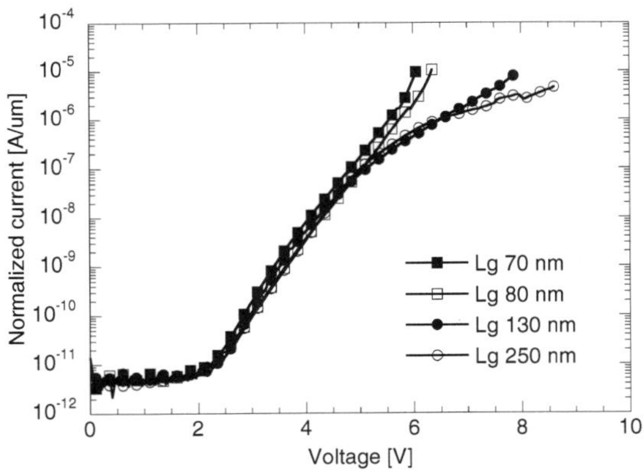

Figure 7.11. Measured breakdown characteristics normalized to W_{intr} for gated diodes with floating gate, W_{fin} 1000 nm and N 64 fins and varying L_g.

local burnout. This means that even within a single wide fin there can still exist a degree of non-uniformity.

In contrast to wide fin NMOS devices, Fig. 7.8, for PMOS devices I_{t2} is decreasing significantly for the largest L_g, Fig. 7.9. This can be attributed to their high holding voltage (5–6 V) needed for bipolar action as seen in Fig. 7.7 and Fig. 7.10. As such, these devices are failing because of gate-oxide breakdown at the drain-gate overlap region instead of thermal failure of the fins. This is described in more

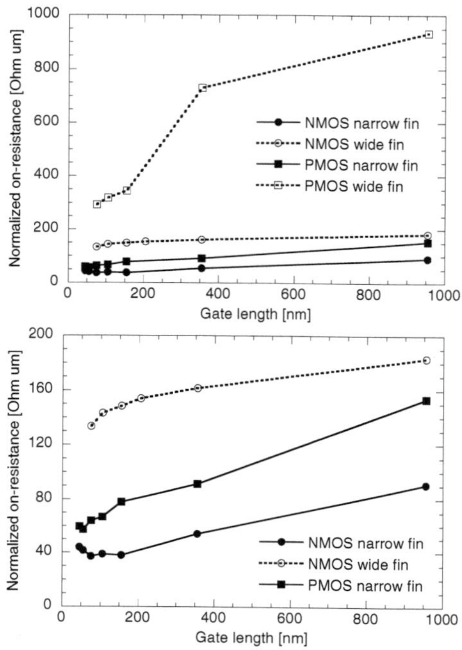

Figure 7.12. High current on-resistance normalized to intrisinc silicon width as a function of gate length for narrow and wide fin FinFET devices in bipolar mode (left: full scale, right: zoom).

detail in Section 7.4.1.3 where several parallel blocks of devices are considered. In case of thermal failure, scaling of the failure level with the number of parallel blocks should be obtained, which is not the case for wide PMOS devices with large L_g.

A possible explanation for the current localization, described in [Gossner *et al.* (2006)], could be the existence of local Schottky contacts between the S/D silicide (NiSi) and the body of the FinFETs [Hoffmann *et al.* (2005)]. These results were obtained from similar IMEC silicon samples. Such a Schottky contact is a result of over-silicidation of the fins where the Ni-silicide can overrun the lowly doped extension region and grow into the channel region. The ESD robustness is very sensitive to over-silicidation. However, in a more mature technology, the problem of over-silicidation should be greatly reduced. Many arguments point to the negative impact of the over-silicidation. First, the over-silicidation is worst for narrow fin devices [Collaert *et al.* (2007a)], where much more statistical variation is measured than for wide fin devices. Second, over-silicidation is less problematic for PMOS devices as Boron retards the silicidation [Collaert *et al.* (2007a)] [Dixit *et al.* (2006)]. This can explain the increased I_{t2} for PMOS devices with smallest gate length when compared to NMOS and the reduced L_g dependency, Fig. 7.8 and Fig. 7.9. Also, much less statistical variation in I_{t2} was measured on PMOS than on NMOS devices. The error bars indicating the standard deviation of I_{t2} for NMOS and PMOS devices in Fig. 7.8 and Fig. 7.9 for W_{intr} normalization show the increased variability for NMOS. Finally, over-silicidation is reduced by processing options like silicide blocking and SEG, which directly translates into an increased ESD performance as described further in Section 7.5.

For wide fin NMOS devices, I_{t2} is equal to 2 mA/um and independent of L_g, Fig. 7.8. The ESD robustness for narrow fin NMOS devices is 0.5 to 1 mA/um when normalized to W_{layout}. However, the robustness regarding W_{intr} is 5 to 8 mA/um, representing an even higher intrinsic I_{t2} than the results reported for planar SOI devices [Keppens *et al.* (2006)]. This is explained by looking at the fin width dependence of I_{t2} in Section 7.4.1.2.

Holding voltage V_h

The condition for the onset of parasitic bipolar action (at low current levels) [Amerasekara and Duvvury (2002)] is

$$\beta(M - 1) \geq 1, \tag{7.5}$$

where β is the common-emitter bipolar current gain and M the multiplication factor. M depends on the breakdown voltage V_{bd} according to [Miller (1957)]:

$$M = \frac{1}{1 - \left(\frac{V_j}{V_{bd}}\right)^n}, \tag{7.6}$$

with V_j the junction voltage and n a fitting parameter ranging from 2 to 6 depending on the type of junction. As can be seen, the holding voltage V_h (V_j where (7.5) is fulfilled) depends on both β and V_{bd}. V_h is extracted according to Fig. 7.6, and increases with increasing L_g (Fig. 7.10) because the base width of the parasitic bipolar is increased which decreases β. Therefore, higher M is needed to satisfy condition (7.5) and thus higher voltages are obtained. V_h saturates with increasing L_g since M increases exponentially with junction voltage. V_h of PMOS is higher when compared to NMOS due to the reduced hole versus electron mobility and the lower avalanche multiplication factor of the hole- versus electron-current [Trémouilles (2004)].

We have verified that the breakdown characteristic is independent of L_g in the range of electric fields which correspond to the holding voltages measured in Fig. 7.10. These results were obtained by performing breakdown measurements on gated diodes (P+/Intrinsic/N+) with floating gate, 1 um W_{fin} and different L_g, see Fig. 7.11. This same result was also measured for narrow fin devices of 20 nm with varying L_g.

As such, V_h can be tuned for narrow fin devices between 2.6 and 3.6 V for NFETs and between 3.5 and 4.6 V for PFETs. The holding voltage is clearly determined as almost no statistical variation was measured.

On-resistance R_{on}

The high current on-resistance R_{on}, normalized to W_{intr} is shown in Fig. 7.12 as a function of L_g. For narrow fin NMOS devices, the on-resistance is relatively independent of L_g for small gate lengths, giving a measure for the access resistance of the device, which is determined by the resistance of the source/drain landing pads, the interconnects and amorphization of the silicon [Collaert *et al.* (2007a)]. Due to OPC fin widening for narrow fins with smallest L_g a lower resistance is expected, however this impact is masked by the access resistance. When further increasing L_g, the additional bipolar transistor voltage drop in the base region becomes visible. Very little statistical variation was measured. Wide fin devices exhibit the same gate length dependency but at a much higher R_{on}. This width dependence of R_{on} is further discussed in Section 7.4.1.2. The resistance of the PMOS increases with increasing L_g and is larger than for the NMOS, which is partly due to the lower hole mobility. In [Dixit *et al.* (2006)], the difference in silicide formation between NMOS and PMOS devices was studied. It was found that for NMOS devices, the sidewalls were completely silicided along the whole height of the S/D region, which was not the case for the PMOS, again

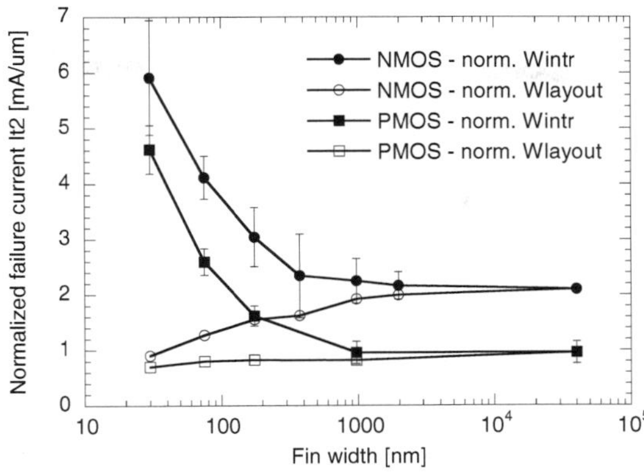

Figure 7.13. Normalized I_{t2} as a function of fin width for FinFET devices with 75 nm gate length in bipolar mode. Devices up to 175 nm fin width consist of 400 fins, up to 2 um of 40 fins and the 40 um wide device has only a single 'fin'.

due to the presence of Boron in the S/D regions. This effect futher explains the increased on-resistance for the PMOS devices.

7.4.1.2 Fin width dependence

The impact of W_{fin} is investigated on the different ESD performance parameters I_{t2}, V_h and R_{on}.

Failure current I_{t2}

In Fig. 7.13, the normalized I_{t2} as a function of W_{fin} is shown for NMOS and PMOS devices with a gate length of 75 nm. The largest statistical variations were measured for the narrowest fins and in general for NMOS. This again can be attributed to their higher sensitivity to over-silicidation, which has a direct negative impact on I_{t2}. When normalizing I_{t2} versus W_{intr} and versus W_{layout}, different trends are observed. An increased intrinsic performance is measured for decreased fin width. This increase in I_{t2} can be attributed to the higher effective heat capacity of the 3D-gate, which fully surrounds the fin. Narrow fins act as regular 'cooling fins'. For wider fins, this 3D-nature of the gate disappears and the device becomes very similar to a planar device, leading to a decrease in I_{t2}. The same dependency and relative difference in I_{t2} versus fin width between NMOS and PMOS is observed. However, when normalizing to W_{layout}, the trend becomes opposite. This is because for smaller fins, there is relatively more area overhead due to the fin-to-fin spacing, making them less area efficient. For wider fins, the difference between the two normalization techniques obviously disappears because of the reduced fin-to-fin spacing overhead. From Fig. 7.13 and all subsequent figures which include fin width dependency, it can be concluded that from a 1 um wide fin onwards (for the given fin height and fin spacing), the devices can be treated as 2D planar SOI instead of 3D FinFET devices.

Holding voltage V_h

V_h as a function of W_{fin} for both NMOS and PMOS devices with short and long L_g is shown in Fig. 7.14. For NMOS devices with 75 nm L_g, V_h is almost independent of W_{fin}. A slight increase in V_h is measured for the narrowest W_{fin}, which can be attributed to two effects: first, the absence of free carriers due to the full depletion of the fin and second, the possible but undesirable oversilicidation of the narrowest fins which increases carrier recombination [Hoffmann *et al.* (2005)]. For PMOS devices with 75 nm L_g, V_h is almost constant with W_{fin} but decreases for the narrowest fins.

For NMOS and PMOS devices with large L_g, only two fin widths were available in the testchip (Fig. 7.14), but their holding voltage

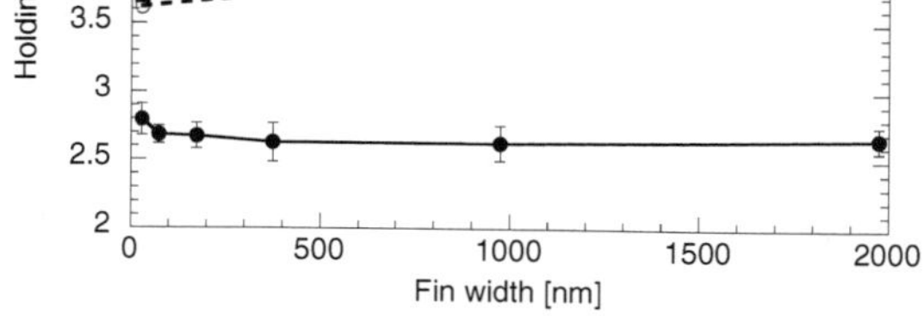

Figure 7.14. Holding voltage as a function of fin width for FinFET devices with 75 nm gate length or 955 nm gate length in bipolar mode.

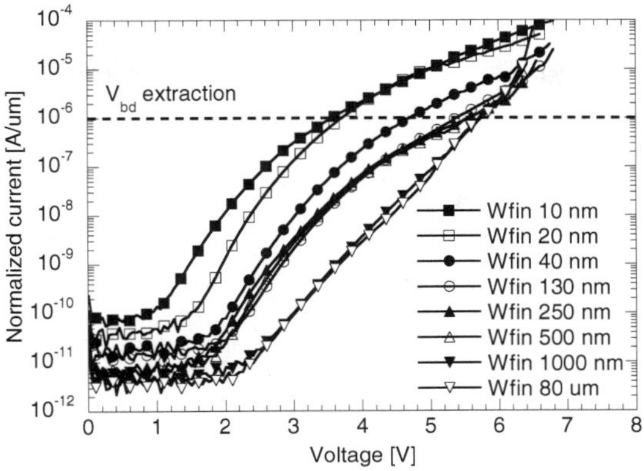

Figure 7.15. Measured breakdown characteristics normalized to W_{intr} for gated diodes with floating gate, L_g 80 nm and varying N and W_{fin}. The number of fins N depends on W_{fin}, ranging from 1 to 400. The breakdown voltage is extracted at 1 μA/um and is shown in Fig. 7.16.

is expected first to remain constant and then to decrease with decreasing W_{fin} as well.

This behavior is explained by measuring the breakdown characteristics on gated diodes with floating gate of 80 nm L_g. A large dependence on W_{fin} is measured even at low voltage levels (Fig. 7.15). At a normalized current level of 1 μA/um, the junction breakdown voltage can be extracted as a function of W_{fin} (Fig. 7.16). When W_{fin} decreases, V_{bd} is seen to remain constant and eventually decrease which is similar to the V_h behavior. This V_{bd} behavior points to a complex 3D-doping profile dependency on W_{fin}.

Further, the impact of W_{fin} on V_h for PMOS devices is larger, which can be explained by the different dependency of the multiplication factor on the junction voltage for electron current M_n (NMOS case) and hole current M_p (PMOS case) as shown in Fig. 7.17 where an analytically calculated value is plotted [Trémouilles (2004)]. M_p increases abruptly around the breakdown voltage, while for NMOS devices a smoother variation of M_n with voltage is obtained. Therefore a shift in V_{bd} for PMOS devices translates almost entirely into a V_h shift, which explains the larger dependence for PMOS devices.

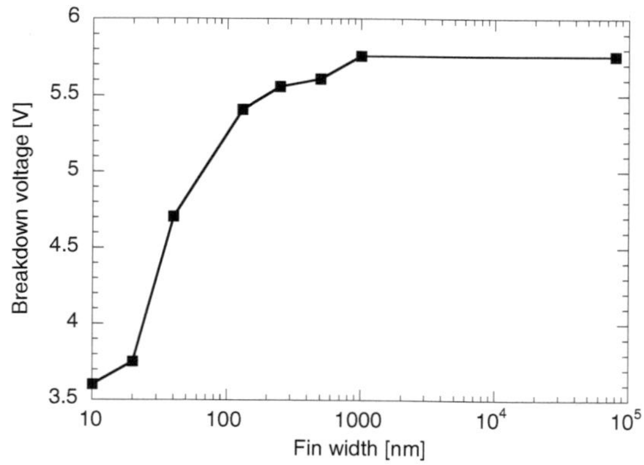

Figure 7.16. Extracted breakdown voltage for gated diodes with floating gate, L_g 80 nm and varying N as a function of W_{fin}. The breakdown voltage is extracted at 1 μA/um.

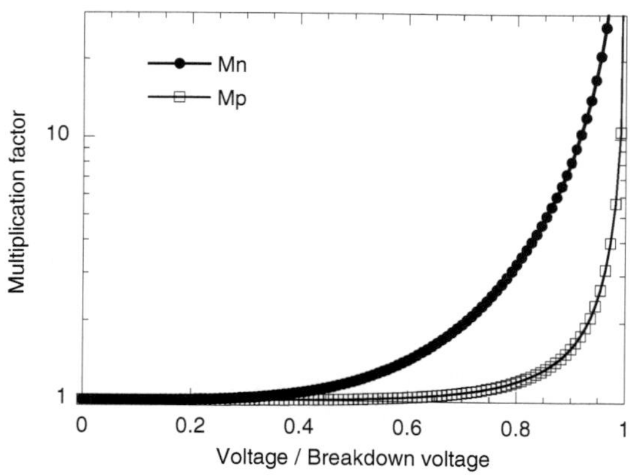

Figure 7.17. Comparison of calculated electron (Mn) and hole (Mp) multiplication factors as a function of voltage normalized to the breakdown voltage, according to [Trémouilles (2004)].

On-resistance R_{on}

R_{on} decreases with decreasing W_{fin} for both NMOS and PMOS devices when normalized to W_{intr}, as seen in Fig. 7.18, for devices with a fixed L_g of 75 nm. For narrow fins, NiSi grows from both the sidewalls and the top, so that the devices can become fully silicided, hence the lower R_{on} [Hoffmann *et al.* (2005)]. A simplified schematic of

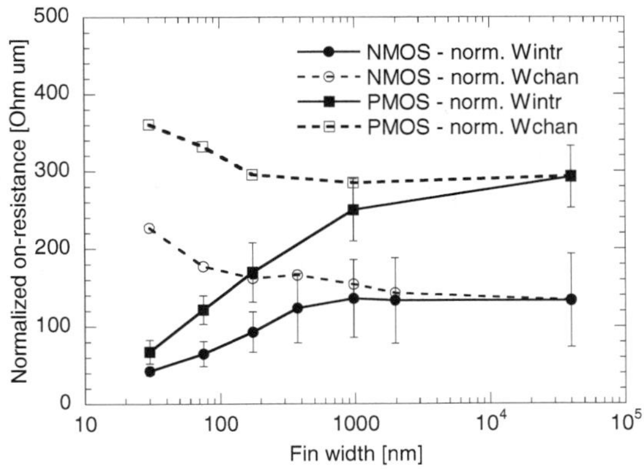

Figure 7.18. ESD on-resistance as a function of fin width for FinFET devices with 75 nm gate length in bipolar mode.

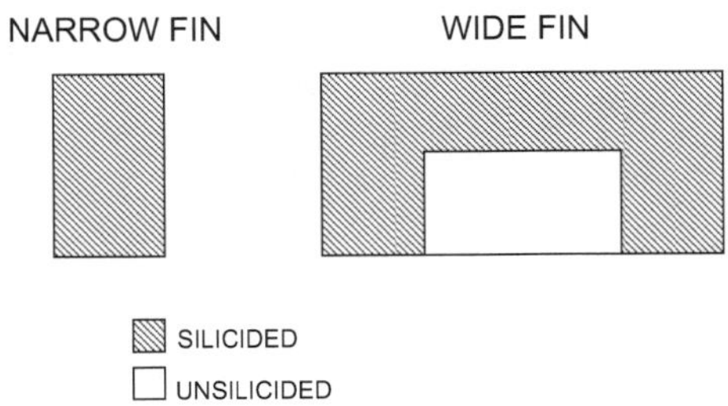

Figure 7.19. Simplified schematic fin cross section, through the fin access region of a fully silicided narrow fin (left) and a partly silicided wide fin (right).

the width-dependent silicidation is shown in Fig. 7.19. The statistical variation of R_{on} increases a lot when increasing the fin width. Since these devices have a gate length of 75 nm, the devices with the largest fin width lack control of SCE. Current starts to conduct already at very low voltages (Fig. 7.6), which makes extraction of the pure bipolar on-resistance very sensitive. For reference, also the normalized R_{on} versus W_{chan} is shown, which is more commonly used in technology-oriented papers. This normalization illustrates the gravity of the problem of series resistance for normal operation in FinFET devices [Dixit *et al.* (2005)], as the resistance increases rapidly for the smallest W_{fin}.

Table 7.1. Measured HBM results on 'large' NMOS and PMOS FinFET devices in bipolar mode. The HBM robustness is normalized to W_{intr}. The shaded cells indicate unexpected low performance

Type	L_g [nm]	W_{fin} [nm]	Number of fins × number of rows	V_{HBM} [kV]	V_{HBM} [V/μm]
NMOS	75	30	400×16	2.4	12.5
NMOS	75	75	400×16	2.7	5.6
NMOS	75	155	400×16	3.5	3.5
NMOS	75	40000	1×16	2	3.1
NMOS	205	40000	1×16	2	3.1
PMOS	75	30	400×16	1.75	9.11
PMOS	75	75	400×16	2.4	5
PMOS	75	155	400×16	3.75	3.8
PMOS	75	40000	1×16	2	3.1
PMOS	205	40000	1×16	**0.7**	**1.1**

7.4.1.3 Number of fins dependence

The scaling of the ESD robustness with the number of fins is verified through both TLP and HBM measurements. Besides changing the number of fins in a single 'finger' device, also a number of different device blocks, *nblocks*, can be placed in parallel, creating a 'multi-finger' device, where the total amount of fins is $N*nblocks$. HBM measurements were performed on 16 parallel blocks of NMOS and PMOS devices with L_g of 75 nm and different W_{fin} ranging from 30 nm to 40 um. The measurement results are summarized in Table 7.1. HBM withstand values of up to 3.75 kV were obtained, indicating scalability of the ESD performance up to levels as required by products. The same trends in terms of HBM performance normalized by W_{intr} as a function of W_{fin}, indicated in the last column of Table 7.1, were obtained as for TLP, see Fig. 7.13. Linear HBM scalability with *nblocks* is demonstrated in Fig. 7.20 for N-type devices where each block consists of 400 fins of each 30 nm W_{fin} and 75 nm L_g. No direct comparison between NMOS and PMOS HBM failure levels should be made in this case as the measurements originate from different wafers. A clear comparison between NMOS and PMOS was already made in the two previous subsections.

As can be seen in Table 7.1, the HBM robustness stays constant for wide fin NMOS devices with increasing L_g, while it suddenly

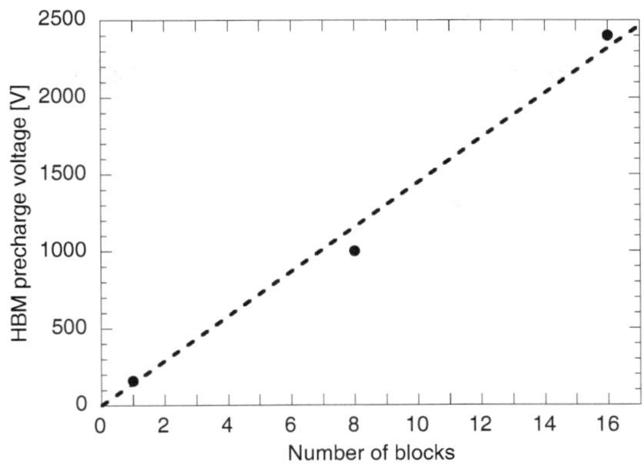

Figure 7.20. HBM robustness scaling as a function of number of blocks for N-type FinFET in bipolar mode with 400 fins of 30 nm W_{fin} and 75 nm L_g.

drops for PMOS, indicated by the shaded cells. These observations are matching the trends obtained from TLP results on single 40 um NMOS and PMOS devices in Fig. 7.8 and Fig. 7.9 respectively, excluding non-uniform failure of the different device blocks of the PMOS devices to be the cause for this sudden decrease in robustness. In Section 7.4.1.1, gate-oxide breakdown at the drain-gate overlap region was put forward as the possible cause for failure for wide fin PMOS devices with large L_g due to their larger holding voltage.

To further substantiate this finding, electrical failure signatures are shown in Fig. 7.21 for NMOS (left) and PMOS (right) devices. The devices have 205 nm L_g and consist of 16 blocks of a 40 um fin. In Fig. 7.21 (left), the NMOS fails during a 2250 V HBM pulse at a current level around 0.2 A. This current level is about 15% of the peak current value. On contrary, for the PMOS device, Fig. 7.21 (right), it fails during a 800 V HBM pulse at a current level of about 67% of the peak current value. This corresponds to a time to failure of roughly 300 ns for the NMOS device and 70 ns for the PMOS. This means that the NMOS fails almost at the end of the pulse, which is typical for power-related failures, while the PMOS fails at the beginning of the pulse, which is typical for voltage-related failures. Further, when analyzing the energy dissipated in the device as a

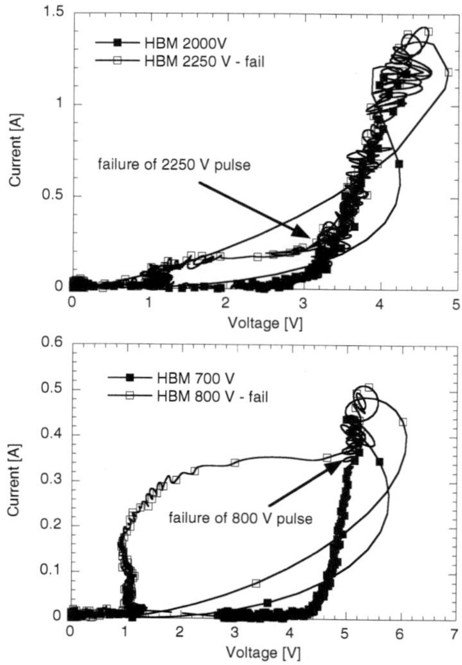

Figure 7.21. HBM-IV curves showing typical failure signatures for NMOS (left) and PMOS (right) in bipolar mode. The devices have 205 nm L_g and 16 blocks of a 40 um fin.

function of time during the HBM pulse according to

$$E(t) = \int V(t)I(t)dt, \tag{7.7}$$

it is found that the total energy dissipated at the end of the pulse increases for the failure pulse compared to previous non-failing pulse in case of NMOS, Fig. 7.22 (left). On the other hand, for the PMOS, Fig. 7.22 (right), the total energy dissipated during the failing pulse is lower than during the previous passing pulse, indicating voltage-failure for the PMOS device.

A different number of parallel blocks of 40 um wide single fin NMOS devices was stressed using TLP in bipolar condition to investigate the current uniformity of multi-block wide fin devices. Increasing the number of blocks from 1 to 4 and 16 reduces the normalized I_{t2} per W_{intr} (Fig. 7.23) which could indicate that some blocks did not turn on. Applying strain by tCESL improves the

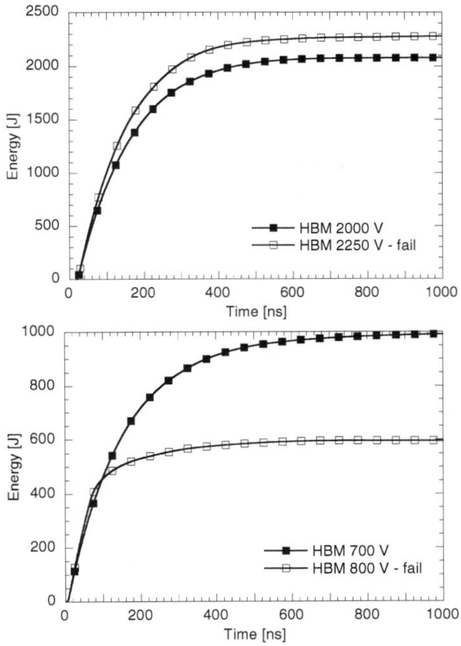

Figure 7.22. Energy dissipated in the device as a function of time during HBM pulses before and after failure, for NMOS (left) and PMOS (right) in bipolar mode. The maximum value at the end of the pulse corresponds to the total energy dissipated in the device during the stress. The devices have 205 nm L_g and 16 blocks of a 40 um fin.

ESD performance. When applying additional ballasting resistance by increasing L_{SD} with 0.4 um each, an increase in I_{t2} is noticed for the 16 parallel blocks. This ballasting resistance improves current uniformity. Strain was found in general to improve the ESD robustness, as described in more detail in Section 7.5.3. Further, when using silicide blocking, as described in Section 7.5.2, not only the robustness of a single fin device improves from 2 mA/um to 3 mA/um, but also the 16 parallel blocks maintain the same normalized ESD performance.

7.4.2 *Gated Diodes*

A cross section of a gated diode is shown in Fig. 7.24 (left) and compared to the MOS-diode (right). The gated diode is sometimes

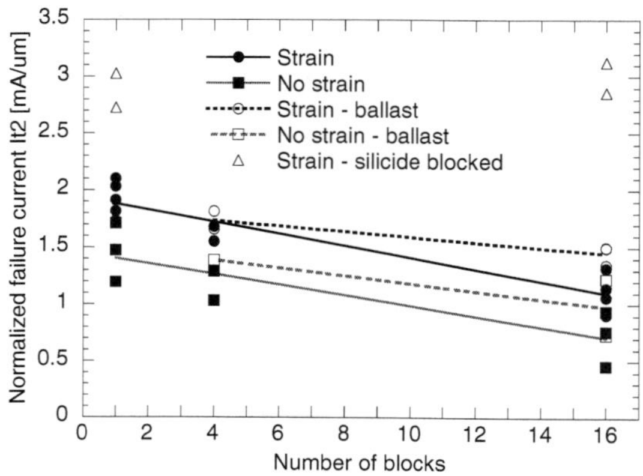

Figure 7.23. Intrinsic normalized failure current of N-type FinFET in bipolar mode as a function of number of blocks of 40 um wide fin devices with 205 nm gate length.

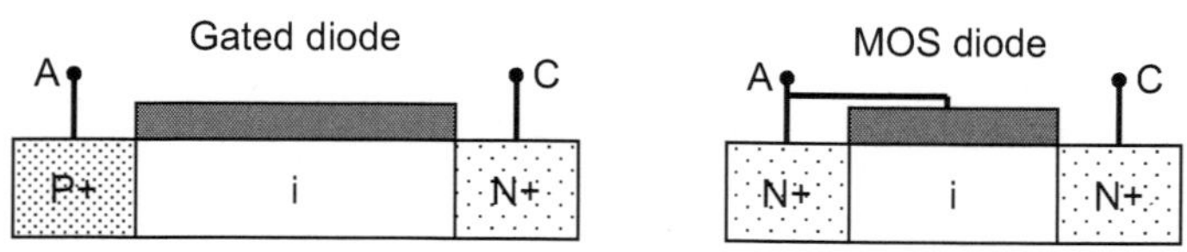

Figure 7.24. Cross-section of gated diode (left) compared to MOS diode (right).

also referred to as poly-diode. The gate of the gated diode is left floating to reduce gate leakage current and parasitic capacitance. The floating gate is also better with respect to the CDM threat [Putnam *et al.* (2004)].

7.4.2.1 Gate length dependence

TLP-IV curves of gated diodes as a function of L_g are compared in Fig. 7.25 with the MOS diode mode. It is clear that gated diodes exhibit an improved I_{t2} and R_{on}, which is optimal for smallest L_g. Note that the gate lengths used for the gated diodes are larger than what can be used for the MOS devices to accommodate for the N+ and P+ doping overlap on the gate due to mask misalignment.

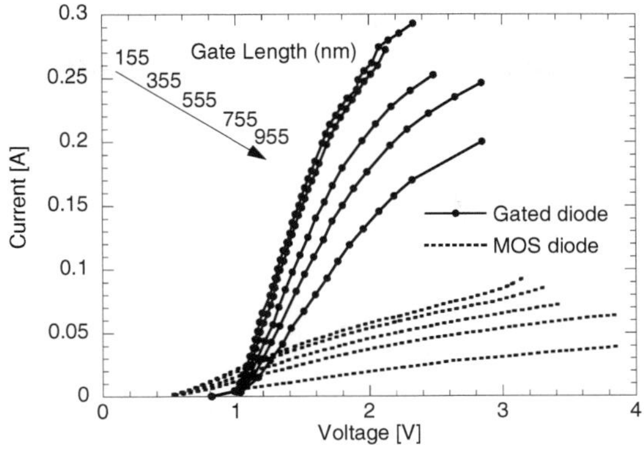

Figure 7.25. TLP-IV curves for different gate lengths of gated diodes in comparison with MOS diode mode. The devices have a fin width of 30 nm and 400 fins in parallel.

7.4.2.2 Fin width dependence

When increasing W_{fin}, I_{t2} normalized per intrinsic silicon width decreases while it increases when considering layout Fig. 7.26, similarly as for the MOS diode mode. Since the leakage current is small for the gated diodes due the larger gate lengths needed, the optimum diode configuration in terms of ESD performance and area consumption is a wide fin diode with the smallest gate length possible.

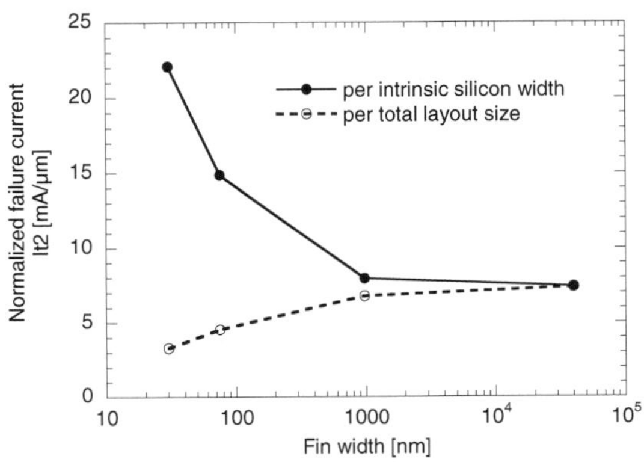

Figure 7.26. Normalized measured I_{t2} as a function of fin width for gated diodes with 555 nm gate length.

7.5 Process Technology Dependencies

The FinFET technology has to cope with some challenges such as a reduced mobility, high S/D access resistance, V_T variability, SCE control. Different process options are introduced to improve these parameters. These process options will also have an impact on the ESD robustness. Therefore, it is important to investigate their influence upfront. In this subsection, the impact of Selective Epitaxial Growth (SEG), Silicide Blocking (SB) and strain is discussed.

7.5.1 *Selective Epitaxial Growth*

For the technology nodes at and below 32 nm, fin widths smaller than 10 nm will be needed to maintain good short channel behavior [Collaert *et al.* (2007a)]. For these narrow fin devices, the access resistance, which is the resistance from the source/drain landing pad to the region underneath the gate, is very high. SEG on source and drain areas is typically used to reduce the contact resistance [Kedzierski *et al.* (2003)] by almost 50%. Due to the increased silicon volume, also the problem of over-silicidation (particularly NMOS) is greatly reduced, because the SEG gets silicided instead of the fin. This leads to a decrease in leakage current by 4 orders of magnitude [Collaert *et al.* (2007b)].

As can be seen in Fig. 7.27, silicon is grown by SEG selectively on all exposed silicon surfaces, i.e., on top of the fins, at the sidewalls of the fin access regions, and on top of the S/D landing pad regions. Where the gate covers the fin (i.e., the channel region), obviously no growth of SEG takes place. Also, SEG does not grow on the gate electrode, since it is protected by a hard mask to avoid bridging between source and drain.

Figure 7.28 and Fig. 7.29 show the influence on narrow fin N- and P-type FinFETs respectively, for different L_g. For both NMOS and PMOS, SEG increases I_{t2} drastically and lowers R_{on}, while the dependency on L_g remains similar. The improved robustness can be mainly attributed to the better heat removal and storage from the drain-body junction of the fin due to the larger fin dimensions in the source and drain access region. The PMOS behavior is less improved by SEG because in general for PMOS FinFET devices the

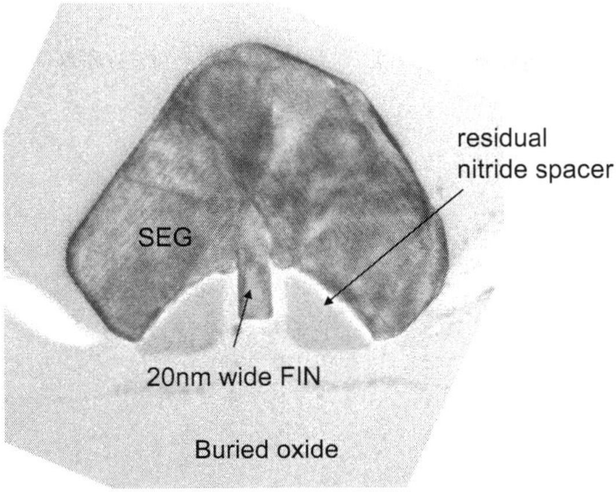

Figure 7.27. Selective Epitaxial Growth (SEG) over one fin.

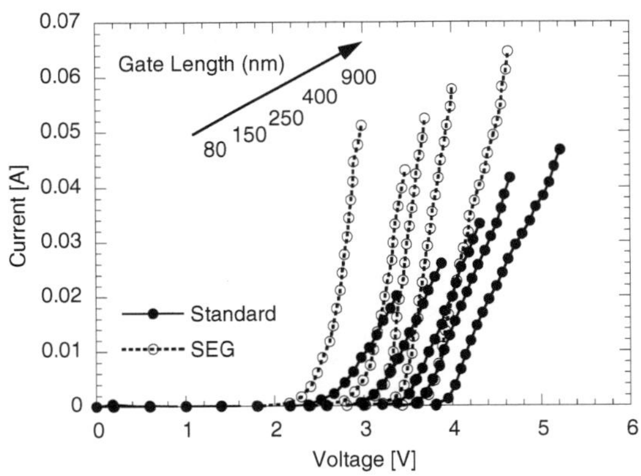

Figure 7.28. TLP-IV curves of N-type FinFET in bipolar mode as a function of gate length for wafers processed with and without SEG. The devices have a fin width of 25 nm and 225 fins in parallel.

contact resistance is not the limiting factor but the lower carrier mobility.

Also the reduction of over-silicidation is a factor which increases I_{t2} for SEG devices due to improved current uniformity. The result is lower measurement variation for SEG devices and a decrease of V_h (Fig. 7.28). The Schottky contact created during over-silicidation

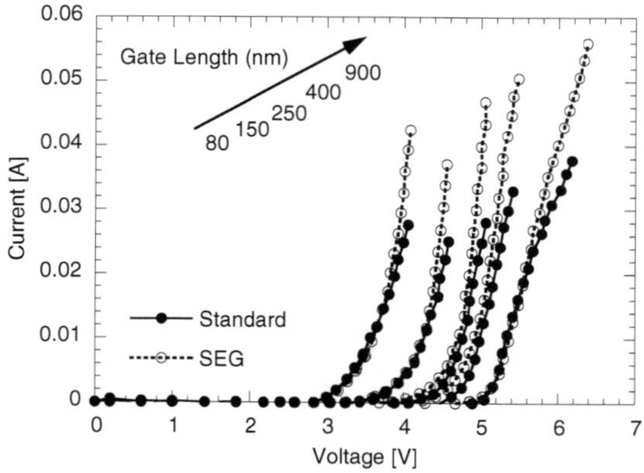

Figure 7.29. TLP-IV curves of P-type FinFET in bipolar mode as a function of gate length for wafers processed with and without SEG. The devices have a fin width of 25 nm and 225 fins in parallel.

is a source for recombination of the carriers generated by impact ionization during turn-on of the parasitic bipolar, lowering its β [Hoffmann *et al.* (2005)]. As a consequence, the required voltage to sustain bipolar operation is lower than when over-silicidation would have occurred. Since the PMOS has less problems with over-silicidation due to the presence of Boron in the P+ S/D regions which slows down the silicidation process, the decrease in V_h is much less pronounced.

Figure 7.30 shows intrinsic normalized I_{t2} for NMOS in bipolar mode from a recent 300 mm FinFET device lot with SEG included in the standard process flow. The devices have a gate length of 45 nm. With SEG, the improved intrinsic I_{t2} due to the 3D-cooling of the fins remains clearly visible as described in Section 7.4.1.2.

However, for this last set of data, two additional process constraints make a direct evaluation of the impact of SEG very difficult. First, due to the testchip design rules, the fin spacing S depends on W_{fin}. For $W_{fin} \leq 40$ nm, the fin pitch is constant at 200 nm, giving a fin spacing of:

$$S = 200\ \text{nm} - W_{fin} \tag{7.8}$$

When $W_{fin} > 50$ nm, the fin spacing itself is constant instead of the fin pitch:

$$S = 300\ \text{nm} \tag{7.9}$$

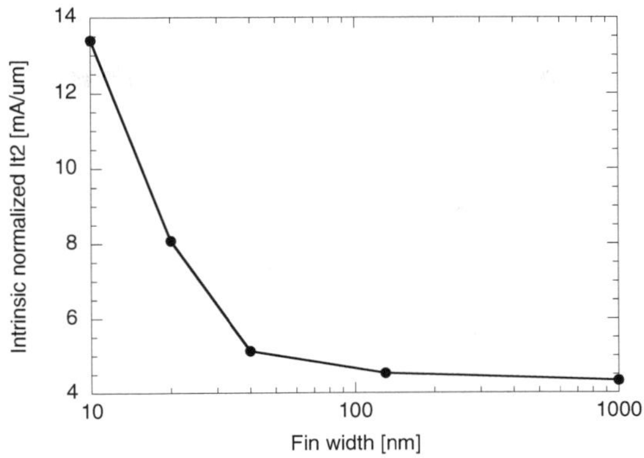

Figure 7.30. Failure current I_{t2} normalized to W_{intr} for NMOS with SEG in bipolar mode. The devices have 45 nm L_g. Narrow fins have intrinsic better I_{t2} performance.

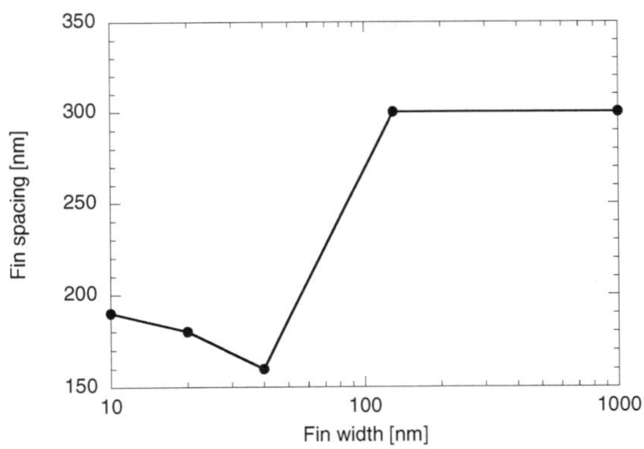

Figure 7.31. Dependence of fin spacing S on W_{fin}.

A graphical representation of the dependence of S on W_{fin} for the devices in Fig. 7.30 is shown in Fig. 7.31. For example, when W_{fin} is decreasing from 40 nm to 10 nm, the fin spacing increases from 160 nm to 190 nm respectively. This increased S will lead to roughly 10% increased intrinsic I_{t2}. This means that the improved performance for narrow fin devices in Fig. 7.30 is not solely due to improved cooling of the fins, but also due to increased fin spacing.

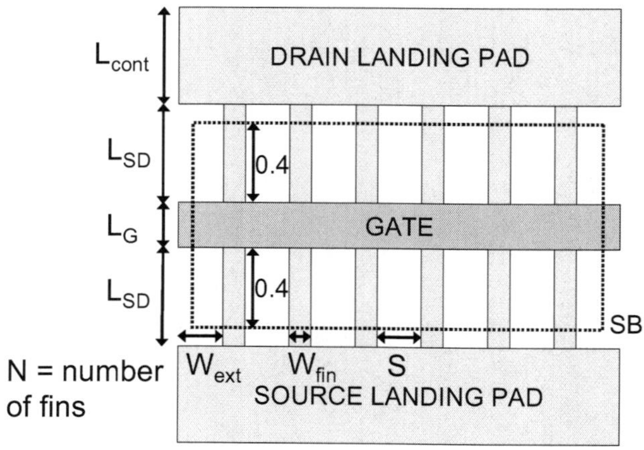

Figure 7.32. Top layout view of a FinFET device including silicide blocking (SB) mask.

Second, the amount of SEG growth depends on the fin width, since it is depending on crystal orientation [Collaert *et al.* (2008)]. In this case, the sidewalls have a {110} orientation with <110> current direction. The actual amount of Si grown on a narrow fin will be smaller than on a wide active area. All these combined elements have to be taken into account when studying the impact of SEG based on the data shown in Fig. 7.30.

7.5.2 *Silicide Blocking*

Silicide Blocking (SB) is known as a technique to improve ESD robustness [Amerasekara and Duvvury (2002)]. A silicide blocking region is applied in the current work to FinFETs which extends 0.4 um over the gate in both direction of source and drain (Fig. 7.32). L_{SD} was increased to accommodate the silicide blocking region. TLP-IV curves are shown in Fig. 7.33 for narrow (left) and wide (right) N-type FinFET devices with and without silicide blocking and in Fig. 7.34 for P-type devices. In the case of NMOS, I_{t2} increases for both narrow and wide devices. For narrow fin devices, the silicide blocking ensures more current uniformity at high current levels among the different fins. However, the leakage current increases progressively, making an accurate determination of I_{t2} difficult. This

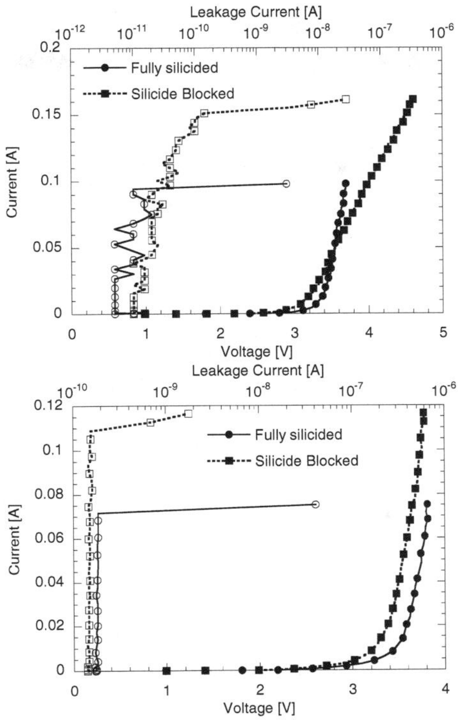

Figure 7.33. TLP-IV curves for narrow (left) and wide (right) fin N-type FinFET devices with and without silicide blocking in bipolar mode with 355 nm gate length. The narrow fin device consists of 400 fins of 30 nm width, while the wide fin device has a single 40 um fin.

could be caused by an increasing number of failed fins. For wide fin NMOS devices, I_{t2} is increased due to the improved uniformity within the single fin, and both the fully silicided and silicide blocked devices fail abruptly. Further, the removal of over-silicidation due to silicide blocking can be seen by the measured decrease in V_h for silicide blocked devices, similar as for SEG, (see Section 7.5.1). Also some over-silicidation seems to be present for wide fin devices, based on their decrease in V_h. On the other hand, SB does not seem to improve I_{t2} for both narrow and wide PMOS devices as seen in Fig. 7.34. A possible explanation could be the occurrence of gate-oxide breakdown as described earlier in Section 7.4.1.1.

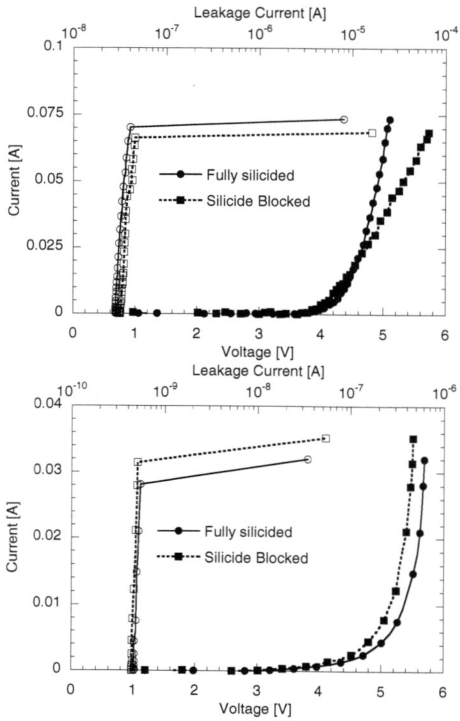

Figure 7.34. TLP-IV curves for narrow (left) and wide (right) fin P-type FinFET devices with and without silicide blocking in bipolar mode with 355 nm gate length. The narrow fin device consists of 400 fins of 30 nm width, while the wide fin device has a single 40 um fin.

7.5.3 *Strain*

TLP measurements are used to provide new insights into the high-current behavior of strained FinFET devices during an ESD event. Using TLP measurements, strain is found to improve the ESD robustness up to 20% in NMOS FinFET devices.

When starting from a {100} silicon wafer with [110] current direction, the electron mobility in narrow fin devices is degraded as the current flows mainly in the sidewalls of the device [Shenai (1991)] [Yang *et al.* (2003)]. These sidewalls have a less favorable crystal orientation compared to the top channel. In order to improve the performance, strain is introduced. For both nMOS and pMOS,

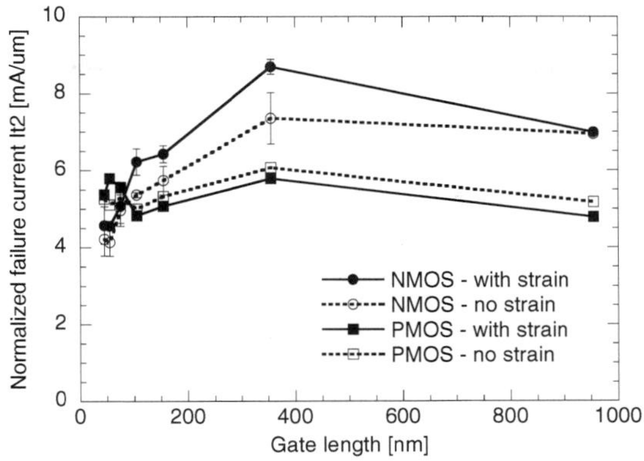

Figure 7.35. Normalized I_{t2} to intrinsic silicon width as a function of gate length for FinFET devices in bipolar mode for wafers with and without tCESL. The devices have a fin width of 30 nm and 400 fins in parallel.

a 100 nm-thick tensile and compressively strained nitride layer with an intrinsic stress of 0.8 GPa were respectively, deposited [Collaert *et al.* (2008)]. A NMOS drive current improvement up to 20% was measured with tensile contact etch stop layer (tCESL). The improvement seen for pMOS due to compressive strain is lower, about 10% [Collaert *et al.* (2008)] [Shin *et al.* (2005)]. Since the PMOS improvement due to compressive strain is only moderate and almost no degradation of the PMOS due to tCESL is measured, a more simple process scheme with only tCESL can be used [Collaert *et al.* (2005)].

The intrinsic normalized I_{t2} for narrow NMOS and PMOS devices with and without tCESL as a function of L_g is shown in Fig. 7.35. An improvement up to 20% in I_{t2} is measured for NMOS devices with medium L_g. Only a slight reduction in I_{t2} is measured for PMOS due to the tCESL. While V_h is unchanged for PMOS, a decreased V_h is measured for NMOS devices with the smallest L_g as seen in Fig. 7.36. This improvement is due to improved electron mobility and is most pronounced for small to medium gate lenghts because they are more impacted by CESL. This improved mobility leads to reduced electric fields, which further improves the high field mobility. The explanation for the most improved I_{t2} for medium L_g for NMOS devices can be found in the extraction of the ESD

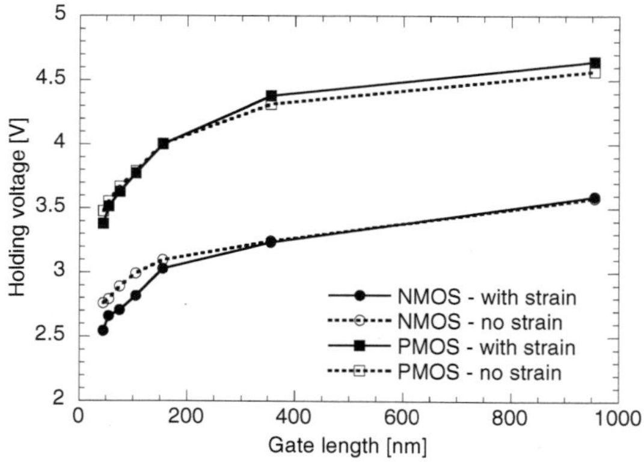

Figure 7.36. Holding voltage of FinFET in bipolar mode as a function of gate length for wafers processed with and without tCESL. The devices have a fin width of 30 nm and 400 fins in parallel.

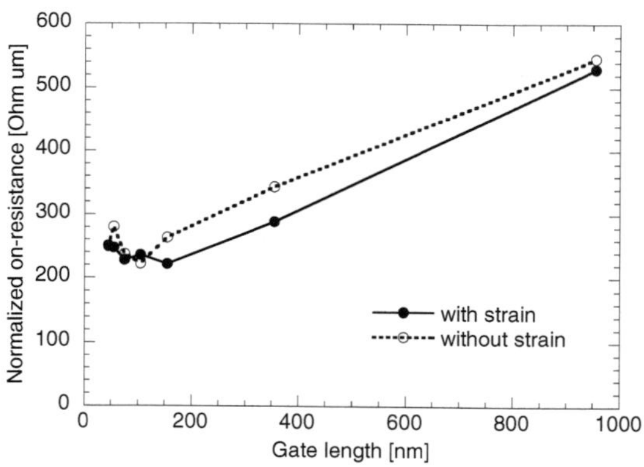

Figure 7.37. ESD on-resistance normalized to total channel width as a function of gate length for narrow N-type FinFET devices with and without tCESL in bipolar mode.

on-resistance R_{on} normalized per W_{chan}, Fig. 7.37. A decrease in R_{on} is measured for NMOS devices with medium L_g, which can be attributed to the mobility improvement due to strain. Since the strain is transferred to the channel via the sides of the source and drain landing pads, for the largest L_g the impact of strain is minimal which results in an unchanged R_{on}. On the other hand, for smallest

L_g, R_{on} is dominated by the access resistance and not by the channel resistance. No difference in heat conduction capability of the strain layer is expected due to the relative low strain level of 800 MPa. Note that SEG will reduce this mobility improvement, since the additional epitaxial grown silicon on the fin increases the distance of the SiN liner to the channel [Collaert *et al.* (2005)] and hence reduces its impact. Yet the advantages of SEG have become very obvious in Section 7.5.1.

7.6 Conclusions

This chapter provides insights into the behavior of FinFET devices under ESD conditions for various layout and process conditions.

Special care has to be taken when normalizing the ESD performance parameters. For physical understanding of ESD behavior in FinFETs, intrinsic silicon width W_{intr} (7.1) should be used. Layout efficiency can be studied using W_{layout} (7.2). ESD robustness of drivers is evaluated using W_{chan} (7.3). For comparison with other technologies, the effective width W_{eff} (7.4) is preferred.

Uniform current conduction is guaranteed in grounded gate MOS devices due to their floating base (no snapback), yielding kV HBM levels for multi-finger multi-fin devices. Some degree of non-uniform failure exists at high current levels which can be improved by increasing gate length and various ballasting techniques. Gated diodes should be drawn as planar-like structures instead of using narrow fins because they have the best performance in terms of I_{t2} per layout due to absence of fin-to-fin spacing overhead. In general, narrow fin devices have improved cooling properties but suffer from reduced area efficiency.

SEG drastically improves I_{t2} and R_{on} and removes any oversilicidation problems. Also Silicide Blocking removes the oversilicidation effect. It further improves I_{t2} due to improved failure current uniformity at the expense of increased R_{on}. Strain also increases I_{t2} by improving the carrier mobility and by improving failure uniformity. FinFET technology development is still facing a lot of process challenges which have a direct impact on the ESD performance of the devices.

All the results demonstrate that the possible extreme sensitivity of FinFET devices would not be a showstopper for the advanced nanotechnologies if ESD is considered during the technology development. However, even with this knowledge, the design of ESD protection for FinFET technology appears to be a challenging task in the future.

References

Vashchenko, V. A. and Sinkevitch, V. F. (2008). *Physical Limitations of Semiconductor Devices* (Springer).

Amerasekara, A. and Duvvury, C. (2002). *ESD in Silicon Integrated Circuits*, 2nd edn. (J. Wiley & Sons).

Collaert, N., Keersgieter, A. D., Anil, K., Rooyackers, R., Eneman, G., Goodwin, M., Eyckens, B., Sleeckx, E., de Marneffe, J., Meyer, K. D., Absil, P., Jurczak, M. and Biesemans, S. (2005). Performance improvement of tall triple gate devices with strained sin layers, *IEEE Electron Dev. Lett*, **26,11**, pp. 820–822.

Collaert, N., Keersgieter, A. D., Dixit, A., Ferain, I., Lai, L., Lenoble, D., Mercha, A., Nackaerts, A., Pawlak, B., Rooyackers, R., Schulz, T., San, K., Son, N., Dal, M. V., Verheyen, P., von Arnim, K., Witters, L., Meyer, K. D., Biesemans, S. and Jurczak, M. (2007a). Multi-gate devices for the 32 nm technology node and beyond, 37th European Solid State Device Research Conference, 2007. ESSDERC 2007, pp. 143–146.

Collaert, N., Rooyackers, R., Dilliway, G., Iyengar, V., Augendre, E., Leys, F., Cayrefourq, I., Ghyselen, B., Loo, R., Jurczak, M. and Biesemans, S. (2007b). Optimization of the mugfet performance on super critical-strained SOI (SC-SSOI) substrates featuring raised source/drain and dual CESL, in *International Symposium on VLSI Technology, Systems and Applications*, pp. 1–2.

Collaert, N., Rooyackers, R., Hikavy, A., Dixit, A., Leys, F., Verheyen, P., Loo, R., Jurczak, M. and Biesemans, S. (2008). Multi-gate devices for the 32nm technology node and beyond: Challenges for selective epitaxial growth, *Thin Solid Films*, **517,1**, pp. 101–104.

Dixit, A., Anil, K., Collaert, N., Goodwin, M., Jurczak, M. and Meyer, K. D. (2005). Analysis of the parasitic source/drain resistance in multiple gate field effect transistors, *IEEE Trans. Electron Dev.* **52,6**, pp. 1132–1140.

Dixit, A., Anil, K., Collaert, N., Zimmerman, P., Jurczak, M. and Meyer, K. D. (2006). Minimization of mugFET source/drain resistance using wrap-around NiSi contacts, *IEEE J. Solid-State Electron.* **50, 7–8**, pp. 1466–1471.

Gossner, H., Russ, C., Siegelin, F., Schneider, J., Schruefer, K., Schulz, T., Duvvury, C., Cleavelin, C. and Xiong, W. (2006). Unique ESD failure mechanism in a MuGFET technology, *IEDM 2006*, pp. 101–104.

Hoffmann, T., Doornbos, G., Ferain, I., Collaert, N., Zimmerman, P., Goodwin, M., Rooyackers, R., Kottantharayil, A., Anil, K., Yim, Y., Jurczak, M. and Biesemans, S. (2005). GIDL and parasitic Schottky barrier leakage elimination in aggressively scaled HfO_2/TiN finFET devices, *IEDM 2005*, pp. 725–728.

Kedzierski, J., Ieong, M., Nowak, E., Kanarsky, T., Zhang, Y., Roy, R., Boyd, D., Fried, D. and Wong, H. P. (2003). Extension and source/drain design for high performance finFET devices, *IEEE Trans. Electron. Dev.* **50,4**, pp. 952–958.

Keppens, B., Wybo, G., Vermont, G. and Camp, B. V. (2006). Concept for body coupling in soi mos transistor to improve multi-finger triggering, EOS/ESD 2006, pp. 172–178.

Maloney, T. and Khurana, N. (1985). Transmission line pulse technique for circuit modeling and ESD phenomena, *EOS/ESD 1985*, pp. 49–54.

Miller, S. L. (1957). Ionization rates for holes and electrons in silicon, *Phys. Rev.* **105**, p. 1246–1249.

Putnam, C., Woo, M., Gauthier, R., Muhammad, M., Chatty, K., Seguin, C. and Halbach, R. (2004). An investigationh of esd protection diode options in SOI, *in Proceedings of the IEEE International SOI Conference*, pp. 24–26.

Russ, C., Gossner, H., Schulz, T., Chaudhary, N., Xiong, W., Marshall, A., Duvvury, C., Schrüfer, K. and Cleavelin, C. (2005). ESD evaluation of the emerging mugFET technology *EOS/ESD 2005*, pp. 280–289.

Russ, C., Gossner, H., Schulz, T., Chaudhary, N., Xiong, W., Marshall, A., Duvvury, C., Schrüfer, K. and Cleavelin, C. (2007). ESD evaluation of the emerging mugFET technology, *IEEE Transaction on Device and Materials Reliability*, **7**, pp. 152–161.

Shenai, K. (1991). Electron mobilities in MOS channels formed along anisotropically dry etched (110) silicon trench sidewalls, *IEEE Electron. Lett.* **27,9**, pp. 715–717.

Shin, K., Chui, C. and King, T. (2005). Dual stress capping layer enhancement study for hybrid orientation nFET CMOS technology, *IEDM 2005*, pp. 1009–1101.

Trémouilles, D. (2004). *Optimisation et modélisation de protections intégrées contre les décharges électrostatiques, par l'analyse de la physique mise en jeu*, Ph.D. thesis, Institut National des Sciences Appliquées de Toulouse, France.

Yang, M., Gusev, E., Ieong, M., Gluschenkov, O., Boyd, D., Chan, K., Kozlowski, P., D'Emic, C., Sicina, R., Jamison, P. and Chou, A. (2003). Performance dependence of CMOS on silicon substrate orientation for ultrathin oxynitride and HfO_2 gate dielectrics, *IEEE Electron Dev. Lett*, **24,5**, pp. 339–341.

Part III

Exploratory Devices and Characterization Tools

Chapter 8

The Junctionless Nanowire Transistor

Bart Sorée,[a,b] Anh-Tuan Pham,[a] Dries Sels,[c] and Wim Magnus[a,b]

[a] *IMEC, Nano Confined Applications and Systems (NCAIS) Department, Physics Modeling and Simulation (MSP) Group, Kapeldreef 75, B-3001 Leuven, Belgium*

[b] *Universiteit Antwerpen, Physics Department, Condensed Matter Theory (CMT) Group, Groenenborgerlaan 171, B-2020 Antwerpen, Belgium*

[c] *Universiteit Antwerpen, Physics Department, Theory of Quantum Systems and Complex Systems (TQS), Universiteitsplein 1, B-2610 Antwerpen, Belgium*

bart.soree@imec.be

In this chapter, the junctionless nanowire transistor is introduced as an alternative device concept to the inversion mode nanowire MOSFET. We first discuss the basic working principle based on an analytical model for long thick nanowires. Then, we scale down the wire radius and discuss the impact of size quantization on the low-field mobility. Next, we also scale down the gate length to investigate the purely ballistic junctionless nanowire and its equivalence to the inversion mode MOSFET nanowire in this regime. Finally, we consider an advanced transport model to investigate the short-channel junctionless nanowire including strain.

CMOS Nanoelectronics: Innovative Devices, Architectures, and Applications
Edited by Nadine Collaert

ISBN 978-981-4364-02-7 (Hardcover), 978-981-4364-03-4 (eBook)
www.panstanford.com

8.1 Introduction

Nanowire field effect transistors are considered to be good candidates to provide at least a partial solution to the scaling problem in micro- and nanoelectronics, in particular gate all around nanowire field effect transistors because the surrounding gate provides the strongest electrostatic control of the channel when compared to other geometries. Due to this strong electrostatic control of the channel it is expected that one can further scale down the gate length before detrimental short channel effects start to kick in. Until recently [1], the main focus was on inversion mode MOSFET nanowires where the source and drain where n^+ doped, while the channel was either intrinsic or p^+ doped for nMOSFET nanowires. Although the nanowire MOSFET holds the promise of excellent scaling properties, there are still some very important stumbling blocks that need to be considered. First of all, when the nanowire MOSFET is in the ON-state the carriers in the channel reside in an inversion layer close to the interface between the substrate and the insulator. As a result surface dominated interactions such as surface roughness scattering will depress the mobility in this regime. When a high-κ insulator is considered one must also account for interface phonons also called "remote phonon" scattering which are detrimental for the mobility [2]. Second, when scaling down the channel or gate length, the fabrication requires very abrupt doping profiles that complicate the production of short channel MOSFET devices.

The first problem involving surface interactions can be solved when one manages to move the charge carriers away from the interface. One possible solution could be to consider a radial heterojunction core-shell GaAs/AlGaAs nanowire [3], but this requires the introduction of advanced processing techniques. Moreover, for such a structure the problem of the abrupt doping profiles would still be still present when considering ultra short gate lengths.

Surprisingly, a rather straightforward solution to the two aforementioned stumbling blocks was already formulated in 1952 when Shockley [4] proposed the junction Field Effect Transistor (JFET) illustrated in Fig. 8.1. The JFET consists of a uniformly doped source, channel and drain region. The gate is a p-type semiconductor

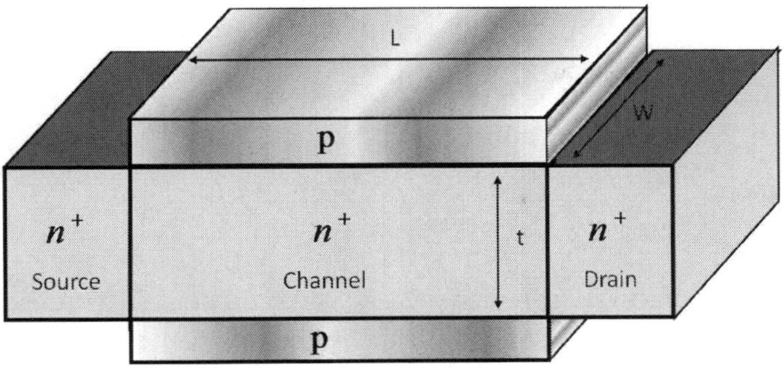

Figure 8.1. Schematic illustration of the junction field effect transistor (JFET). L is the length of the channel under the gate region, W is the width of the device, while t is the body thickness.

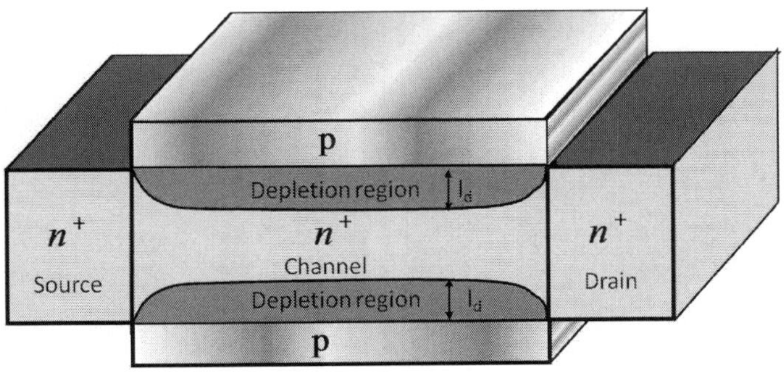

Figure 8.2. Schematic illustration of the junction field effect transistor (JFET) where the depletion region is indicated. The depletion length is denoted by l_d.

in direct contact with the channel region. As a result, a p-n junction is realized at the channel-gate region and the resulting built-in potential provides the barrier that prevents electrons from leaking into the gate. The presence of the built-in potential originating from the p-n junction together with an applied gate voltage will deplete the channel of the JFET as illustrated in Fig. 8.2. Thus, the JFET is essentially a voltage controlled resistor. When no gate bias is applied together with a small source-drain bias V_D the current through the JFET device is given by [4, 5]

$$I_\mathrm{SD} = \frac{q\mu_n N_\mathrm{D} W}{L}(2t - 2l_\mathrm{d})V_\mathrm{D} \tag{8.1}$$

where μ_n is the bulk mobility for the electrons, N_D the positively ionized donors, while l_d is the depletion length. In equilibrium, when no source-drain voltage is applied, the depletion length as a function of gate voltage is determined as

$$l_\mathrm{d} = \left[\frac{2\epsilon_\mathrm{s}(V_\mathrm{bi} - V_\mathrm{G})}{qN_\mathrm{D}}\right]^{1/2}. \tag{8.2}$$

Applying a negative gate voltage ($V_\mathrm{G} < 0$) increases the depletion length l_d. The threshold or pinch-off voltage V_T is easily obtained as the gate voltage for which full depletion occurs, i.e., when $l_\mathrm{d} = t/2$:

$$V_\mathrm{T} = V_\mathrm{bi} - \frac{eN_\mathrm{D}t^2}{2\epsilon_\mathrm{s}}. \tag{8.3}$$

Clearly the JFET provides a solution to both the interface interaction and doping junction problem but this device is not tailored to the current needs for transistor operation. Historically, the main reason for choosing a MOSFET device over a JFET device was the poor gate control over the charge in the channel region of the JFET because the charge carriers are mainly residing in the bulk of the channel and not at the interface in an inversion region close to the gate as is the case in a MOSFET. When the JFET was conceived the typical dimensions and doping densities that were used for this device required gate voltages of several volts in order to switch off (pinch-off) the device. However, when the channel thickness t or the doping density becomes sufficiently small, the required gate voltage to pinch-off the channel becomes comparable to modern standards. Today, the production of nanowire devices with radial dimensions in the nanometre regime has become feasible and the JFET concept may again play a more prominent role as a low power device. Instead of the JFET which contains a p-n junction as the channel-gate interface we instead consider an insulator between the channel and the gate. Initially, this idea was designated the name iJFET (insulator JFET) and was first reported in [1] where the basic working principle was explained by means of an analytical model. Since then, other research groups have been working on this novel device concept [6–11]. In 2010, the first junctionless transistor was fabricated [9] and the new device was eventually designated with the name "junctionless transistor."

8.2 Basic Working Principles of the Junctionless Nanowire Transistor

The junctionless nanowire transistor consists of a uniformly doped source, drain and channel with surrounding oxide and gate as illustrated schematically in Fig. 8.3. Before discussing the operation of the junctionless nanowire under source-drain bias, we first explain how the majority charge carriers in the channel behave when a gate voltage is applied in the absence of a source-drain voltage, i.e., we are considering the junctionless nanowire in equilibrium. In Fig. 8.4 the bandstructure of the cylindrical junctionless nanowire in the radial direction of a cross section in the middle of the channel is schematically depicted for different gate voltages. In order to simplify the discussion we assume that there is no workfunction difference between the metal gate and semiconducting channel material. For zero gate voltage (Fig. 8.4(a)) the Fermi level in the channel is determined by the doping density N_D through the charge neutrality condition. The wire is in the ON-state and the majority carriers are electrons delivered by the ionized donors. When applying a negative gate voltage greater than the threshold or pinch-off voltage the channel will be depleted as

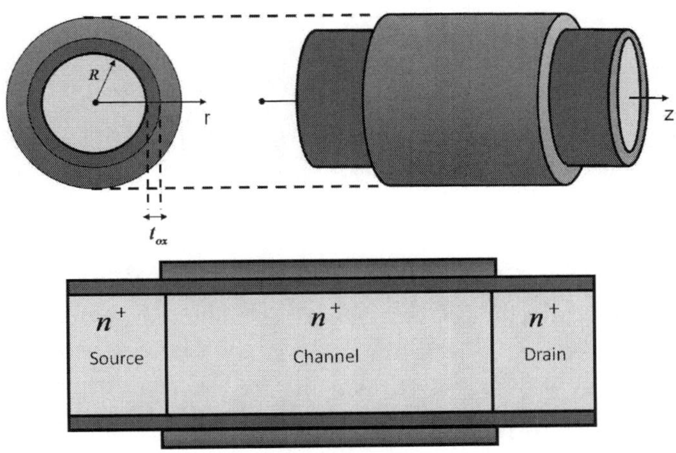

Figure 8.3. Schematic representation of the cylindrical junctionless nanowire.

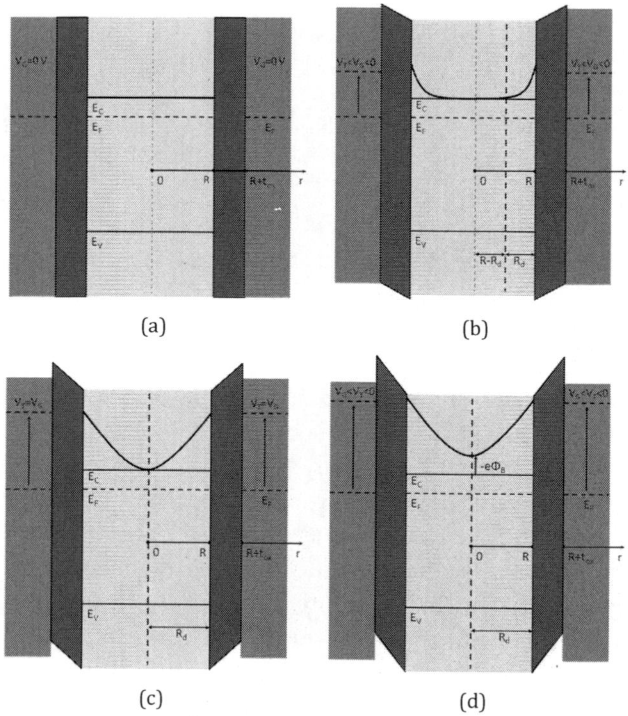

Figure 8.4. Band diagrams for the junctionless nanowire transistor in the radial direction. (a) Flatband. (b) Partial depletion. (c) Full depletion or pinch-off. (d) Subthreshold.

depicted in Fig. 8.4(b) where R_d represents the radial depletion length. For sufficient negative gate voltage equal to the threshold voltage the channel will be fully depleted or pinched off as illustrated in Fig. 8.4(c). The gate voltage V_G at which full depletion occurs will be called the threshold or pinch-off voltage V_T. Further decreasing the gate voltage as indicated in Fig. 8.4(d) creates a potential barrier Φ_B with respect to the source and drain and the wire will operate in the subthreshold regime. In Fig. 8.5 we have also schematically depicted the charge density distribution for the case where the wire is fully open (Fig. 8.5(a)), partially depleted (Fig. 8.5(b)), fully depleted or pinched off (Fig. 8.5(c)) and in subthreshold mode (Fig. 8.5(d)).

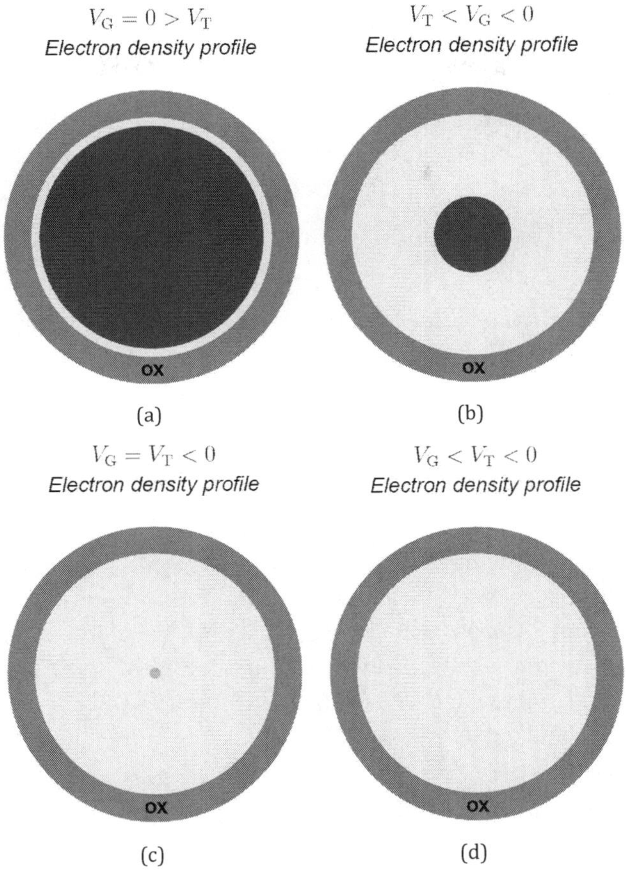

Figure 8.5. Schematic representation of the charge density profile in a cross section of the junctionless nanowire transistor. (a) Flatband (ON-state). (b) Partial depletion. (c) Full depletion or pinch-off. (d) Subthreshold (OFF-state).

When a source-drain bias is applied, the majority carriers in the channel will move under the influence of the generated electric field in the transport direction. For $V_G = 0$, the entire channel is available for the majority carriers because no depletion region is present and the wire is in the ON-state. In this case, the current flows throughout the entire cross section of the channel region. As the gate voltage is decreased, the majority carriers are pushed to the center of the wire leaving behind the fixed positively ionized donors. Now, the current flows mainly in the middle of the wire. Further decreasing the gate voltage will eventually fully deplete or pinch off the wire and when $V_G \leq V_T$ the majority carriers encounter a potential energy barrier $-e\Phi_B$ and the junctionless nanowire transistor is in the OFF or subthreshold state.

8.3 Analytical Model for Long and Thick Nanowires

For long, thick nanowires and a not too large source-drain bias, one can resort to the usual approximations where the charge density profile in the radial direction in the channel is assumed to be abrupt. Furthermore, we assume that the variation of the electrostatic potential profile in the transport direction being the z-direction is sufficiently smooth to make the gradual channel approximation. These approximations yield a great amount of information of how the junctionless nanowire transistor operates in the "classical" regime. It will also bring insight into a number of constraints one needs to keep in mind with regard to doping density, wire radius and threshold voltage.

8.3.1 *The Abrupt Depletion Approximation*

In equilibrium, when no source-drain bias is applied, but where a gate bias can modulate the charge density in the channel, we can assume, in the long-channel approximation, that the electrostatic potential and, hence, the charge density only depends on the radial coordinate. Furthermore, we adopt the abrupt depletion approximation as schematically depicted in Fig. 8.6 for the space charge in the channel, i.e., the charge density is given by

$$\rho(r) = \begin{cases} qN_D, & R - R_d \leq r \leq R \\ 0, & 0 \leq r \leq R - R_d \end{cases} \tag{8.4}$$

where N_D represents the density of ionized donors in the channel, R_d is the depletion length, while $q = +1.602 \times 10^{-19}$ C. We solve the corresponding Poisson's equation assuming long channel and

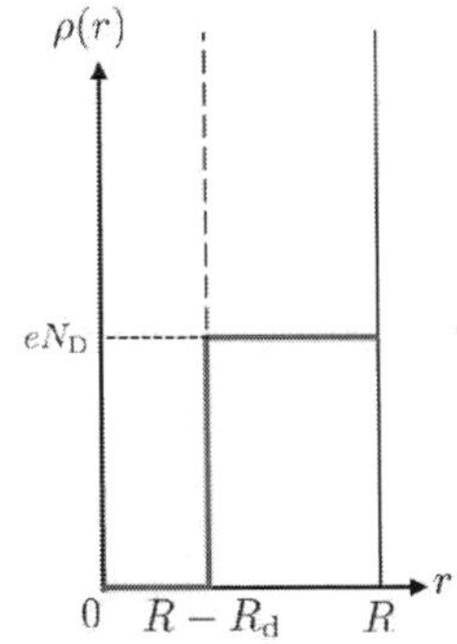

Figure 8.6. Charge density profile in the abrupt depletion approximation.

no source-drain voltage which renders the electrostatic potential $\Phi(r)$ a function of the radial coordinate only, and Poisson's equation reduces to

$$\nabla^2\Phi = \frac{1}{r}\frac{d}{dr}\left(r\frac{d\Phi}{dr}\right) = -\frac{\rho(r)}{\epsilon_{\mathrm{si}}} \tag{8.5}$$

where ϵ_{si} is the permittivity of the silicon channel. The general solution to Eq. (8.5) in the undepleted or neutral region $0 \leq r \leq R - R_{\mathrm{d}}$ of the channel, and in the oxide and gate region is given by

$$\begin{aligned}\Phi(r) &= 0 \quad 0 \leq r \leq R - R_{\mathrm{d}}\\ \Phi(r) &= -\frac{qN_{\mathrm{D}}}{4\epsilon_{\mathrm{si}}}(r^2 - (R - R_{\mathrm{d}})^2)\\ &\quad + \frac{qN_{\mathrm{D}}}{2\epsilon_{\mathrm{si}}}(R - R_{\mathrm{d}})^2 \ln\frac{r}{R - R_{\mathrm{d}}} \qquad R - R_{\mathrm{d}} \leq r \leq R\end{aligned} \tag{8.6}$$

while in the oxide region

$$\begin{aligned}\Phi_{\mathrm{ox}}(r) &= \frac{qN_{\mathrm{D}}}{2\epsilon_{\mathrm{ox}}}(R_{\mathrm{d}}^2 - 2RR_{\mathrm{d}})\ln\frac{r}{R} + \frac{qN_{\mathrm{D}}}{2\epsilon_{\mathrm{si}}}(R_{\mathrm{d}} - R_{\mathrm{d}})^2 \ln\frac{R}{R - R_{\mathrm{d}}}\\ &\quad + \frac{qN_{\mathrm{D}}}{4\epsilon_{\mathrm{si}}}(R_{\mathrm{d}}^2 - 2RR_{\mathrm{d}}) \quad R \leq r \leq R + t_{\mathrm{ox}}\end{aligned}$$

where ϵ_{ox} is the oxide permittivity. To connect the electrostatic gate potential with the depletion length we make use of the boundary condition $V_{\mathrm{G}} = \Phi_{\mathrm{ox}}(R + t_{\mathrm{ox}})$ which results in

$$V_{\mathrm{G}} = -\gamma(R^2 - (R - R_{\mathrm{d}})^2) + 2\alpha(R - R_{\mathrm{d}})^2 \ln\frac{R}{R - R_{\mathrm{d}}} \tag{8.7}$$

where

$$\gamma = \alpha + \beta \ln \frac{R + t_{\mathrm{ox}}}{R}, \quad \alpha = \frac{q N_{\mathrm{D}}}{4\epsilon_{\mathrm{si}}} \quad \text{and} \quad \beta = \frac{q N_{\mathrm{D}}}{2\epsilon_{\mathrm{ox}}}. \tag{8.8}$$

Solving Eq. (8.7) for $R - R_{\mathrm{d}}$ then yields the following expression for the radius of the conducting part of the channel:

$$R - R_{\mathrm{d}} = \left[-\frac{V_{\mathrm{G}} + \gamma R^2}{\alpha W\left(-\dfrac{V_{\mathrm{G}} + \gamma R^2}{\alpha R^2 e^{\gamma/\alpha}} \right)} \right]^{1/2} \tag{8.9}$$

where $W(z)$ is the Lambert W-function which is the inverse of the function $f(W) = We^W$ [12]. The depletion length R_{d} is a function of the gate voltage V_{G}, radius R, oxide thickness t_{ox}, doping density N_{D} and permittivities of the channel and insulator ϵ_{Si} and ϵ_{ox}. The required gate voltage for full depletion when no source-drain bias is applied is obtained by setting $R - R_{\mathrm{d}} = 0$ in Eq. (8.9) resulting in the following expression for the threshold or pinch-off voltage:

$$V_{\mathrm{T}} = -\gamma R^2. \tag{8.10}$$

In Fig. 8.7 we show a plot of the pinch-off or threshold voltage for different wire radii as a function of doping density. As expected, when the wire radius increases for fixed doping density, or when the doping density increases for fixed radius, a more negative gate voltage is required in order to fully deplete (pinch-off) the wire.

8.3.2 *The Gradual Channel Approximation: Current Above Threshold*

In this section we calculate and discuss the current–voltage characteristics in the gradual channel approximation, which requires the channel length to be sufficiently large. Considering a nanowire device where the source is at ground potential $V_{\mathrm{S}} = 0$, while the drain end is at positive potential V_{D}, the channel will be subject to a potential profile $V(z)$ in response to the applied source-drain voltage. In the gradual channel approximation [5], the depletion

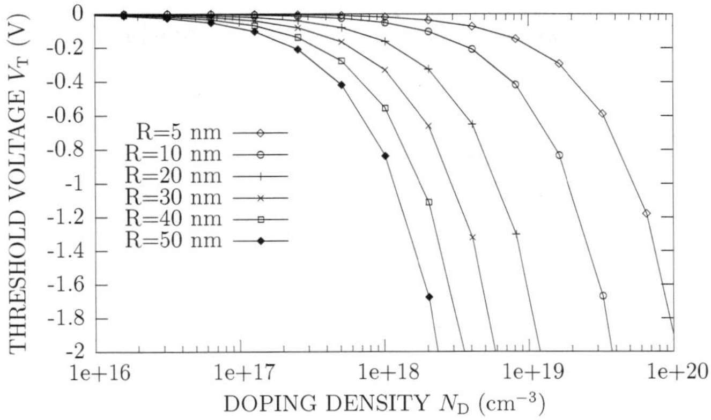

Figure 8.7. Threshold or pinch-off voltage as a function of doping density for different wire radii.

length (8.9) then also becomes a function of z by replacing V_G with $V_G - V(z)$:

$$R - R_d(z) = \left[-\frac{V_G + \gamma R^2 - V(z)}{\alpha W \left(-\frac{V_G + \gamma R^2 - V(z)}{\alpha R^2 e^{\gamma/\alpha}} \right)} \right]^{1/2} \quad (8.11)$$

For positive $V_D > 0$, the junctionless nanowire transistor is turned off when pinch off (full depletion) occurs at the source, i.e., when $R - R_D(0) = 0$. This is realized when $V_G = V_T = -\gamma R^2$. When $V_D > 0$ is sufficiently large such that the drain end is pinched off, i.e., $R - R_d(L)$, the current saturates.

To calculate the source-drain current I_{SD} above threshold we start with the observation that the infinitesimal contribution to the resistance of a volume element with length dz is given by:

$$\frac{dz}{q\mu_n N_D \pi (R - R_d(z))^2} \quad (8.12)$$

where the z-dependent depletion length $R_d(z)$ is, of course, given by Eq. (8.11) Making use of the infinitesimal voltage drop $dV(z) =$

$I_{\mathrm{SD}} d R(z)$ we obtain after integration:

$$I_{\mathrm{SD}} = \zeta \int_0^{V_{\mathrm{D}}} dV \left[\frac{V_{\mathrm{G}} - V + \gamma R^2}{\alpha W \left(-\frac{V_{\mathrm{G}} - V + \gamma R^2}{\alpha R^2 e^{\gamma/\alpha}} \right)} \right] \tag{8.13}$$

where we have introduced the parameter $\zeta = q\mu_n N_{\mathrm{D}}\pi/L$. Making use of the following integral identity for the Lambert W-function:

$$\int du \, \frac{u}{W(u)} = \frac{1}{4} e^{2W(u)} (2W(u) + 1) \tag{8.14}$$

we obtain

$$I_{\mathrm{SD}} = \zeta \alpha e^{2\gamma/\alpha} R^4 \frac{1}{4} \left[e^{2W(u)} (2W(u) + 1) \right]_{u_0}^{u_1} \tag{8.15}$$

where the integration boundaries are given by

$$u_0 = -\frac{V_{\mathrm{G}} + \gamma R^2}{\alpha R^2 e^{\gamma/\alpha}}, \quad u_1 = -\frac{V_{\mathrm{G}} + \gamma R^2 - V_{\mathrm{D}}}{\alpha R^2 e^{\gamma/\alpha}} \tag{8.16}$$

8.3.2.1 Flatband condition: $V_{\mathrm{G}} = 0$

In the case where $V_{\mathrm{G}} = 0$ for sufficiently small V_{D}, in particular $|V_{\mathrm{D}}| \ll \gamma R^2$ it is possible to obtain the following straightforward result from Eq. (8.15) after linearization w.r.t. V_{D} (linear response) for the source-drain current:

$$I_{\mathrm{SD}} \approx \zeta R^2 V_{\mathrm{D}} = \frac{q\mu_n N_{\mathrm{D}}}{L} \pi R^2 V_{\mathrm{D}}. \tag{8.17}$$

Of course this result can also be obtained by making the observation that for $V_{\mathrm{G}} = 0$ the channel of the junctionless nanowire transistor is fully open, i.e., no depletion region is present. Assuming that the current density $J = q N_{\mathrm{D}} \mu_n E$ with $E = V_{\mathrm{D}}/L$ is homogeneously distributed throughout the entire channel region for small V_{D}, and making use of the fact that the entire cross-sectional area is available for the charge carriers, the current is obtained as

$$I_{\mathrm{SD}} = J \times \pi R^2 \tag{8.18}$$

which agrees with Eq. (8.17). For sufficiently high V_{D} the current will saturate and becomes:

$$I_{\mathrm{SDsat}} = -\zeta \frac{R^4}{4} (-2\gamma + \alpha) = -\frac{q\mu_n N_{\mathrm{D}} \pi}{4L} R^4 (-2\gamma + \alpha) \tag{8.19}$$

which for small oxide thickness relative to the wire radius ($t_{ox} \ll R$) approximately reduces to

$$I_{\mathrm{SDsat}} = \frac{q\mu_{\mathrm{n}} N_{\mathrm{D}}\pi}{4L}\alpha R^4. \tag{8.20}$$

8.3.2.2 Depletion: $V_{\mathrm{G}} < 0$

When the gate potential is nonzero the current in the linear and saturation regime can be expressed in terms of the Lambert W-function. In the linear regime this yields

$$I_{\mathrm{SD}} \approx -\zeta R^2 e^{\gamma/\alpha} \frac{u_0}{W(u_0)} V_{\mathrm{D}} \tag{8.21}$$

where

$$u_0 = -\frac{V_{\mathrm{G}} + \gamma R^2}{\alpha R^2 e^{\gamma/\alpha}} \tag{8.22}$$

while in saturation we obtain

$$I_{\mathrm{SDsat}} = -\zeta \alpha e^{2\gamma/\alpha} R^4 \frac{1}{4} \left[e^{2W(u_{\mathrm{sat}})}(2W(u_{\mathrm{sat}}) + 1)\right] \tag{8.23}$$

where due to $V_{\mathrm{Dsat}} = V_{\mathrm{G}} - V_{\mathrm{T}}$

$$u_0(V_{\mathrm{G}} = V_{\mathrm{T}} + V_{\mathrm{Dsat}}) = u_{\mathrm{sat}} = -\frac{V_{\mathrm{Dsat}}}{\alpha R^2 e^{\gamma/\alpha}}. \tag{8.24}$$

8.3.3 *Subthreshold Current*

The subthreshold current is obtained by assuming that only the diffusion component contributes to the current. The current density is then obtained from

$$J = qD_n \frac{\partial n(r, z)}{\partial z} \approx qD_n \frac{n_1(r) - n_2(r)}{L} \tag{8.25}$$

where D_n is the diffusion constant and n_1, n_2 are the electron densities at $z = 0$ and $z = L$, respectively. The total current is then obtain by integrating over the cross section:

$$I = \frac{qD_n}{L} 2\pi \int_0^R dr\, r[n(r, 0) - n(r, L)] \tag{8.26}$$

where $n(r, z)$ is the electron density with

$$n(r, 0) = N_{\mathrm{D}} \exp(-q|\Phi_B|/kT)) \exp\left(\frac{-q^2 N_{\mathrm{D}}}{4kT\epsilon_{\mathrm{Si}}} r^2\right) \tag{8.27}$$

$$n(r, L) = N_\mathrm{D} \exp(-q(|\Phi_B| + |V_D|)/kT) \exp\left(\frac{-q^2 N_\mathrm{D}}{4kT\epsilon_\mathrm{Si}} r^2\right) \tag{8.28}$$

The integration in Eq. (8.26) is straightforward and for $\xi R^2 \gg 1$ the following result is obtained:

$$I_\mathrm{SD} \approx \frac{\pi \mu_n kT}{\xi L} e^{-e|\Phi_\mathrm{B}|/kT} \left[1 - e^{-|V_\mathrm{D}/kT}\right] \tag{8.29}$$

where $\xi = e^2 N_\mathrm{D}/4kT\epsilon_\mathrm{si}$ and the Einstein relation $D_n = kT\mu_n/q$ is used. From the expression (8.29) for the subthreshold current we can easily derive the subthreshold slope:

$$SS = \left[\frac{d \log_{10} I_\mathrm{SD}}{dV_\mathrm{G}}\right]^{-1}. \tag{8.30}$$

In order to do so, it is important to realize that the dependence of the subthreshold current on V_G is hidden in the barrier potential Φ_B. The relation between the potential energy barrier Φ_B and the gate voltage is given by

$$\Phi_\mathrm{B} = V_\mathrm{G} - V_\mathrm{T}, \quad V_\mathrm{G} \leq V_\mathrm{T}. \tag{8.31}$$

Taking the derivative of log I_SD w.r.t. V_G then yields:

$$\begin{aligned} \left(\frac{d \log_{10} I_\mathrm{SD}}{dV_\mathrm{G}}\right)^{-1} &= \left[\frac{d}{dV_\mathrm{G}} \log_{10}\left(e^{-q|\Phi_\mathrm{B}|/kT}\right)\right]^{-1} \\ &= \left[\frac{q}{kT} \log_{10} e \frac{d\Phi_\mathrm{B}}{dV_\mathrm{G}}\right]^{-1} \\ &= \frac{kT}{q \log_{10} e} = 60 \text{ mV/dec} \end{aligned} \tag{8.32}$$

at room temperature.

8.3.4 *Discussion*

The analytical model described above for thick and long junctionless nanowires yields a great deal of insight into the basic working principle of the junctionless nanowire transistor. The current–voltage characteristics are schematically depicted in Fig. 8.8. First of all, it is rather striking to see that the typical current–voltage characteristics are very similar to a MOSFET transistor. Both the junctionless and MOSFET nanowire transistor exhibit a linear

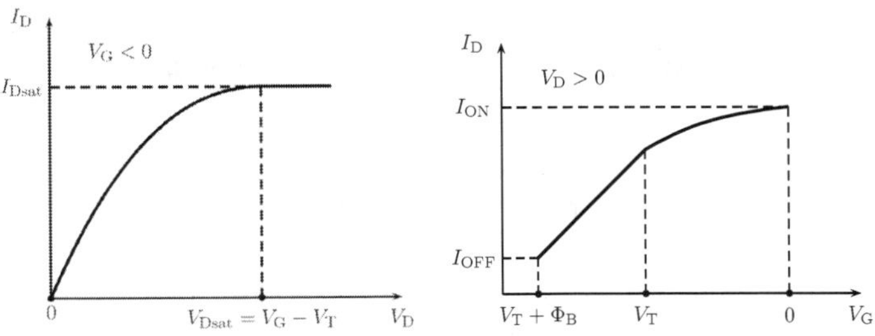

(a) (b)

Figure 8.8. Schematic representation of the current versus (a) source-drain voltage and (b) gate voltage. In (b) the current scale is logarithmic resulting in a constant 60 mv/dec slope for the subthreshold regime.

regime for V_D sufficiently small and saturate when $V_D = V_G - V_T$. In the case of the junctionless transistor the threshold voltage V_T is given by Eq. (8.10) representing the required gate voltage to fully deplete the wire, while in the case of a nanowire MOSFET the threshold voltage is defined as the gate voltage at which an inversion layer starts to be formed. Second, note that both the above threshold and subthreshold current are proportional to the bulk mobility μ_n of the charge carriers in the nanowire. The bulk mobility of course depends on the amount of doping in the channel. For an intrinsic silicon nanowire the bulk mobility of the charge carriers (electrons) is approximately 1300 cm^2/Vs. Increasing the doping density to about 10^{19} cm^{-3} reduces the intrinsic bulk mobility to about 100 cm^2/Vs. The current in the junctionless nanowire transistor thus depends on the amount of doping through the mobility. On the other hand the current above threshold is proportional to the doping density N_D. Increasing the doping by from intrinsic (10^{14} cm^{-3}) to 10^{19} cm^{-3}, i.e., by five orders of magnitude, only decreases the mobility by a factor of 10. At a first glance, one would be tempted to dope the wire as heavily as possible. However, the threshold voltage V_T is also a function of doping density. In particular, the absolute value of the threshold voltage $|V_T|$ increases as the doping density is increased. Because we have neglected the work function difference between the gate region and the channel, the threshold voltage corresponds to the required gate voltage sweep required to go from flatband (ON) to full depletion (subthreshold, OFF). Obviously, one would like to keep this gate sweep limited (typically smaller than 1 V). Increasing the doping density thus results in a larger required gate sweep to turn the device from ON to OFF. In order to keep the V_T constant one may decrease the wire radius R, but this will in turn have an impact on the current. In particular, the flatband current (8.17) for the ON-state of the junctionless nanowire transistor is proportional to R^2 and will decrease correspondingly when the doping is increased while keeping the threshold voltage fixed.

8.4 Low-Field Mobility Modeling for Long Thin Junctionless Nanowires

Now that we have obtained some insight into the macroscopic behavior of the junctionless nanowire transistor we turn our attention to the properties of this device when one or more dimensions are scaled down. Here, we will focus on ultrathin nanowires whose radius becomes so small that quantum mechanical size quantization becomes important. Due to size quantization, a number of essential properties change. In the first instance, the electronic structure now consists of energy subbands with associated eigenfunctions obtained from a self-consistent Poisson–Schrödinger problem. This will impact the charge density profile such that the abrupt depletion approximation is not valid anymore. Also the low-field mobility will be influenced by size quantization. In addition, the bulk mobilities obtained as a function of donor doping density no longer hold. First of all, because of the inherent change of the electronic structure when size quantization is important, as well as due to an additional scattering mechanism: surface roughness scattering. Whereas for the macroscopic junctionless nanowire the surface roughness scattering component could be neglected because the majority of the charge carriers are residing throughout the volume of the channel and not at the interface between the channel and insulator, the ultrathin nanowire will be affected quite strongly depending on the radius of the wire and the parameters that characterize surface roughness.

8.4.1 Quantum Mechanical Electronic Structure of the Junctionless Nanowire

In order to calculate the low-field mobility, we need the electronic structure of the cylindrical nanowire in equilibrium when no source-drain voltage is applied. The corresponding energy eigenvalues or subband spectrum together with the eigenfunctions are are a solution to the self-consistent Poisson–Schrödinger problem. The Schrödinger equation can be expressed in cylindrical coordinates for electrons and holes:

$$-\frac{\hbar^2}{2m_{\alpha\perp}}\left[\frac{1}{r}\frac{d}{dr}\left(r\frac{d}{dr}\right)+\frac{1}{r^2}\frac{\partial^2}{\partial\phi^2}\right]\Psi \\ -\frac{\hbar^2}{2m_{\alpha z}}\frac{\partial^2}{\partial z^2}\Psi+U_{\mathrm{e}}(r)\Psi=\epsilon\Psi \tag{8.33}$$

$$-\frac{\hbar^2}{2m_{\beta}}\left[\frac{1}{r}\frac{d}{dr}\left(r\frac{d}{dr}\right)+\frac{1}{r^2}\frac{\partial^2}{\partial\phi^2}+\frac{\partial^2}{\partial z^2}\right]\Psi+U_{\mathrm{h}}(r)\Psi=\epsilon\Psi \tag{8.34}$$

where $m_{\alpha\perp} = 2m_{\alpha x}m_{\alpha y}/(m_{\alpha x} + m_{\alpha y})$, $m_{\alpha i}$ $(i = x, y, z)$ are the effective masses of the twofold degenerate conduction band valleys $(\alpha = 1, 2, 3)$ of silicon in the x, y and z directions, while m_β $(\beta = 1, 2, 3)$ are the effective masses of the hole valence bands (light, heavy and split-off band) of silicon. Equations (8.33) and (8.34) also contain potential energy terms $U_{\mathrm{e}}(r, z) = -e\Phi(r, z)$ and $U_{\mathrm{h}}(r, z) = e\Phi(r, z)$ which are determined self-consistently with Poisson's equation:

$$\nabla^2\Phi = -\frac{\rho}{\epsilon_{\mathrm{Si}}} = -\frac{1}{\epsilon_{\mathrm{Si}}}[N_{\mathrm{D}}^{+}(r) - N_{\mathrm{A}}^{-}(r) + p(r) - n(r)]. \tag{8.35}$$

Throughout the present calculation we again adopt the long-channel approximation and as a result, the potential energy term as well as the charge density do not depend on the axial coordinate z and are only dependent on the radial coordinate. Due to axial symmetry, the wave functions can be factorized as $\Psi_{k\nu\alpha}(r, \phi, z) = F_{\nu\alpha}(r)e^{im\phi}e^{ikz}$ with $m = 0, \pm1, \pm2, \ldots$, while ν is shorthand for $\nu = n, m$. The self-consistent Poisson–Schrödinger problem then reduces to calculating the radial part $F_{\nu\alpha}(r)$ of the wave function. The electron and hole densities are obtained from

$$n(r) = 2 \times \sum_{k\nu\alpha} g_\alpha |F_{\nu\alpha}(r)|^2 f_{\mathrm{e}}(E_{\mathrm{C}} + E_{\nu\alpha}(k)) \tag{8.36}$$

$$p(r) = 2 \times \sum_{k\nu\beta} |G_{\nu\beta}(r)|^2 f_{\rm h}(E_{\rm V} + E_{\nu\beta}(k)) \qquad (8.37)$$

where $f_{\rm e}(E) = 1/(1 + \exp(\beta_{\rm e}(E - E_{\rm F})))$ and $f_{\rm h}(E) = 1 - f_{\rm e}(E)$ are the Fermi–Dirac distributions for electrons and holes respectively, while $E_{\rm C}$ and $E_{\rm V}$ denote the conduction and valence band minima and $g_\alpha = 2$ is the valley degeneracy factor for the conduction band valleys of silicon. The Fermi level $E_{\rm F}$ is determined by requiring global charge neutrality in the wire, that is

$$\int_0^R dr\, r[n(r) + N_{\rm A}^-(r)] = \int_0^R dr\, r[p(r) + N_{\rm D}^+(r)]. \qquad (8.38)$$

In Figs. 8.9 and 8.10 a plot of the electronic structure and electron density for the junctionless nanowire transistor is depicted for $R =$ 5 nm for gate voltages ranging from flatband ($V_{\rm G} = 0$ V) to pinch-off ($V_{\rm G} = V_{\rm T}$). The pinch-off voltage is approximately $V_{\rm T} \approx -0.95$ V corresponding to a doping density of $N_{\rm D} = 10^{20}$ cm^{-3}.

8.4.1.1 Flatband condition

When the junctionless nanowire FET is in the flatband condition, i.e., $V_{\rm G} = 0$ the solution of the self-consistent Poisson–Schrödinger problem turns into the well known standard mathematical problem when we make the approximation that the electrostatic potential $\Phi = 0$. Moreover, because we are considering a nanowire channel with considerable doping density $N_{\rm D}$, the hole density can be neglected and we only need to consider the electrons. In this case the solutions to the Schrödinger equation for the electrons are Bessel functions and the discrete energy spectrum and eigenfunctions are given by

$$\Psi_{mn\alpha}(r, \phi, z) = C_{mn} e^{ikz} e^{im\phi} J_n\left(\frac{x_{mn} r}{R}\right) \qquad (8.39)$$

$$E_{nm\alpha}(k) = \frac{\hbar^2 k^2}{2m_{\alpha z}} + \frac{\hbar^2 x_{mn}^2}{2m_{\alpha\perp} R^2} \qquad (8.40)$$

where the x_{mn} are the Bessel zeroes and where the C_{mn} are normalization constants. Note that this is an approximation in the sense that we assume there exists a flatband state. The reader will immediately notice that although the Fermi level in the gate region

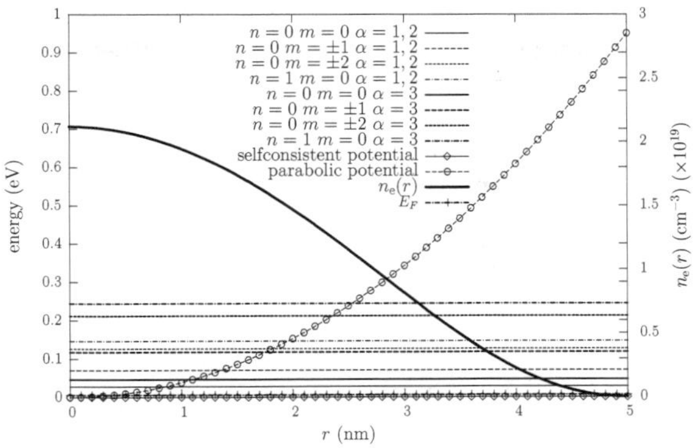

Figure 8.9. Electronic structure of a junctionless nanowire with radius $R = 5$ nm for $V_G = 0$ V (fully open, no depletion). Shown in the figure is the sub band structure for a limited amount of energy eigenvalues, the self-consistent potential energy and the electron density profile.

is aligned with the Fermi level in the channel, hard wall confinement of the charge carriers which is reflected in the boundary condition that the wave function vanish at the interface $r = R$ will make both the electron and hole density inhomogeneous. As a result, the electrostatic potential which can be derived from Poisson's equation can never by constant for $0 \leq r \leq R$. Nevertheless, we persist on using the flatband as an approximation of the real electrostatic potential. It turns out that the numerical result obtained when $V_G = 0$ agrees very well with the flatband approximation. In Fig. 8.9 a plot of the energy eigenvalues as well as the self-consistent potential energy and the parabolic potential energy corresponding with the "classical" calculation performed with the analytical model when $V_G = 0$ from Section 8.3 are depicted. There are several important conclusions that can be drawn from this figure. First of all, as mentioned earlier the energy spectrum is not continuous, but discrete due to size confinement. In this plot a limited number of energy eigenvalues (subbands) is plotted. Second, the electron density is not constant, but shows a peak in the middle of the wire while it is zero at the wire channel edge ($r = R$). This is due to quantum mechanical confinement where the vanishing of the wave function is required as a boundary condition to the Schrödinger

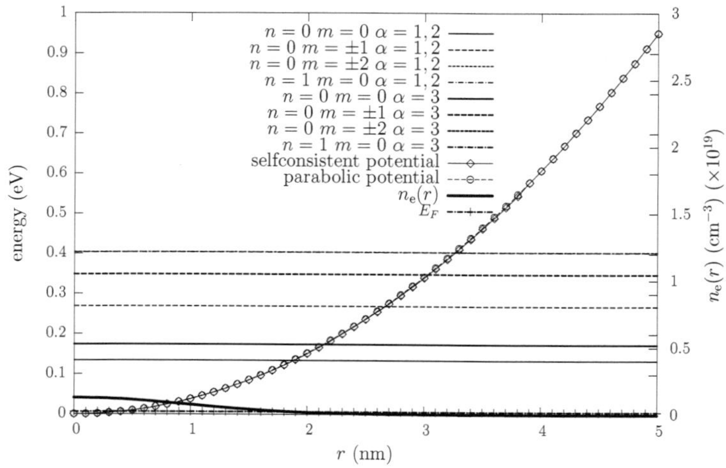

Figure 8.10. Electronic structure of a junctionless nanowire with radius $R = 5$ nm for $V_G = V_T$ (pinched off, full depletion). Shown in the figure is the sub band structure for a limited amount of energy eigenvalues, the self-consistent potential energy and the electron density profile.

equation (if we neglect wave function penetration into the insulator, which will not alter this conclusion qualitatively).

8.4.1.2 Full depletion or pinch-off condition

When we make the gate voltage equal to the classical threshold voltage obtained from Section 8.3, i.e., Eq. (8.10), we first of all observe from Fig. 8.10 that the electron density is again mainly localized in the center of the wire while being zero at $r = R$ due to quantum confinement but now the peak of electron density is of course much lower than obtained in flatband condition due to depletion. Second, due to the additional confining potential energy, not only the electron density is lowered, but energy quantization has increased, i.e., the distance between the different subbands has increased. Finally, we also observe that the self-consistent potential energy almost exactly coincides with the classical potential energy obtained from the analytical model from Section 8.3 when the wire is fully depleted ($V_G = V_T$ or $R - R_d = 0$) where the electrostatic potential can be obtained from Eq. (8.6) and is readily shown to be purely parabolic:

$$\Phi(r) = -\frac{qN_{\mathrm{D}}}{4\epsilon_{\mathrm{si}}} r^2, \quad 0 \le r \le R. \tag{8.41}$$

8.4.2 *Low Field Mobility and Scattering Mechanisms*

We use the following expression for the low-field mobility:

$$\mu = \frac{4e}{2kTn} \sum_{\nu\alpha} g_\alpha \int_{E_{\nu\alpha}}^{\infty} dE\ \rho_{1\mathrm{D}}^{\nu\alpha}(E) \tau_{\nu\alpha}(E) \mathrm{v}_{\nu\alpha}^2(E) f_{\nu\alpha}(E)[1 - f_{\nu\alpha}(E)] \tag{8.42}$$

where $f_{\nu\alpha}(E)$ is the equilibrium Fermi–Dirac distribution function, while

$$n = \frac{2}{L} \sum_{\nu\alpha k} g_\alpha f_{\nu\alpha}(k) \tag{8.43}$$

is the linear electron density. In Eq. (8.42) the quantity $v_{\nu\alpha}(k)$ refers to the group velocity:

$$v_{\nu\alpha}(k) = \frac{1}{\hbar} \frac{dE_{\nu\alpha}(k)}{dk} \tag{8.44}$$

while $\tau_{\nu\alpha}(k)$ is the relaxation time and $f_{\nu\alpha}(k)$ is the equilibrium distribution function all related to the ν-th subband and the α-th valley. The function $\rho_{1\mathrm{D}}^{\nu\alpha}(E)$ is the one-dimensional density of states

$$\rho_{1\mathrm{D}}^{\nu\alpha}(E) = \frac{1}{\pi\hbar} \sqrt{\frac{m_\alpha}{2(E - E_{\nu\alpha})}} \tag{8.45}$$

for $E > E_{\nu\alpha}$. The relaxation rate $\tau_{\nu\alpha}(E)$ is obtained from the Boltzmann equation in the relaxation time approximation:

$$\frac{1}{\tau(k\nu)} = \sum_{k'\nu'} S(k'\nu', k\nu) \frac{1 - f(E')}{1 - f(E)} \left(1 - \frac{v_z^{\nu'}(k')\tau_{\nu'}(k')}{v_z^{\nu}(k)\tau_\nu(k)}\right). \tag{8.46}$$

The microscopic scattering rate $S(k'\nu', k\nu)$ is obtained from Fermi's golden rule and we consider acoustic phonon scattering, optical phonon scattering, surface roughness and ionized impurity scattering as the main scattering agents [13].

In Fig. 8.11 the mobilities limited by phonon scattering, surface roughness and ionized impurity scattering are shown for a wire of radius $R = 2.5$ and 5 nm. The parameters describing the electron-phonon interaction, in particular the deformation potentials were

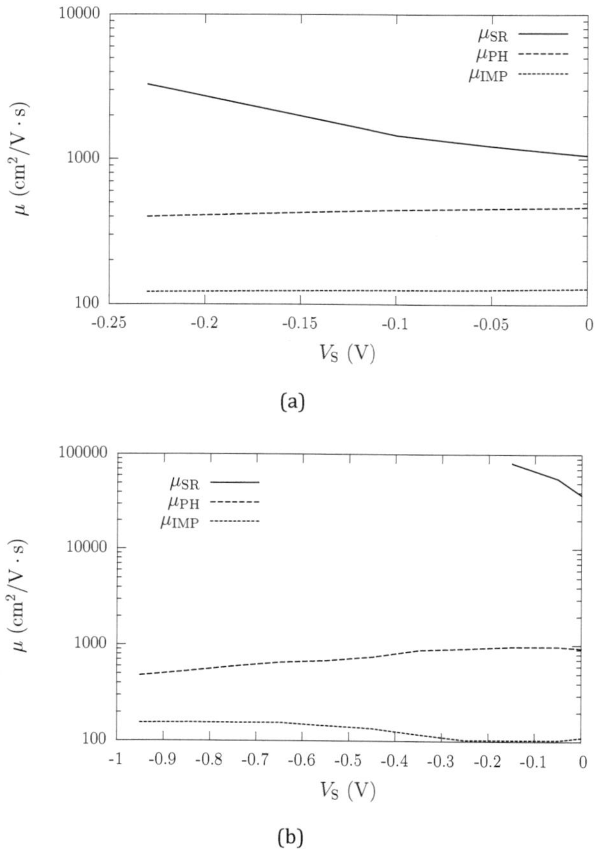

Figure 8.11. Phonon, surface roughness and ionized impurity limited mobilities as a function of surface voltage V_S for a junctionless nanowire transistor with doping density $N_D = 10^{20}$ cm^{-3} corresponding to a threshold voltage of $V_T = -0.95$ V. (a) $R = 2.5$ nm, (b) $R = 5.0$ nm.

taken from reference [13], while the parameters describing surface roughness, namely the correlation length and average step height have been assigned the typical values of 1.3 nm and 0.5 nm respectively. In Fig. 8.11(a) the lowest mobility is limited by ionized impurity scattering due to the heavy doping $N_D = 10^{20}$ cm^{-3}. Phonon and surface rougness scattering are much lower, thus yielding higher corresponding mobilities, and according to

Mathiessen's rule the total mobility will be mainly limited by ionized impurity mobility. For a wire with radius $R = 5$ nm the conclusion is identical: ionized impurity scattering is the main reason for depressing the mobility as can be seen from Fig 8.11(b). It is interesting to note that surface roughness scattering becomes completely negligble in this case. This was to be expected because, as noted in the beginning of this chapter, surface effects play a minor role in the junctionless nanowire. Of course, when the wire radius becomes too small, say 2–3 nm, surface roughness will become dominant.

8.5 Ballistic Transport in Ultrashort Thin Junctionless Nanowires

In this section we address the ultimately scaled junctionless nanowire transistor. Both the radius of the nanowire and the channel length are scaled down to such small dimensions that both size quantization due to confinement in the radial direction as well as potential energy variation in the z-direction can not be neglected. Moreover, we will scale down the gate length to a size sufficiently small to bring the wire in the "ballistic" transport regime. We will show that the ultra-short channel junctionless nanowire transistor and the inversion mode MOSFET nanowire become equivalent devices in this regime. The discussion in this section will be limited to ballistic transport in the GaAs nanowire.

8.5.1 *Schrödinger–Poisson Problem*

Because the electron Hamiltonian (8.33) is rotationally invariant, we factorize the wave function in the usual manner:

$$\psi(r, \phi, z) = \frac{1}{\sqrt{2\pi}} e^{im\phi} \zeta(r, z) \tag{8.47}$$

where $m = 0, \pm 1, \pm 2, \ldots$. Considering the fact that the energy associated with the confinement of the particle in the wire is usually substantially larger than the kinetic energy associated with the motion of the particle along the wire, we expand $\zeta(r, z)$ in the following multi-mode basis [14]:

$$\zeta(r, z) = \sum_n \phi_n(z)\chi_n(r; z) \tag{8.48}$$

where the $\chi_n(r; z)$ are solutions of the following eigenvalue problem

$$-\frac{\hbar^2}{2m_\perp}\left[\frac{\partial^2}{\partial r^2} + \frac{1}{r}\frac{\partial}{\partial r} - \frac{m^2}{r^2}\right]\chi_n(r; z)$$
$$+U(r, z)\chi_n(r; z) = E_n(z)\chi_n(r; z). \tag{8.49}$$

The envelope function $\phi_n(z)$ has to satisfy the following coupled Schrödinger equation:

$$-\frac{\partial^2\phi_n(z)}{\partial z^2} - 2\sum_{j=1}^{\infty} c_{nj}^1(z)\frac{\partial\phi_j(z)}{\partial z} - \sum_{j=1}^{\infty} c_{nj}^2(z)\phi_j(z)$$
$$= \frac{2m_z^*}{\hbar^2}(\epsilon - E_n(z))\phi_n(z) \tag{8.50}$$

where the z dependent coefficients c_{nj}^1 and c_{nj}^2 are defined as

$$c_{nj}^1(z) = \int_0^R rdr\ \chi_n(r; z)\frac{\partial}{\partial z}\chi_j(r; z) \tag{8.51}$$

$$c_{nj}^2(z) = \int_0^R rdr\ \chi_n(r; z)\frac{\partial^2}{\partial z^2}\chi_j(r; z). \tag{8.52}$$

Note that the eigenvalues of the "confinement Schrödinger equation," Eq. (8.49), serve as the effective potential for the envelope functions. The above decomposition into subbands has two advantages. First, the large number of wavefunctions $\zeta(r, z)$ required to calculate the charge density all involve the same basis functions $\chi_n(r; z)$. These functions, which are the solutions of Eq. (8.49), need to be computed only once for a given potential. Second, the coupled Schrödinger equation only needs to be solved for the number of relevant modes, that decreases with decreasing wire radius and increasing confinement. The subband decomposition approach is expected to be computationally less demanding and quicker than the full dimensional one [14]. The quantum transmitting boundary method (QTBM) [15] supplies the boundary conditions for the coupled Schrödinger equation. The source and drain are considered to be infinitely long, ideal electron reservoirs where the potential will be a function of the radial coordinate only, i.e., $U(r, z) = U(r, z_c)$ where z_c stands for the z-coordinate of the contact-device interface.

This makes it possible to find an exact solution for the envelope functions in the leads. Imposing continuity of the wavefunction and its derivative at the interface between the lead and the active region gives the boundary condition for Eq. (8.50). The current density in the subband decomposition method can be written as

$$J(r, z) = \sum_{c}\sum_{i}\int d\epsilon \frac{e\hbar}{m_z^*}\mathrm{Im}\left(\overline{\zeta}_{c,i,\epsilon}(r, z)\nabla\zeta_{c,i,\epsilon}(r, z)\right) f(\epsilon - \mu_c), \tag{8.53}$$

where f is the Fermi–Dirac distribution and μ_c is the chemical potential associated with the source if $z_c = z_s$ or the drain if $z_c = z_d$. The wavefunction $\zeta_{c,i,\epsilon}(r, z)$ represents the solution of the Schrödinger equation where a particle with energy ϵ is injected in the ith mode from contact c. Similarly, the electron density is defined as

$$n(r, z) = \sum_{c}\sum_{i}\int d\epsilon |\zeta_{c,i,\epsilon}(r, z)|^2 f(\epsilon - \mu_c). \tag{8.54}$$

Given the density, the electrostatic potential can be calculated by Poisson's equation:

$$\nabla\epsilon(r)\nabla\Phi = e(n(r, z) - N_d). \tag{8.55}$$

where N_d represents the doping density while the potential energy for Eq. (8.49) is simply $U = -e\Phi$. As the QTBM requires the potential to be constant in the leads, we impose Neumann boundary conditions at the contact-device interface

$$\frac{\partial\Phi}{\partial z}\,|_{z=z_s} = 0, \quad \frac{\partial\Phi}{\partial z}\,|_{z=z_d} = 0. \tag{8.56}$$

The potential is furthermore assumed to be known at a radius $R + t_{ox}$ and symmetry requires the axial derivative of the potential to vanish in the center, resulting in the following radial boundary conditions:

$$\frac{\partial\Phi}{\partial r}\,|_{r=0} = 0, \quad \Phi(R + t_{ox}, z) = V_G. \tag{8.57}$$

8.5.2 *Equivalence of the Junctionless (Pinch-Off) and Inversion Mode MOSFET Nanowire*

Figure 8.12 shows simulations results for both the junctionless (pinch-off) and inversion mode MOSFET GaAs nanowires with a

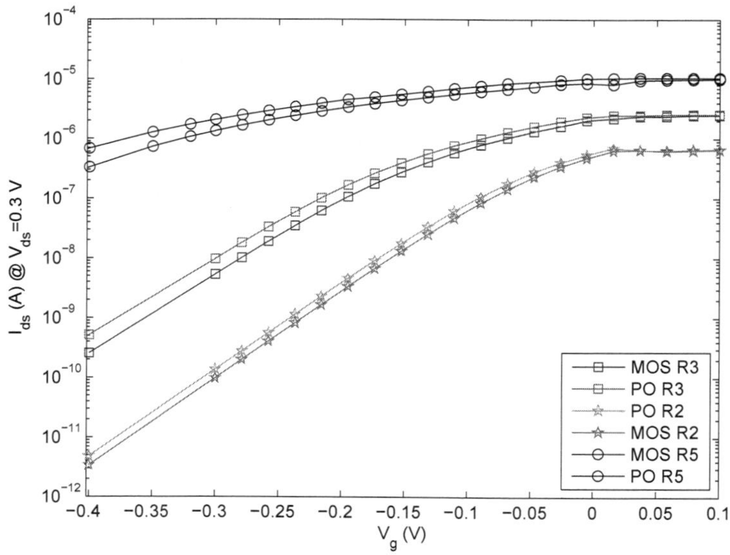

Figure 8.12. Drain current as a function of gate voltage for a junctionless (pinch-off) FET nanowire and inversion mode MOSFET nanowire for $R = 2, 3$ and 5 nm with $L_G = 5$ nm, $V_D = 0.3$ V and $N_D = 10^{19}$ cm^{-3}. See also Color Insert.

radius R of 2, 3 and 5 nm are shown. A gate insulator of 1 nm thickness consisting of SiO_2 was chosen and we have neglected the workfunction difference between the GaAs channel and the metal gate. The gate length was chosen to be $L_G = 5$ nm, while the source and drain are assumed to extend to infinity as implied by the QTBM. We furthermore consider the doping density in the wire to be $N_D^+ = 10^{19}$ cm^{-3} and the temperature of the system is $T = 300$ K. Fig. 8.12 clearly illustrates that the current–voltage characteristics of the junctionless and MOSFET GaAs nanowire are almost identical for ultra-short nanowire channels where the ballistic transport regime is valid. The small difference between the current–voltage characteristics is due to the small built-in potential which is still present in the MOSFET nanowire. Research has indeed shown that the built-in voltage of the short-channel n-i-n GaAs nanowire MOSFET is indeed negligible [16]. As a consequence, one can indeed

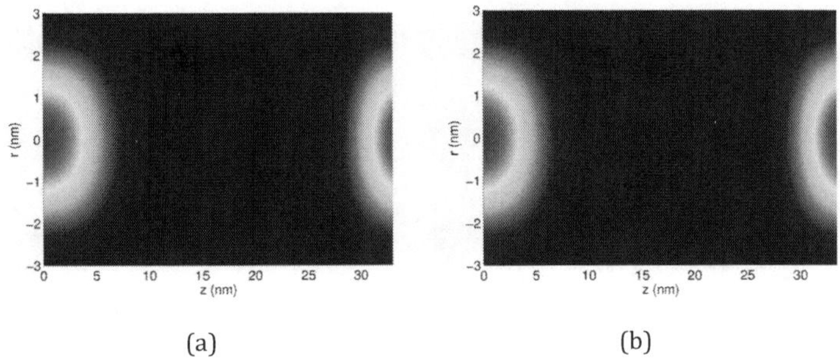

Figure 8.13. Density contour plot with $V_G = -0.3$ V, $L_G = 15$ nm, $R = 3$ nm, $V_D = 0.3$ V, $N_D = 10^{19}$ cm^{-3}. (a) Junctionless nanowire, (b) MOSFET nanowire.

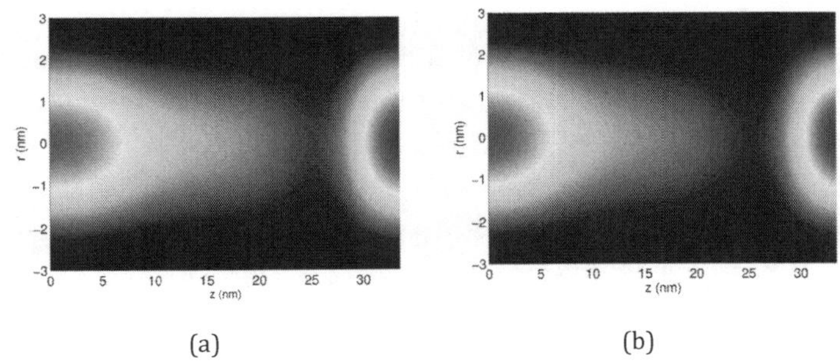

Figure 8.14. Density contour plot with $V_G = -0.075$ V, $L_G = 15$ nm, $R = 3$ nm, $V_D = 0.3$ V, $N_D = 10^{19}$ cm^{-3}. (a) Junctionless nanowire (b) MOSFET nanowire.

conclude that the junctionless and MOSFET GaAs nanowire are equivalent devices. This is further illustrated by the charge density profiles plotted in Figs. 8.13–8.15 for which we considered a GaAs nanowire with gate length $L_G = 15$ nm and radius $R = 3$ nm with fixed source-drain voltage $V_D = 0.3$ V. Again a doping density of $N_D = 10^{19}$ cm^{-3} was used for the junctionless nanowire and for the source-drain regions of the MOSFET nanowire. The left figures are the junctionless nanowires, while the right hand side figures are the inversion mode MOSFET nanowires. Going from Fig. 8.13 to 8.15 the gate voltage is gradually increased from the full depletion

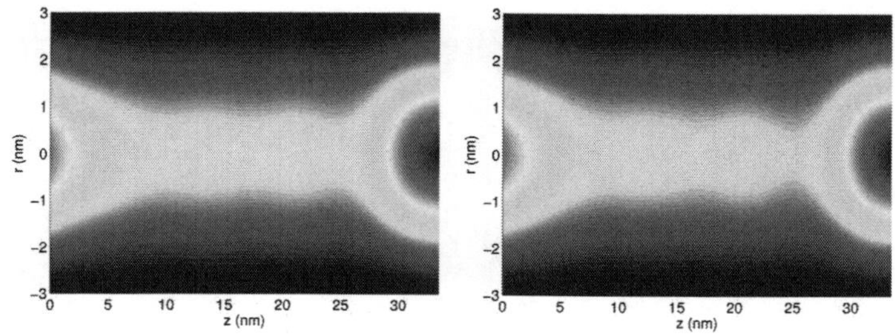

(a) (b)

Figure 8.15. Density contour plot with $V_G = 0.06$ V, $L_G = 15$ nm, $R = 3$ nm, $V_D = 0.3$ V, $N_D = 10^{19}$ cm^{-3}. (a) Junctionless nanowire, (b) MOSFET nanowire.

(OFF) state ($V_G = -0.3$ V) to almost flatband (ON) state ($V_G = -0.06$ V). The charge densities for both the junctionless nanowire and inversion mode MOSFET GaAs nanowire are almost identical.

8.6 Advanced Transport Modelling of the Junctionless Nanowire Transistor

8.6.1 *The Poisson–Schrödinger Problem*

In order to describe transport in short gate length junctionless nanowire transistors without resorting to purely ballistic transport but taking into account scattering we need to solve the self-consistent Poisson–Schrödinger problem together with the Boltzmann transport equation. Moreover, because we are also interested in the junctionless pFET transistor including the effect of strain, we need to deal with the hole band structure in more detail. Whereas for the low-field mobility calculations and ballistic transport model we only considered the junctionless nFET where electrons are the (majority) charge carriers we were able to solve the transport problem using the effective mass approximation. However, in the previous sections, we also needed the hole density to obtain the equilibrium Fermi level position in the nFET junctionless nanowire and we made the crude approximation that the hole valence bands can be approximated by spherically symmetric energy bands where each band can be characterized by a single effective mass. In reality, these bands are warped and non-parabolic and applying stress or strain will deform the hole bands considerably. To this end, we here calculate the hole band structure using the $6 \times 6\ \mathrm{k} \cdot \mathrm{p}$ Schrödinger equation for the junctionless pFET nanowire, while for the junctionless nFET we rely on the effective mass approximation. The starting point of the calculation is to write the wave function of sub band ν associated with band μ using the following ansatz:

$$\psi_\nu^\mu(r, \phi, z, k) = \zeta_\mu^\nu(r, \phi, k)e^{ikz} \quad (8.58)$$

where ζ is the envelope function, while k is the wave number in the z-direction. For the nFET we employ the effective mass approximation and the number of bands for each valley of the conduction band is limited to $\mu = 1$, while for the three valence bands of the pFET we consider $\mu = 1, \ldots, 6$ bands. The wave function (8.58) is a solution to the self-consistent Poisson–Schrödinger problem which involves solving a two-dimensional Schrödinger equation. However, if we expand the envelope function ζ_μ^ν into Fourier harmonics $Y_m(\phi)$ we can reduce the problem to a two-dimensional effective Schrödinger problem depending only on the radial coordinate r. Expanding the wave function (8.58) as follows:

$$\zeta_\mu^\nu(r, \phi, k) = \sum_m \zeta_{\mu,m}^\nu(r, k)Y_m(\phi) \quad (8.59)$$

with $\zeta_{\mu,m}^\nu$ the expansion coefficient and $Y_m(\phi) = e^{im\phi}/\sqrt{2\pi}$ the Fourier harmonic of order m. Substitution into the Schrödinger equation and multiplying with $Y_m^*(\phi)$ and integration over the angle ϕ the yields the following eigen value problem for both the nFET and pFET junctionless nanowire:

$$\sum_{\mu',m'} \left[H_{m,m'}^{\mu,\mu'}(-i\nabla_\mathrm{r}, k) + e\Phi(r)\delta_{m,m'}\delta_{\mu,\mu'} \right] \zeta_{\mu',m'}^\nu = \epsilon^\nu(k)\zeta_{\mu,m}^\nu(r, k) \quad (8.60)$$

where $\Phi(r)$ is the electrostatic potential, while $\epsilon^\nu(k)$ is the eigen energy associated with subband ν as a function of k. The Hamiltonian operator $H_{m,m'}^{\mu,\mu'}(-i\nabla_\mathrm{r}, k)$ is given by

$$H^{\mu,\mu'}_{m,m'}(-i\nabla_{\mathrm{r}}, k) = \int_0^{2\pi} d\phi\ Y^*_m(\phi) H^{\nu,\nu'}(-i\nabla_{\mathrm{r}}, k) Y_m(\phi) \qquad (8.61)$$

with $H^{\nu,\nu'}$ the ν, ν' element of the $N \times N$ Hamiltonian.

Making an initial guess for the electrostatic potential $\Phi(r)$, the eigen energies and associated wave functions are obtained from which the charge density can be calculated using the Fermi–Dirac distribution function. Using the Poisson equation with the obtained charge density as a source term, the electrostatic potential is updated and agains enters the Schrödinger equation. This self-consistent iteration process continues until convergence is reached.

The influence of strain on the band structure can be considered by the Pikus–Bir model [17]. The Pikus–Bir strain Hamiltonian can be constructed based on the strain tensor and must be included into the Hamiltonian.

8.6.2 *The Boltzmann Transport Equation*

A deterministic method is used to solve the multisubband Boltzmann transport equation. The method is based on the Fourier expansion of the distribution function in the 1D k-space, which is analogous to the spherical harmonic expansion method for the bulk case [18].

In the semiclassical framework stationary transport of carriers within a device can be described by a distribution function $f^{\nu}(\mathrm{r}, \mathrm{k})$, which is a function of position in the phase space (r, k) and depends also on the subband index ν. Having a 1D k-space the wave vector on which the distribution function depends is given by $\mathrm{k} = \pm k\mathrm{e}_z$. In real space the junctionless FET is assumed to be homogeneous in (x, y) plane. Therefore, the distribution function depends only on z in the real space. The distribution function $f^{\nu}(z, \mathrm{k})$ fulfills the stationary BTE [19, 20] for subband ν:

$$\frac{1}{\hbar}\mathrm{F}^{\nu} \cdot \nabla_{\mathrm{k}} f^{\nu} + \mathrm{v}^{\nu} \cdot \nabla_{\mathrm{r}} f^{\nu} = \hat{S}^{\nu}\{f\}. \qquad (8.62)$$

Here, $\hat{S}^{\nu}\{f\}$ is the scattering integral. The total force F due to a gradient in the total energy is given by

$$\mathrm{F}^{\nu}(z, \mathrm{k}) = \mathrm{F}^{\nu}_{E}(z, \mathrm{k}). \qquad (8.63)$$

In terms of the total subband energy $\varepsilon^{\nu}(z, \vec{k})$, which is the eigenenergy of the $\mathrm{k} \cdot \mathrm{p}$ Schrödinger equation, $\mathrm{F}^{\nu}_{E}(z, \mathrm{k})$ is given by

$$\mathrm{F}^{\nu}_{E}(z, \mathrm{k}) = -\nabla_{\mathrm{r}} \left[\varepsilon^{\nu}(z, \mathrm{k})\right] = -\frac{\partial}{\partial z} \left[\varepsilon^{\nu}(z, \mathrm{k})\right] \mathrm{e}_{z}. \qquad (8.64)$$

The Pauli exclusion principle is included in the scattering integral. Taking into account the assumption that scattering events are local in the real space, the scattering integral reads [21, 22]

$$\hat{S}\{f\} = 2\frac{1}{2\pi} \sum_{\nu'} \left\{ \int (1 - f^{\nu}(z, k)) S^{\nu,\nu'}(z, \mathrm{k}|\mathrm{k}') f_{e}^{\nu'}(z, k') dk' - \int (1 - f_{e}^{\nu'}(z, k')) S^{\nu',\nu}(z, \mathrm{k}'|\mathrm{k}) f^{\nu}(z, k) dk' \right\} \qquad (8.65)$$

where the transition rate $S^{\nu',\nu}(z, \mathrm{k}'|\mathrm{k})$ is given by

$$S^{\nu',\nu}(z, \mathrm{k}'|\mathrm{k}) = \sum_{\eta,\mp} c^{\nu',\nu}_{\eta,\mp}(z, \mathrm{k}'|\mathrm{k}) \delta(\varepsilon^{\nu'}(z, k') - \varepsilon^{\nu}(z, k) \mp \hbar\omega_{\eta}). \quad (8.66)$$

η is the scattering mechanism index, c the transition coefficient from the initial state (ν', k') to the final state (ν, k), and $\hbar\omega_{\eta}$ the energy transfer due to scattering. For an elastic scattering mechanism η, $\hbar\omega_{\eta} = 0$, $c_{\eta,+} = c_{\eta}$, and $c_{\eta,-} = 0$. Three important scattering mechanisms are considered: acoustic phonon scattering, optical phonon scattering and surface roughness scattering. The scattering matrix elements of phonon scattering [22] are approximated such that they can be considered as velocity randomizing.

We solve the Boltzmann transport equation within the relaxation time approximation where it is assumed that only linear response of the distribution function due to lateral electric field along the channel is included, that is

$$f^{\nu}_{\pm}(z, k) = f^{\nu}_{eq}(z, \varepsilon^{\nu}(z, k)) + \delta f^{\nu}_{\pm}(z, k) \qquad f_{eq} \gg \delta f_{\pm}. \qquad (8.67)$$

Here, the first-order term δf does not disturb the particle density.

8.6.3 *Results*

Figure 8.16 shows I_{D}–V_{GS} curves in a junctionless nanowire POFET and in a nanowire MOSFET for $V_{\mathrm{DS}} = 1$ mV. The two devices have the same short gate length of 16 nm. For two devices the subthreshold

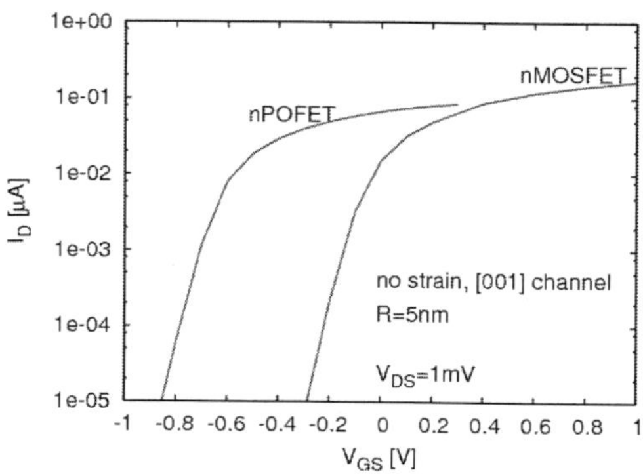

Figure 8.16. I_D–V_{GS} curves in a junctionless nanowire POFET and in a nanowire MOSFET. $V_{DS} = 1$ mV. $L_g = 16$ nm.

slope of the I_D–V_{GS} curves is shown to be nearly the same (about 60 mV/dec).

Figure 8.17 shows the ohmic channel conductance of a junctionless nanowire FET and nanowire MOSFET with 16 nm gate length evaluated based on the Boltzmann–Poisson–Schrödinger equation solution or based on the drift-diffusion approximation. It is shown that the drift-diffusion approximation overestimates the ohmic channel conductance, especially for the high V_{GS} range. In such short channels the gradient of subband potential energy at the interface between the channel and the source or drain is much higher than the gradient of subband potential energy in the middle of the channel. This is the main reason for the failure of the drift-diffusion approximation in sub-100 nm gate length devices. As a consequence, the drift-diffusion approximation can not capture the quasi ballistic transport effects in the short channel devices, whereas the Boltzmann–Poisson–Schrödinger equation approach can. The mobility variation due to uniaxial stress in a junctionless nanowire nFET or pFET with a homogenous channel is shown in Fig. 8.18. Here, the uniaxial stress direction is [110] (parallel to the channel direction). The simulation results are shown to be in excellent agreement with the experimental data [11] using the wafer bending

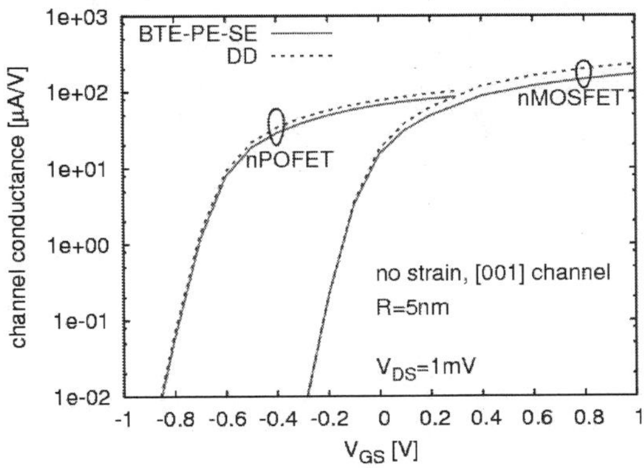

Figure 8.17. Ohmic channel conductance of a junctionless nanowire POFET and of a nanowire MOSFET evaluated based on the Boltzmann transport, Poisson and Schrödinger equation solution or based on the drift-diffusion approximation. $V_{DS} = 1$ mV. $L_G = 16$ nm.

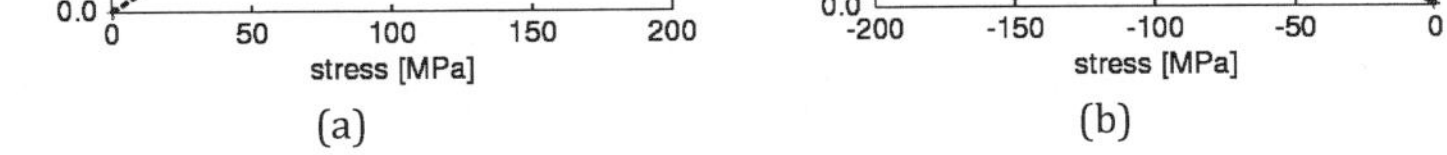

Figure 8.18. Simulation results and experimental data for mobility variation due to uniaxial stress in a junctionless nanowire nPOFET (a) or pPOFET (b) with a homogenous channel. The experimental data are from [11]. The uniaxial stress direction is [110] (parallel to the channel direction).

technique. The tensile stress results in a higher mobility for nPOFET, whereas compressive stress results in a higher mobility for pPOFET. A mobility variation up to 5% can be achieved for an 150 MPa stress for both the n- and p-type junctionless FET.

References

1. B. Sorée, W. Magnus, and G. Pourtois, Analytical and self-consistent quantum mechanical model for a surrounding gate mos nanowire operated in jfet mode, *J. Comput. Phys.* **7**, 380–383, (2008).
2. M. Fischetti, D. Neumayer, and E. Cartier, Effective electron mobility in Si inversion layers in metal–oxide–semiconductor systems with a high-k insulator: the role of remote phonon scattering, *J. Appl. Phys.* **90**, 4587, (2001).
3. M. Tambe, S. Lim, M. Smith, L. Allard, and S. Gradecak, Realization of defect free epitaxial core-shell gaas/algaas nanowire heterostructures, *Appl. Phys. Lett.* **93**, 151917, (2008).
4. W. Shockley, A unipolar field effect transistor, *Proc. IRE.* **40**, 1365, (1952).
5. S. Sze and K. Ng, *Physics of Semiconductor Devices* (John Wiley & Sons, Hoboken, New Jersey, 2007).
6. B. Sorée, W. Magnus, M. Szepieniec, W. Vandenberghe, A. Verhulst, G. Pourtois, G. Groeseneken, S. D. Gendt, and M. Heyns, Novel device concepts for nanotechnology: the nanowire pinch-off fet and graphene tunnelFET,, *ECS Trans.* **28**, 15–26, (2010).
7. B. Sorée and W. Magnus, Silicon nanowire pinch-off fet: basic operation and analytical model, *Proceedings of ULIS 2009*. pp. 245–248, (2009).
8. C.-W. Lee, A. Afzalian, N. D. Akhavan, R. Yan, I. Ferain, and J.-P. Colinge, Junctionless multigate field effect transistor, *Appl. Phys. Lett.* **94**, 053511, (2009).
9. J. Colinge, C. Lee, A. Afzalian, N. Akhavan, R. Yan, I. Ferain, P. Ravazi, B. O'Neill, A. Blake, M. White, A. Kelleher, B. McCarthy, and R. Murphy, Nanowire transistors without junctions, *Nat. Nanotechnol.* **5**, 225–229, (2010).
10. L. Ansari, B. Feldman, G. Fagas, J. Colinge, and J. Greer, Simulation of junctionless Si nanowire transistors with 3 nm gate length, *Appl. Phys. Lett.* **97**, 062105, (2010).
11. J. Raskin, J. Colinge, I. Ferain, A. Kranti, C. Lee, N. Akhavan, R. Yan, P. Razavi, and R. Yu, Mobility improvement in nanowire junctionless transistors by uniaxial strain, *Appl. Phys. Lett.* **97**, 042114, (2010).
12. F. Chapeau-Blondeau, Numerical evaluation of the lambert w-function and application to generation of generalized gaussian noise with exponent 1/2, *IEEE Transactions on Signal Processing*. pp. 2160–2165, (2002).

13. S. Jin, M. Fischetti, and T.-W. Tang, Modeling of electron mobility in gated silicon nanowires at room temperature: surface roughness scattering, dielectric screening and band nonparabolicity, *J. Appl. Phys.* **102**, 083715, (2007).
14. E. Polizzi and N. Abdallah, Subband decomposition approach for the simulation of quantum electron transport in nanostructures, *J. Comput. Phys.* **202**, 150–180, (2004).
15. C. Lent and D. Kirkner, The quantum transmitting boundary method, *J. Appli. Phys.* **67**, 6353, (1990).
16. D. Sels, B. Sorée, and G. Groeseneken, Quantum ballistic transport in the junctionless nanowire pinch-off field effect transistor, *J. Comput. Electron.* **10**, (2011).
17. G. Bir and G. Pikus, *Symmetry and Strain-Induced Effects in Semiconductors* (New York: John Wiley & Sons, New York, 1974).
18. C. Jungemann, A. Pham, B. Meinerzhagen, C. Ringhofer, and M. Bollhöfer, Stable discretization of the Boltzmann equation based on spherical harmonics, box integration, and a maximum entropy dissipation principle, *J. Appl. Phys.* **100**, 024502.1–024502.13, (2006).
19. O. Madelung, *Introduction to Solid State Theory* (Springer, Berlin, 1978).
20. C. Jacoboni and P. Lugli, *The Monte Carlo Method for Semiconductor Device Simulation.* (Springer, Wien, 1989).
21. C. Jungemann, A. Emunds, and W. Engl, Simulation of linear and nonlinear electron transport in homogeneous silicon inversion layers, *Solid-State Electron.* **36**, 1529–1540, (1993).
22. M. Fischetti, Z. Ren, P. M. Solomon, M. Yang, and K. Rim, Six-band *kdotp* calculation of the hole mobility in silicon inversion layers: Dependence on surface orientation, strain, and silicon thickness, *J. Appl. Phys.* **94**, 1079–1095, (2003).

Chapter 9

The Variational Principle: A Valuable Ally Assisting the Self-Consistent Solution of Poisson's Equation and Semi-Classical Transport Equations

Wim Magnus,[a,b] **Hamilton Carrillo-Nuñez,**[a] **and Bart Sorée**[a,b]

[a]*Department of Physics, Universiteit Antwerpen, Groenenborgerlaan 171, B-2020 Antwerpen, Flanders, Belgium*
[b]*IMEC, Nano Confined Applications and Systems (NCAIS) Department, Physics Modeling and Simulation (MSP) Group, Kapeldreef 75, B-3001 Leuven, Flanders, Belgium*
wim.magnus@ua.ac.be

Quantifying charged carrier transport in semiconductor devices on a microscopic scale typically amounts to the self-consistent solution of Poisson's equation yielding the electric potential, one or more kinetic equations governing the carrier distribution functions, and a set of constitutive equations relating the potential to the distribution functions and various related quantities.

In this chapter, we show that the variational principle and its well-known toolbox of Lagrangians and action functionals can be successfully translated into an efficient numerical algorithm not only facilitating the above-mentioned self-consistent solution flow, but also monitoring the stability of the latter over all successive iterations.

CMOS Nanoelectronics: Innovative Devices, Architectures, and Applications
Edited by Nadine Collaert

ISBN 978-981-4364-02-7 (Hardcover), 978-981-4364-03-4 (eBook)
www.panstanford.com

9.1 Introduction

Today's miniaturization of semiconductor devices and components not only has led to substantial complications on the side of processing, fabrication and reliability but also has tremendously increased the mathematical complexity encountered when nanoscale devices are to be modeled with acceptable accuracy.

On the one hand, quantum mechanics inevitably determines the behavior of moving charges, either through the transverse quantization of subband energies in narrow conduction channels, or when the device working principle is found to rely on quantum interference effects.

On the other hand, even when electron–electron interactions are treated only up to the level of the Hartree or the random phase approximation, the potential profile becomes strongly dependent on position, especially inside the active device areas. Emerging as a solution to Poisson's equation, the potential profile generally appears both in the Schrödinger equation governing the transverse subband ladders, and the quantum-kinetic equations that account for the quantum effects observed in the transport direction, such as the Wigner–Liouville equation [1] and the Pauli–Van Hove–Van Vliet [2, 3] master equations.

A non-equilibrium average extracted from the solution to the kinetic equations, the charge density in turn enters the right-hand side of Poisson's equation. Consequently, the prediction of transport characteristics of modern nanodevices requires the self-consistent solution of Poisson's equation, the Schrödinger equation and the appropriate transport equations as well as the constitutive equations that provide various non-equilbrium occupation numbers. Although Poisson's equation itself can be considered a linear differential equation — given the potential profile, the self-consistent solution scheme reveals a highly nonlinear dependence of the distribution functions, wave functions, etc. on the local potential. Hence, the numerical iteration loops swapping back and forth between Poisson's equation and the kinetic/constitutive equations are still burdening the computational efficiency as well as the stability of the numerical results obtained.

As is well known, the calculus of variations is based on the principle of least or, more generally, stationary action. In the framework of differential equations, the latter amounts to the observation that the exact solution to a differential equation minimizes a properly constructed action functional, while all test functions used to vary the action functional satisfy the required boundary/initial conditions. For instance, being commonly known in the field of electromagnetism [4–6], the action functional and the corresponding Lagrangian underlying the Maxwell equations, has been successfully applied to generate approximate analytical expressions for the electromagnetic potentials by minimizing explicitly the action with respect to a number of tunable, free parameters. However, the use of the variational principle in the context of transport modeling is much less a common practice. In the recent past [7] the action functional related to Poisson's equation and the classical constitutive equations was minimized analytically to study a class of semiconductor devices in quasi-equilibrium.

In this work, we show that the variational principle can be exploited as a numerical tool to self-consistently solve Poisson's equation and a set of semi-classical transport equations whereas the iterative evaluation of the action adds an absolute criterion monitoring the convergence of the iteration scheme. Section 9.2 briefly reviews the action functional associated with Maxwell's equations describing an electromagnetic field in the presence of given charge and current density profiles. In Section 9.3 the action functional is extended to include charge densities which are local functionals of the electrostatic potential and a sufficient condition is provided for the action extremum to be a minimum. Moreover, it is shown that the latter condition is not only met by the charge density functionals extracted from classical transport calculations (e.g., based on drift–diffusion-like equations) but also applies to quantum kinetic equations where the adiabatic approximation is invoked to account for the slowly varying parts of the electrostatic potential. As a benchmark, some calculations on ballistic transport in a Si nanowire field-effect transistor (FET) carried out with the variational scheme are shown and discussed in Section 9.4 and, finally, a few suggestions for future work are given in the outlook Section 9.5.

9.2 The Electromagnetic Field: Lagrangian and Action

In general, an arbitrary electromagnetic field is characterized by a scalar potential $V(\mathbf{r}, t)$ and a vector potential $\mathbf{A}(\mathbf{r}, t)$ from which the electric field and the magnetic induction may be derived at any space–time point $(\mathbf{r}, t)$ according to

$$\mathbf{E}(\mathbf{r}, t) = -\nabla V(\mathbf{r}, t) - \frac{\partial \mathbf{A}(\mathbf{r}, t)}{\partial t}, \quad \mathbf{B}(\mathbf{r}, t) = \nabla \times \mathbf{A}(\mathbf{r}, t). \tag{9.1}$$

From elementary electromagnetism [4, 6], the Lagrangian density of the electromagnetic field interacting with a given charge density $\rho(\mathbf{r}, t)$ and a current density $\mathbf{J}(\mathbf{r}, t)$ is known to be

$$\mathcal{L} = \frac{1}{2}\left(\epsilon\,|\nabla V|^2 - \frac{1}{\mu}|\nabla \times \mathbf{A}|^2\right) + \mathbf{J}\cdot\mathbf{A} - \rho V, \tag{9.2}$$

where ϵ (μ) denotes the electric permittivity (magnetic permeability) of the environment. The appropriate action S appears to be a functional of the electromagnetic potentials V and $\mathbf{A}$, obtained as a composed time and volume integral:

$$S[V, \mathbf{A}] = \int_{t_0}^{t_1} \mathrm{d}t \int_{\Omega} \mathrm{d}^3 r\ \mathcal{L}\big[V(\mathbf{r}, t), \mathbf{A}(\mathbf{r}, t), \mathbf{r}, t\big]. \tag{9.3}$$

t_0 and t_1 delimit the time interval during which the electromagnetic field flow is to be examined while Ω is a closed volume in 3D configuration space. For general purposes, one may take Ω to encompass the entire 3D Euclidean space and assert that all potentials become vanishingly small at $\partial\Omega$, the boundary surface of Ω - under the assumption that ρ and $\mathbf{J}$ are strictly localized in 3D space. In the context of device modeling, however, Ω is usually restricted to the device volume, in which case the lacking information on the potential values outside Ω calls for a proper set of boundary conditions specifying V and $\mathbf{A}$ (and/or their derivatives) on $\partial\Omega$.

Making S stationary, i.e., imposing $\delta S = 0$ w.r.t. arbitrary variations δV and $\delta\mathbf{A}$ that vanish at the integration limits is equivalent to solving the Euler–Lagrange equations leading to the four Maxwell equations

$$\nabla\cdot\mathbf{E} = \frac{\rho}{\epsilon}, \quad \nabla\cdot\mathbf{B} = 0, \tag{9.4}$$

$$\nabla \times \mathbf{E} = -\frac{\partial \mathbf{B}}{\partial t}, \quad \nabla \times \mathbf{B} = \mu\left(\mathbf{J} + \epsilon\frac{\partial \mathbf{E}}{\partial t}\right). \tag{9.5}$$

Since the remainder of this chapter merely involves the effect of static (irrotational) electric fields on the charge distribution in singly connected device regions (of genus 0), from hereof we ignore the vector potential and the associated magnetic field to focus exclusively on Poisson's equation

$$\nabla^2 V = -\frac{\rho}{\epsilon} \tag{9.6}$$

where ϵ refers to the static permittivity of either the semiconductor (ϵ_s) or the oxide layer (ϵ_{ox}) characterizing the devices under investigation.

Correspondingly, the time integral in the action functional can be removed and the effective action reduces to

$$S[V] = \int_\Omega \mathrm{d}^3 r \left(\frac{1}{2}\epsilon |\nabla V|^2 - \rho V \right). \tag{9.7}$$

If the charge density is externally specified on a mesh $\mathbf{r}_1, \ldots \mathbf{r}_n$ as $\rho_i \equiv \rho(\mathbf{r}_i)$, $1 \leqslant i \leqslant n$, the numerical solution to Poisson's equation may be obtained by discretizing $\nabla V(\mathbf{r})$ in Eq. (9.7) and solving

$$\frac{\partial S}{\partial V_i} = 0, \quad 1 \leqslant i \leqslant n, \tag{9.8}$$

while treating the array $\rho_1, \ldots, \rho_n$ as a set of independent parameters.

9.3 The Principle of Least Action for Self-Consistent Solutions

As anticipated in the introduction, the potential and charge profiles in a realistic semiconductor device are self-consistently intertwined because, apart from the fixed charges arising from ionized donors and acceptors, the concentration of mobile electrons and holes depends on the potential in a complicated way. Therefore, we first modify the action functional of Eq. (9.7) to include charge density functionals that exhibit a highly non-linear dependence on $V(\mathbf{r})$. As an explicit restriction, we further neglect any non-local behavior of $\rho[V]$, i.e., we assume that the value of ρ at any point $\mathbf{r}$ is determined solely by $V(\mathbf{r})$. This way, we may generalize the original functional (9.7) in which $\rho(\mathbf{r})$ is a fixed profile, to the following expression:

$$S[V] = \int_\Omega \mathrm{d}^3 r \left(\frac{1}{2}\epsilon |\nabla V|^2 - \int_{V_0}^{V(\mathbf{r})} \mathrm{d}V' \rho[V'] \right), \tag{9.9}$$

where V_0 is an arbitrary reference potential that does not contribute to the variations of S w.r.t. variations of $V(\mathbf{r})$.

First, we prove that the function $V(\mathbf{r})$ that makes S stationary is a solution to the nonlinear Poisson equation

$$\nabla^2 V(\mathbf{r}) = -\frac{1}{\epsilon}\,\rho[V(\mathbf{r}), \mathbf{r}], \tag{9.10}$$

where the local, but nonlinear dependence of ρ on $V(\mathbf{r})$ is in accordance with the constitutive equations that are invoked in the model under study. To this end, we calculate the variation of S caused by an arbitrary variation $\delta V(\mathbf{r})$ of the potential profile, which vanishes at the boundary surface $\partial\Omega$.

Secondly, we show that the extremum of S is a genuine minimum - and not a saddle point, as will also be reflected in the stability of the numerical minimization algorithm that is built on these findings.

The variation of S can be extracted straightforwardly from

$$\begin{aligned}\delta S &\equiv S[V + \delta V] - S[V]\\ &= \int_\Omega \mathrm{d}^3 r \left[\frac{1}{2}\epsilon\left(\left|\nabla\left(V(\mathbf{r}) + \delta V(\mathbf{r})\right)\right|^2 - \left|\nabla V(\mathbf{r})\right|^2\right)\right.\\ &\qquad \left. - \int_{V(\mathbf{r})}^{V(\mathbf{r})+\delta V(\mathbf{r})} \mathrm{d}V' \rho[V']\right].\end{aligned} \tag{9.11}$$

Using Gauss's theorem

$$\int_\Omega \mathrm{d}^3 r\; \nabla\cdot\left(\delta V(\mathbf{r})\nabla V(\mathbf{r})\right) = \int_{\partial\Omega} \mathbf{d\,S}\cdot\nabla V(\mathbf{r})\,\delta V(\mathbf{r}), \tag{9.12}$$

where the right-hand side equals zero as $\delta V(\mathbf{r})$ vanishes when $\mathbf{r} \in \partial\Omega$. Inserting therefore

$$\int_\Omega \mathrm{d}^3 r\, \nabla\delta V(\mathbf{r})\cdot\nabla V(\mathbf{r}) = -\int_\Omega \mathrm{d}^3 r\, \delta V(\mathbf{r})\nabla^2 V(\mathbf{r}) \tag{9.13}$$

into Eq. (9.11) and expanding $\rho(V')$ in a second-order Taylor series around $V' = V(\mathbf{r})$, we find

$$\begin{aligned}\delta S = \int_\Omega \mathrm{d}^3 r &\left[-\delta V(\mathbf{r})\left(\epsilon\nabla^2 V(\mathbf{r}) + \rho[V(\mathbf{r})]\right) + \right.\\ &\left.\frac{1}{2}\left(\epsilon\left|\nabla\delta V(\mathbf{r})\right|^2 - \left.\frac{\partial\rho[V']}{\partial V'}\right|_{V'=V(\mathbf{r})}\cdot\left(\delta V(\mathbf{r})\right)^2\right)\right].\end{aligned} \tag{9.14}$$

Ignoring first the second-order contributions, we observe that putting $\delta S = 0$ for all $\delta V(\mathbf{r})$ that vanish on $\partial\Omega$ eventually requires that $V(\mathbf{r})$ solve Eq. (9.10), as expected. Next, substituting the formally exact solution into Eq. (9.14), we conclude that

$$\frac{\partial \rho[V]}{\partial V} \leqslant 0, \quad \forall V \tag{9.15}$$

is a sufficient condition for the second-order variation to become positive definite, thus ensuring that the extremal value of the action functional is a minimum indeed.

Next we need to find out in which relevant cases we can concretely use the criterion formulated in (9.15), bearing in mind that the charge density inside a semiconductor device generally builds up from mobile electrons and holes as well as fixed dopant charges:

$$\rho(\mathbf{r}) = e\left[p(\mathbf{r}) - n(\mathbf{r}) + N_{\mathrm{D}}^{+}(\mathbf{r}) - N_{\mathrm{A}}^{-}(\mathbf{r})\right]. \tag{9.16}$$

where $e = +1.602 \times 10^{19}$ C represents the absolute value of the electron charge; $p(\mathbf{r})$ and $n(\mathbf{r})$, respectively, denote the concentrations of the mobile holes and electrons; $N_{\mathrm{D}}^{+}(\mathbf{r})$ and $N_{\mathrm{A}}^{-}(\mathbf{r})$ refer to the contributions arising from the ionized donors and acceptors. Treating the latter as fixed charges, not depending on the potential profile, one may characterize the electron and hole concentrations of a non-degenerate semiconductor [7] by the classical Boltzmann relations

$$n(\mathbf{r}) = n_{\mathrm{i}} \exp\left(\frac{\mu_n + eV(\mathbf{r})}{k_{\mathrm{B}}T}\right), \quad p(\mathbf{r}) = n_{\mathrm{i}} \exp\left(-\frac{\mu_p + eV(\mathbf{r})}{k_{\mathrm{B}}T}\right), \tag{9.17}$$

where n_{i} is the intrinsic carrier concentration and μ_n and μ_p, respectively, denote the electron and hole quasi-chemical potentials. Clearly, $\rho(\mathbf{r})$ not only appears to be a local functional of $V(\mathbf{r})$ but also seems to satisfy condition (9.15) as can be seen from

$$\frac{\partial \rho}{\partial V} = -\frac{en_{\mathrm{i}}}{k_{\mathrm{B}}T}\left[\exp\left(\frac{\mu_n + eV}{k_{\mathrm{B}}T}\right) + \exp\left(-\frac{\mu_p + eV}{k_{\mathrm{B}}T}\right)\right] < 0. \tag{9.18}$$

Moreover, the integral over V' in (9.9) can be done analytically, leading to

$$S[V] = \int_{\Omega} \mathrm{d}^3 r \left[\frac{1}{2}\epsilon |\nabla V(\mathbf{r})|^2 - e\Big(N_{\mathrm{D}}^{+}(\mathbf{r}) - N_{\mathrm{A}}^{-}(\mathbf{r}) \Big) V(\mathbf{r}) \right.$$
$$+ n_{\mathrm{i}} k_{\mathrm{B}} T \left(\exp\left(-\frac{\mu_p}{k_{\mathrm{B}} T} \right) \left(\exp\left(\frac{\mu_n + eV}{k_{\mathrm{B}} T} \right) \right. \right.$$
$$\left. \left. \left. + \exp\left(-\frac{\mu_p + eV}{k_{\mathrm{B}} T} \right) \right) \right) \right], \tag{9.19}$$

which is directly applicable to numerical processing. However, as explained in the following section, it is also possible to extend the variational approach to semi-classical transport that, nevertheless, accounts for quantum confinement effects.

9.4 Ballistic Current in a Si Nanowire Transistor

As a benchmark for the variational approach, we study the electrostatic potential profile and the electron distribution in an (100) n-channel metal–oxide–semiconductor field-effect transistor (MOSFET), which takes the form of a thin Si nanowire with an allround gate, as illustrated in Fig. (9.1) The nanowire device consists of two heavily doped n^+ source and drain regions that are connected by an unintentionally doped p-type region.

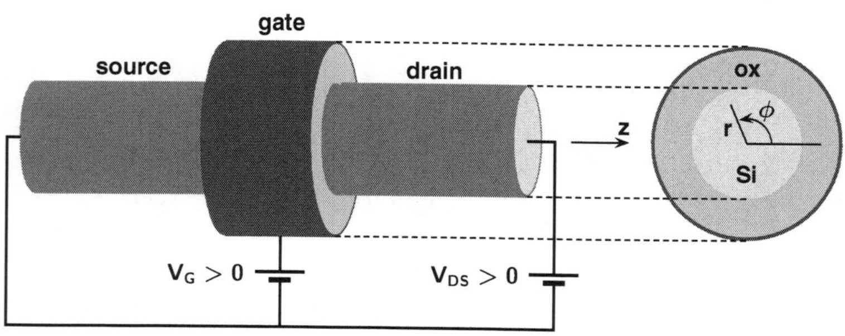

Figure 9.1. Cylindrical n-channel Si nanowire FET with an allround gate.

9.4.1 *Hamiltonian and Electronic Structure*

Considering the Si nanowire a perfect cylinder and adopting the effective-mass approximation, we may express the one-electron Hamiltonian in terms of cylindrical coordinates (r, ϕ, z) as

$$H_\alpha = -\frac{\hbar^2}{2m_{\alpha\perp}}\left(\frac{\partial^2}{\partial r^2} + \frac{1}{r}\frac{\partial}{\partial r} + \frac{1}{r^2}\frac{\partial^2}{\partial \phi^2}\right) - \frac{\hbar^2}{2m_{\alpha z}}\frac{\partial^2}{\partial z^2} + U(r, z). \tag{9.20}$$

The index α represents one of the six conduction band valleys of Si, whereas $m_{\alpha x}, m_{\alpha y}, m_{\alpha z}$ are the effective masses in the principal, crystallographic directions and the "perpendicular" effective mass in a planar cross section is given by

$$m_{\alpha\perp} = \frac{2m_{\alpha x}m_{\alpha y}}{m_{\alpha x} + m_{\alpha y}}. \tag{9.21}$$

Assuming full cylindrical symmetry, we may ignore any angular dependence of the electron and hole concentrations and the potential energy $U(r, z)$. The latter essentially combines the abrupt potential barrier U_B separating the Si body with radius R from the oxide layer of thickness t_{ox} with the electrostatic energy $-eV(r, z)$:

$$U(r, z) = U_B\theta(R < r < R + t_{ox}) - eV(r, z), \tag{9.22}$$

where the logic step function is given by

$$\theta(x) = \begin{cases} 1 & \text{if } x \text{ is true,} \\ 0 & \text{else.} \end{cases} \tag{9.23}$$

The source, channel and drain lengths are, respectively, denoted by L_S, L_{CH} and L_D, whereas the total wire length equals $L = L_S + L_{CH} + L_D$. Incorporating the electron–electron interaction in the Hartree approximation, the electrostatic potential $V(r, z)$ reflects the built-in potentials characterizing the two *p-n* junctions as well as the applied gate and drain voltages, V_G and V_{ds}. Furthermore, for the sake of simplicity, we have neglected all leakage currents originating from electrons that are able to tunnel from the conduction channel to the gate region which is equivalent to adopting the limit $U_B \to \infty$. Consequently, all electrons are strictly confined to reside inside the Si body, their wave functions being bound to vanish at the interface $r = R$. Following a conventional standard approach, we would next solve the Schrödinger equation for an initial potential profile to obtain the radial and azimuthal subband ladders as a function of V_G and V_{ds} and other tunable parameters. Then, after having inserted the resulting wave functions and eigenenergies into the constitutive and kinetic equations, we would derive the charge density, use it to upgrade $V(r, z)$ by solving Poisson's equation and complete the whole iteration cycle until convergence has been reached. Here, we have used a simplified method to extract the dependence of the non-equilibrium charge density depends on the electrostatic potential. Following [8], we have adopted the modified local density approach (MLDA) to describe the charge density and potential profiles in the nanowire FET. Doing so, we first make the bold assumption that the potential $V(r, z)$ takes a constant value V_0 throughout the entire device. Then, accounting for the huge, abrupt oxide barrier ($U_B \to \infty$), we may express the normalized one-electron wave functions and the corresponding eigenenergies, respectively, as

$$\begin{aligned}
\psi_{\alpha ml}(k; r, \phi, z) &= \frac{J_m\left(\dfrac{x_{ml} r}{R}\right) e^{im\phi} e^{ikz}}{\sqrt{2\pi^2 R^2}\,|J_{m+1}(x_{ml})|}, \\
E_{\alpha ml}(k) &= \frac{\hbar^2 k^2}{2m_{\alpha z}} + \frac{\hbar^2 x_{ml}^2}{2m_{\alpha\perp} R^2} + V_0, \\
m &= 0, \pm 1, \pm 2, \ldots; \quad l = 1, 2, \ldots. \qquad (9.24)
\end{aligned}$$

m and l are the azimuthal and radial quantum numbers labeling the corresponding subband ladders, x_{ml} being the l-th zero of the Bessel function $J_m(x)$, whereas k denotes the 1D wave vector (wave number) along the z-direction. Labeling as well the electron distribution function $f(r, z, k)$ with the single-particle quantum numbers (α, m, l), we may obtain the constitutive equation that provides us with the electron concentration including a spin degeneracy factor 2:

$$\begin{aligned}
n(r, z) &= 2 \sum_{m=-\infty}^{\infty} \sum_{l=1}^{\infty} \sum_{\alpha} \int_{-\infty}^{\infty} dk\, |\psi_{\alpha ml}(k; r, \phi, z)|^2 f_{\alpha ml}(r, z, k) \\
&= \sum_{m=0}^{\infty} \sum_{l=1}^{\infty} C_{ml} J_m^2\left(\frac{x_{ml} r}{R}\right) \sum_{\alpha} \int_{-\infty}^{\infty} dk\, f_{\alpha ml}(r, z, k), \qquad (9.25)
\end{aligned}$$

with

$$C_{ml} = \frac{2 - \delta_{m0}}{\pi^2 R^2 J_{m+1}^2(x_{ml})}. \qquad (9.26)$$

9.4.2 *Distribution Function, Kinetic and Constitutive Equations*

Obeying an appropriate kinetic equation, the distribution function depends on the value of V_0, e.g., through the one-electron energies $E_{\alpha ml}(k)$:

$$f_{\alpha ml}(k) = f_{\alpha ml}(k; V_0). \tag{9.27}$$

Generally, the value V_0 would be irrelevant as the eigenenergies are determined up to a constant, but in the present context, we need to keep its presence explicitly, the reason being that the second step of the MLDA amounts to replacing the — artificial — constant V_0 by the local potential $V(r, z)$, i.e.,

$$V_0 \to V(r, z) \quad \Rightarrow \quad f_{\alpha ml}(k; V_0) \to f_{\alpha ml}(k; V(r, z)). \tag{9.28}$$

As a result, the effect of the *abrupt* oxide barrier is accounted for quantum mechanically through the wave functions vanishing at $r = R$, while the *smooth* variations of the potential are described classically by simply adding $-eV(r, z)$ to the electron energies. Assuming further that the hole concentration is treated classically according to Eq. (9.17), we finally obtain the constitutive equation that expresses $\rho[V]$ in the MLDA approach as a local functional, i.e.,

$$\rho[r, z, V] = e\big(p[r, z, V] - n[r, z, V] + N_{\mathrm{D}}^{+}(r, z) - N_{\mathrm{A}}^{-}(r, z)\big), \tag{9.29}$$

$$p[r, z, V] = n_{\mathrm{i}} \exp\left(-\frac{\mu_p + eV(r, z)}{k_{\mathrm{B}}T}\right), \tag{9.30}$$

$$n[r, z, V] = \sum_{m=0}^{\infty}\sum_{l=1}^{\infty} C_{ml} J_m^2\left(\frac{x_{ml} r}{R}\right) \sum_{\alpha} \int_{-\infty}^{\infty} \mathrm{d}k\, f_{\alpha ml}(r, z, k; V(r, z)), \tag{9.31}$$

from which it becomes clear that condition (9.15) is satisfied.

Next, we make the dependence of $f_{\alpha ml}(r, z, k; V(r, z))$ on $V(r, z)$ explicit by assuming purely ballistic transport described by the collision-free Boltzmann equation (or Vlasov equation)

$$\frac{\partial f_{\alpha ml}(r, z, k, t)}{\partial t} + \frac{\hbar k}{2m_{\alpha z}} \cdot \frac{\partial f_{\alpha ml}(r, z, k, t)}{\partial z} - \frac{e}{\hbar} \cdot \frac{\partial V(r, z)}{\partial k} \frac{\partial f_{\alpha ml}(r, z, k, t)}{\partial k} = 0, \tag{9.32}$$

which obviously ignores all longitudinal reflections and tunneling events. When scattering mechanisms need to be incorporated, an efficient numerical algorithm based on Lagrange–Charpit method [9, 10] can be employed to solve the time-dependent Boltzmann transport equation. In the present case, however, as we are focusing on ballistic transport, we neglect all scattering events and, starting as well from the LC-method, we may derive an analytical solution to Eq. (9.32) yielding the steady-state distribution function [11] provided that, for each $r < R$, the potential energy profile $U(r, z) = -eV(r, z)$ attains a unique maximum $U_{\mathrm{M}}(r)$. Generally, the latter is not too restrictive an assumption for a biased nanowire FET, as illustrated in Fig. 9.2. The resulting distribution function reads

$$f_{\alpha ml}(r, z, k) = F\left(E_{\alpha ml}(k) - eV(r, z), \mu(r, z, \hbar k)\right), \tag{9.33}$$

where

$$F(E, \mu) = \frac{1}{1 + \mathrm{e}^{\beta(E-\mu)}}, \tag{9.34}$$

is the Fermi–Dirac function $\mu(r, z, \hbar k)$ can be interpreted as a non-uniform chemical potential, depending on the drain voltage V_{ds} and

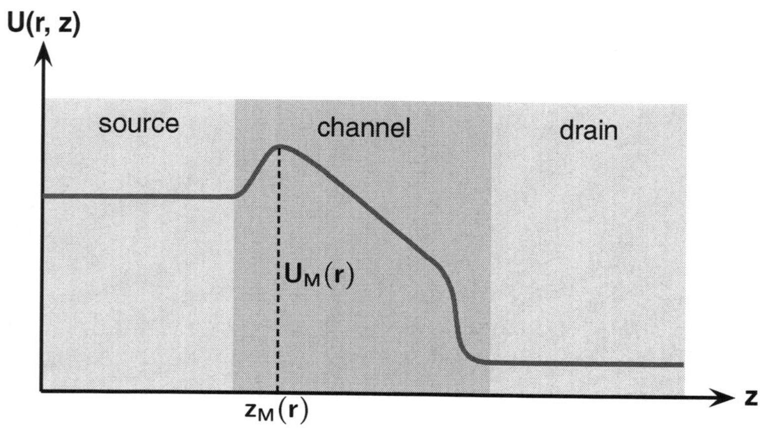

Figure 9.2. Typical potential energy profile inside the inversion layer of a biased n-channel nanowire FET. The dashed line indicates its maximum value $U_{\mathrm{M}}(r)$ located at $z = z_{\mathrm{M}}(r)$.

the equilibrium Fermi energy $E_{\rm F}$ which corresponds to $V_{\rm ds} = 0$, i.e.,

$$\mu(r, z, p) = E_{\rm F} - eV_{\rm ds}\Big[\theta\big(z \leqslant z_{\rm M}(r)\big)\theta\big(p \leqslant -p_{\rm M}(r, z)\big) + \theta\big(z \geqslant z_{\rm M}(r)\big)\theta\big(p \leqslant p_{\rm M}(r, z)\big)\Big], \tag{9.35}$$

with $p_{\rm M}(r, z) = \sqrt{2m_{\alpha z}\big(U_{\rm M}(r) + eV(r, z)\big)}$.

9.4.3 *Action Functional and Numerical Algorithm*

Now, having written the electron distribution function explicitly as a functional of the potential, we may exploit Eqs. (9.29–9.31) to evaluate the corresponding contributions to the action, which will be denoted, respectively, by $S_{\rm doping}$, $S_{\rm p}$ and $S_{\rm n}$. The contribution arising from the fixed dopant ions simply reduces to

$$\begin{aligned} S_{\rm doping}[V] &= -e\int_\Omega {\rm d}^3r\,\left[N_{\rm D}^+(r, z) - N_{\rm A}^-(r, z)\right] V(r, z) \\ &= -2\pi e\int_0^R {\rm d}r\, r\left[N_{\rm D}^+\int_0^{L_{\rm S}} {\rm d}z\, V(r, z) - N_{\rm A}^-\int_{L_{\rm S}}^{L_{\rm S}+L_{\rm CH}} {\rm d}z\, V(r, z) \right. \\ &\quad \left. + N_{\rm D}^+\int_{L-L_{\rm D}}^{L} {\rm d}z\, V(r, z)\right] \end{aligned} \tag{9.36}$$

where the prefactor 2π is due to the trivial integration over the polar angle ϕ. Similarly, the contribution from the holes that is taken from Eq. (9.19) can be expressed as

$$S_{\rm p}[V] = -2\pi e\, k_{\rm B}T\int_0^R {\rm d}r\, r\int_0^L {\rm d}z\, \exp\left(-\frac{\mu_p + eV(r, z)}{k_{\rm B}T}\right) \tag{9.37}$$

Using Eq. (9.31) and integrating $n[r, z, V']$ over V', we further obtain the electron contribution that reflects the inversion layer confinement,

$$\begin{aligned} S_{\rm n}[V] = 2\pi e\, k_{\rm B}T\sum_{m=0}^{\infty}\sum_{l=1}^{\infty} C_{ml}\int_0^R {\rm d}r\, rJ_m^2\left(\frac{x_{ml}r}{R}\right)\int_0^L {\rm d}z\sum_\alpha\int_{-\infty}^{\infty}{\rm d}k \\ \times \ln\left[1 + \exp\left(\frac{\mu(r, z, \hbar k) - E_{\alpha ml}(k) + eV(r, z)}{k_{\rm B}T}\right)\right]. \end{aligned} \tag{9.38}$$

Finally, for the sake of simplicity, we mention the contribution related to the energy of the electric field:

$$S_{\mathrm{E}}[V] = \frac{1}{2}\int_{\Omega} \mathrm{d}^3r\,\epsilon(r)\,|\nabla V(\mathbf{r})|^2$$
$$= \pi \int_{R}^{R+t_{\mathrm{ox}}} \mathrm{d}r\, r\,\epsilon(r) \int_0^L \mathrm{d}z \left[\left(\frac{\partial V(r,z)}{\partial r}\right)^2 + \left(\frac{\partial V(r,z)}{\partial z}\right)^2\right] \tag{9.39}$$

with $\epsilon(r) = \epsilon_{\mathrm{s}}\theta(r \leqslant R) + \epsilon_{\mathrm{ox}}\theta(R < r \leqslant R + t_{\mathrm{ox}})$.

The next step is to discretize the total action $S = S_{\mathrm{E}} + S_{\mathrm{doping}} + S_{\mathrm{p}} + S_{\mathrm{n}}$ on a two-dimensional grid $\{(r_i, z_j),\ 0 \leqslant i \leqslant N_r,\ 1 \leqslant j \leqslant N_z\}$ with $r_0 = 0, r_{N_r} = R + t_{\mathrm{ox}}, z_0 = 0, z_{N_z} = L$ or, equivalently, to introduce $N_r \times N_z$ cells

$$\Omega_{ij} = [r_{i-1}, r_i] \cup [z_{j-1}, z_j]; \quad 1 \le i \le N_r, \quad 1 \le j \le N_z \tag{9.40}$$

covering the entire device. In order to perform the calculation of various contributions to the action appearing as integrations over all cells, we need to specify the shape functions fixing the functional dependence of $V(r, z)$ within each given cell. In view of the cylindrical symmetry, we have used

$$V(r,z) = \begin{cases} V_{1j-1} + (V_{0j} - V_{0j-1})\dfrac{z - z_{j-1}}{z_j - z_{j-1}}, & 1 \leqslant j \leqslant N_z \\[2ex] V_{i-1,j-1} + \dfrac{V_{i,j-1} - V_{i-1,j-1}}{\ell_i}\ln\left(\dfrac{r}{r_{i-1}}\right) & \\[2ex] +(V_{i-1,j} - V_{i-1,j-1})\dfrac{z - z_{j-1}}{z_j - z_{j-1}}, & \\[2ex] \ell_i \equiv \ln\dfrac{r_i}{r_{i-1}}, \quad 2 \le i \le N_r, & 1 \leqslant j \leqslant N_z. \end{cases} \tag{9.41}$$

where $V_{i,j}$ denotes the potential at the mesh point (r_i, z_j). Applying Eq. (9.41) we immediately obtain the contribution to Eq. (9.39) from Ω_{ij},

$$S_{\mathrm{EM}}^{(ij)} = \frac{1}{2}C_{r,ij}\left(V_{i,j-1} - V_{i-1,j-1}\right)^2 + \frac{1}{2}C_{z,ij}\left(V_{i-1,j} - V_{i-1,j-1}\right)^2 \tag{9.42}$$

where the capacitances $C_{r,ij}$ and $C_{z,ij}$ are given by

$$C_{r,ij} = 2\pi\epsilon_{ij}(1-\delta_{i1})\frac{z_j - z_{j-1}}{\ell_i}, \quad C_{z,ij} = \pi\epsilon_{ij}\frac{r_i^2 - r_{i-1}^2}{z_j - z_{j-1}}, \quad (9.43)$$

and ϵ_{ij} equals either ϵ_s or ϵ_{ox} depending on whether the cell Ω_{ij} is located in the Si or oxide region. The contributions related to Ω_{ij}, arising from the other parts of the action, can be treated in a similar way on adopting the Simpson rule for the remaining volume integrals and simple Gauss quadrature to deal with the integral over k in Eq. (9.38). Then, considering S a function of the variables $\{V_{i,j}\}$, we may show by direct evaluation that the equations

$$\frac{\partial S}{\partial V_{i,j}} = 0, \quad 0 \leqslant i \leqslant N_r, \ 0 \leqslant j \leqslant N_z \quad (9.44)$$

which induce the mimimization of S, do coincide with the discretized non-linear Poisson equation representing the simultaneous solution of Poisson's equation and the constitutive equations (9.29–9.31) as well as encompassing the non-equilibrium (ballistic) distribution function. Solving the linear parts of these equations for $V_{i,j}$ we may recast them in the following iterative algorithm:

$$V_{i,j}^{\text{new}} = G\,(V_{i,j}^{\text{old}}, V_{i-1,j}^{\text{old}}, V_{i+1,j}^{\text{old}}, V_{i,j-1}^{\text{old}}, V_{i,j+1}^{\text{old}}), \quad (9.45)$$

which can be straightforwardly recast in the form of a Gauss–Seidel scheme. The computational flow based on the above algorithm roughly evolves as follows:

(1) Insert an educated guess for the potential profile $V_{i,j}$ into the right-hand side of Eq. (9.45) and obtain a new profile from the left-hand side.
(2) Iterate on the previous step and verify whether the updated action S is lower than the previous one.
(3) Terminate the iterations after the n-th iteration when the *relative* convergence criterion

$$\max\left|V_{i,j}^{(n)} - V_{i,j}^{(n-1)}\right| \leqslant \eta \cdot \max\left|V_{i,j}^{(n-1)}\right| \quad (9.46)$$

and the *absolute* convergence criterion

$$S^{(n)} < S^{(n-1)} < S^{(n-2)} < \ldots S^{(1)}, \quad (9.47)$$

are simultaneously met for a prescribed tolerance $\eta > 0$.

Once convergence has been attained, the steady-state ballistic current flowing through the nanowire FET may be calculated [11] from

$$J(r) = \frac{ek_{\mathrm{B}}T}{2\pi\hbar}\sum_{m=0}^{\infty}\sum_{l=1}^{\infty} C_{ml}J_m^2\left(\frac{x_{ml}r}{R}\right) \times \sum_{\alpha} \ln\left[\frac{1+\exp\left(\dfrac{E_{\mathrm{F}}-U_{\mathrm{M}}(r)-W_{\alpha ml}}{k_{\mathrm{B}}T}\right)}{1+\exp\left(\dfrac{E_{\mathrm{F}}-U_{\mathrm{M}}(r)-W_{\alpha ml}-eV_{\mathrm{ds}}}{k_{\mathrm{B}}T}\right)}\right], \quad (9.48)$$

where

$$W_{\alpha ml} = \frac{\hbar^2 x_{ml}^2}{2m_{\alpha\perp}R^2} \quad (9.49)$$

are the subband energies associated with the radial and azimuthal subband ladders.

9.4.4 *Some Results*

As an illustration, we have calculated the self-consistent charge and potential distribution in the MLDA approximation as well as the resulting ballistic current for a biased nanowire. To this end, we have simply treated the source and drain regions as equipotential volumes, i.e., we have taken $V(r,z) = 0$ and $V(r,z) = V_{\mathrm{ds}}$ respectively for $0 \leqslant z \leqslant L_{\mathrm{S}}$ and $L - L_{\mathrm{D}} \leqslant z \leqslant L$. Having further ignored work function differences between Si and the metal gate region for the sake of simplicity, we have imposed $V(R+t_{\mathrm{ox}}, z) = V_{\mathrm{G}}$ for $L_{\mathrm{S}} \leqslant z \leqslant L - L_{\mathrm{D}}$. Finally, we have linearly interpolated the potential $V(R+t_{\mathrm{ox}}, z)$ along the "floating surfaces" $r = R + t_{\mathrm{ox}}$, $0 \leqslant z \leqslant L_{\mathrm{S}}$, $L - L_{\mathrm{D}} \leqslant z \leqslant L$. The simulation results shown in the figures below apply to a nanowire FET with $R = 2.5$ nm, $L_{\mathrm{S}} = L_{\mathrm{D}} = 10$ nm, $L_{\mathrm{CH}} = 20$ nm, $T = 300$ K, $N_{\mathrm{D}} = 10^{20}$ cm^{-3}, $N_{\mathrm{A}} = 10^{18}$ cm^{-3}, $V_{\mathrm{G}} = 0.7$ V, $T = 300$ K and $\eta = 10^{-3}$. The rectangular equidistant grid contains $N_r \times N_z = 120 \times 120$ cells. In Fig. 9.3 the normalized action is plotted against the number of iterations for $V_{\mathrm{ds}} = 0.1$ V and 0.3 V. In order to trace the evolution of the action over subsequent iteration cycles, we have extended the number

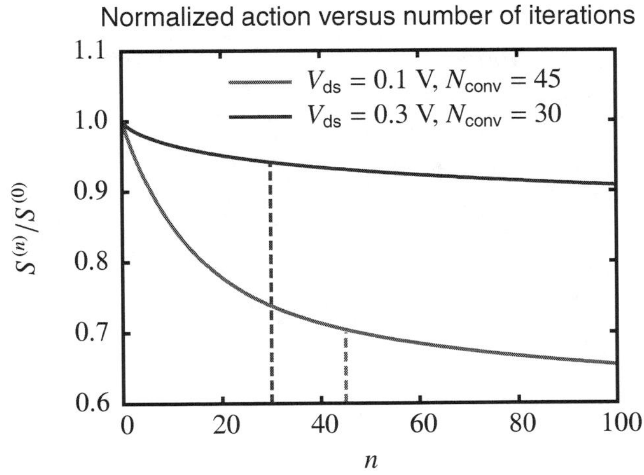

Figure 9.3. Normalized action versus number of iterations for $V_{ds} = 0.1$ V and $V_{ds} = 0.3$ V. N_{conv} is the number of iterations required to reach relative convergence given a tolerance $\eta = 10^{-3}$, as depicted by the dashed lines. Parameters: $R = 2.5$ nm, $L_S = L_D = 10$ nm, $L_{CH} = 20$ nm, $T = 300$ K, $N_D = 10^{20}$ cm^{-3}, $N_A = 10^{18}$ cm^{-3}, $V_G = 0.7$ V, $T = 300$ K, $N_r = N_z = 120$. See also Color Insert.

of iterations far beyond the relative convergence criterion. As a result, both curves of Fig. 9.3 reveal the relatively slow pace of the absolute convergence sequence that monitors the evolution of the action toward its exact minimum. However, the exact minimal action being considerably lower than the value obtained when relative convergence is achieved, should not be a matter of concern. After all, the numerical calculation of the genuine minimum would generally call for quite a large numerical accuracy, say on the level of machine precision, which would substantially exceed moderate tolerances such as 10^{-3} or larger. In other words, the absolute convergence should be rather viewed as an indicator guarding the stability of the numerical solution that could be expected if a new simulation with a smaller tolerance were to be made.

Contour plots of the ballistic distribution functions obtained from minimizing the action functionals and using Eq. (9.33) are depicted in Fig. 9.4 for the ground-state subband ($m = 0, l = 1$) of the lowest valley ($\alpha = 1$) and at $r = 2.2$ nm, which corresponds

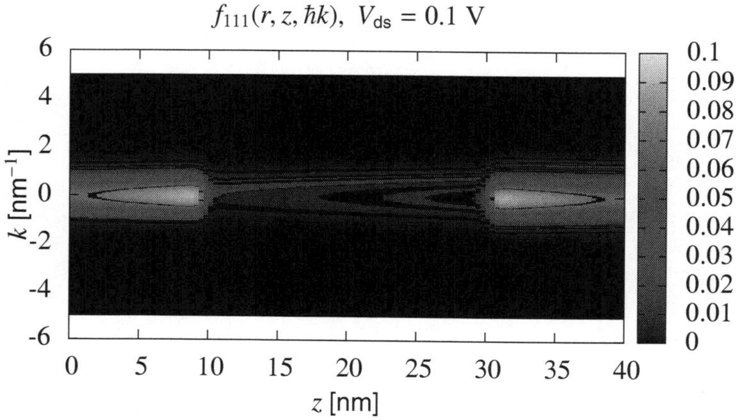

(a)

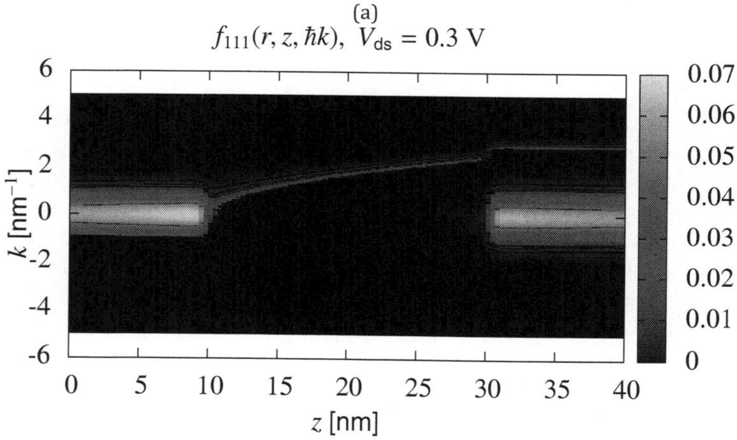

(b)

Figure 9.4. Contour plots of the ground-state ballistic distribution functions for $V_{ds} = 0.1$ V (a) and $V_{ds} = 0.3$ V (b), illustrating the occurrence of ballistic jets. The channel region corresponds to the interval 10 nm $\leqslant z \leqslant$ 30 nm. $m = 0, l = \alpha = 1$ and $r = 2.2$ nm. Other parameters same as in Fig. 9.3. See also Color Insert.

to a spot of high electron density, given a wire radius of $R = 2.5$ nm. Finally, the ballistic currents calculated with the help of the above distribution functions are shown in Fig (9.5) for $V_G = 0.5, 0.6$ and 0.7 V.

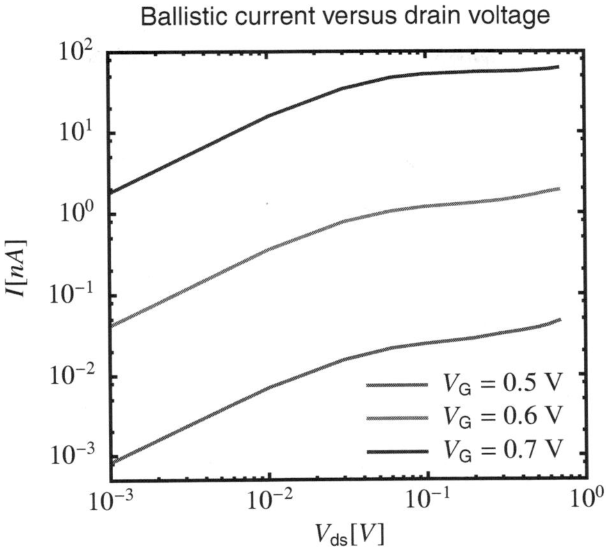

Figure 9.5. Ballistic current versus drain voltage for three different gate voltages. $R = 2.5$ nm. Other parameters same as in Fig. 9.3. See also Color Insert.

9.5 Outlook

In spite of its promising perspective, the variational principle described in this chapter as well as its implementation in numerical programs suffers from two major restrictions: (1) It has been formulated and worked out only for electrostatic fields governed merely by Poisson's equation and (2) it heavily relies on the MLDA, which is the key feature allowing for the introduction of self-consistency in Eq. (9.9) through the charge density, which forcefully takes the form of a strictly local functional of the potential $V(\mathbf{r})$. In this light, we see two possible extensions of the present formalism.

First, numerous applications related to carrier transport in semiconductors interacting with an electromagnetic field in the ultra-high frequency range, only require the classical transport theory, which remains compatible with the MLDA, whereas the real challenge is in writing proper numerical code that is capable of solving Maxwell's equations for 3D structures in the high-frequency range. Numerical code being developed to this end may therefore greatly benefit from an extended variational principle built on the full electromagnetic action discussed in Section 9.2, i.e.,

$$S[V,\mathbf{A}] = \int_{\Omega} \mathrm{d}^3 r \left(\frac{1}{2}\epsilon |\nabla V|^2 - \frac{1}{2\mu} |\nabla \times \mathbf{A}|^2 - \int_{V_0}^{V(\mathbf{r})} \mathrm{d}V' \rho[V',\mathbf{A}'] \right.$$
$$\left. \times \int_{\mathbf{A}_0}^{\mathbf{A}(\mathbf{r})} \mathrm{d}\mathbf{A}' \cdot \mathbf{J}[V',\mathbf{A}'] \right), \tag{9.50}$$

such that $\delta S[V,\mathbf{A}] = 0$ would analogously give rise to the four Maxwell equations self-consistently coupled to the (classical) kinetic and constitutive equations.

Second, a less straightforward approach could be envisaged in order to abandon the MLDA-related restriction while keeping focus on static fields, as would be required when a fully quantum mechanical treatment of transport becomes inevitable. Since the non-local dependence of the constitutive equations is pronouncedly present in the carrier wave functions, though in a very implicit way, an alternative and more transparent route may be provided by the formalism of path integrals.

References

1. F. Brosens and W. Magnus, Newtonian trajectories: A powerful tool for solving quantum dynamics, *Solid St. Commun.* **150**, 2102–2105 (2010).
2. C. M. Van Vliet and A. Barrios, Quantum electron transport beyond linear response, *Physica A.* **315**, 493–536 (2002).
3. C. M. Van Vliet, *Equilibrium and Non-Equilibrium Statistical Mechanics* (World Scientific, London, Singapore, 2010), 2nd edition.
4. J. D. Jackson, *Classical Electrodynamics* (Addison Wesley Publishing Company, New York, USA, 2005), 2nd edition.
5. R. B. Leighton, R. P. Feynman, and M. Sands, *The Feynman Lectures on Physics.* vol. 2 (Addison-Wesley, USA, 1966).
6. W. Magnus and W. Schoenmaker, *Introduction to Electromagnetism,* In *Handbook of Numerical Analysis,* vol. 13, *Special volume: Numerical Methods in Electromagnetics,* pp. 3–103. Elsevier North Holland, Amsterdam, The Netherlands, 1st edition (2005).

7. C.-Y. Lee, K. Lee, C.-K. Kim, and M.-U. Kim, Variational Formulation of Poisson's Equation in Semiconductor at Quasi-Equilibrium and Its Applications, *IEEE Trans. Electron Devices.* **44**(9), 1507–1515, (1997).
8. G. Paasch and H. Übensee, A modified local density approximation. Electron density in inversion layers, *Phys. Stat. Solidi (b).* **113**(1), 165–178 (1982).
9. W. Magnus, F. Brosens, and B. Sorée, Modeling drive currents and leakage currents: a dynamic approach, *J. Comput. Electron.* **8**, 307–323 (2009).
10. W. Magnus, F. Brosens, and B. Sorée, Time dependent transport in 1d micro- and nanostructures: solving the Boltzmann and Wigner — Boltzmann equations, *J. Phys. C: Conf. Series.* **193**, 012004-1 (2009).
11. H. Carrillo-Nuñez, W. Magnus, and F. M. Peeters, A simplified quantum mechanical model for nanowire transistors based on non-linear variational calculus, *J. Appl. Phys.* **108**, 063708-8 (2010).

Chapter 10

New Tools for the Direct Characterisation of FinFETS

G. C. Tettamanzi,[a,b] A. Paul,[c] S. Lee,[c] G. Klimeck,[c,d] and S. Rogge[a,b]

[a] *Kavli Institute of Nanoscience, Delft University of Technology, Lorentzweg 1, 2628 CJ Delft, The Netherlands*
[b] *CQC2T, University of New South Wales, Sydney, NSW 2052, Australia*
[c] *Network for Computational Nanotechnology, Purdue University, West Lafayette, Indiana 47907, USA*
[d] *Jet Propulsion Laboratory, California Institute of Technology, Pasadena, California 91109, USA*
g.tettamanzi@unsw.edu.au

10.1 Introduction

This chapter discusses how classical transport theories such as the thermionic emission (Sze, 1981), can be used as a powerful tool for the study and the understanding of the most complex mechanisms of transport in fin field effect transistors (FinFETs). By means of simple current and differential conductance measurements, taken at different temperatures and different gate voltages (V_G's), it is possible to extrapolate the evolution of two important parameters such as the spatial region of transport and the height of thermionic barrier at the centre of the channel. Furthermore, if the measurements are used in

CMOS Nanoelectronics: Innovative Devices, Architectures, and Applications
Edited by Nadine Collaert

ISBN 978-981-4364-02-7 (Hardcover), 978-981-4364-03-4 (eBook)
www.panstanford.com

conjunction with simulated data, it becomes possible to also extract the interface trap density of these objects. These are important results, also because these parameters are extracted directly on state-of-the-art devices and not in specially designed test structures. The possible characterization of the different regimes of transport that can arise in these ultra-scaled devices having a doped or an undoped channel are also discussed. Examples of these regimes are full body inversion and weak body inversion. Specific cases demonstrating the strength of the thermionic tool are discussed in Sections 10.2, 10.3, and 10.4.

10.2 Transport in Doped N-FinFETs

Non-planar field-effect transistors called FinFETs (Hisamo *et al.*, 2000) have been developed to solve the issues of gate control encountered with the standard planar geometry when the channel length is reduced to a sub-45 nm size. Their triple-gate geometry is expected to have a more efficient gate action on the channel and to solve the leakage problem through the body of the transistor, one of the most dramatic short channel effects (Hisamo *et al.*, 2000). However, their truly three-dimensional (3D) structure makes doping — and thus also potential — profiles very difficult to simulate and to understand using previous knowledge on device technology. Transport studies at low temperature, where the thermally activated transport is suppressed, can bring insight to these questions by measuring local gate action. For these reasons, in a recent work (Sellier *et al.*, 2007), the potential profile of these devices has been investigated by conductance measurements. This has allowed the observation of the formation of a sub-threshold channel at the edge of the silicon nanowire. This corner effect has been proposed (Doyle *et al.*, 2003; Fossum *et al.*, 2003) as an additional contribution to the sub-threshold current in these 3D triple-gate structures, where the edges of the nanowire experience stronger gate action due to the geometric enhancement of the electric field. However, besides extensive simulation work (Doyle *et al.*, 2003; Fossum *et al.*, 2003) — due to the difficulties with these 3D structures — very little experimental work (Xiong *et al.*, 2004) has been published previous

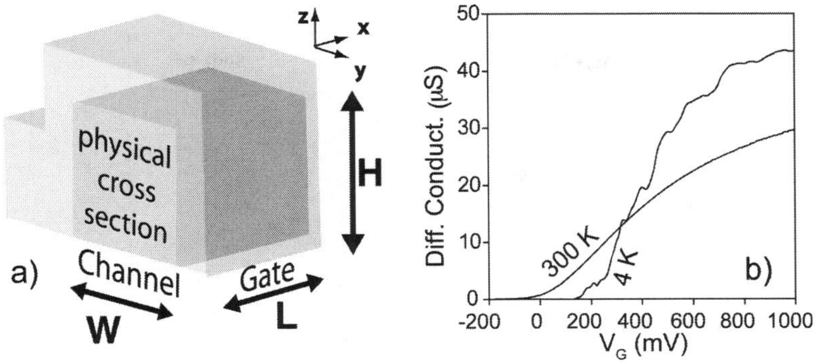

Figure 10.1. (a) Schematic of the FinFET geometry where the gate surrounds the Si nanowire (the fin). (b) Low Bias differential conductance vs. gate voltage for a long and narrow silicon FinFET (L = 950 nm, W = 35 nm).

to the ones discussed in this chapter. This paragraph focusses on the description of the experimental observation of the corner effect on doped devices identical to the ones described in the next chapter (see Fig. 10.1a).

10.2.1 *Thermionic Emission in Doped FinFET Devices*

The aim of this section is to show that, by using a combination of differential conductance ($G = dI_{SD}/dV_{SD}$) versus V_G traces taken at different temperature, and of low temperature Coulomb blockade (CB) (see Sellier *et al.* (2007) and references therein) measurements, it is possible to infer the existence of a dot located at the edge of the fin and thus of the corner effect (Doyle *et al.*, 2003; Fossum *et al.*, 2003).

In the investigated device series the height of the fin wire is always H = 65 nm, while the width ranges from W = 35 nm to 1 μm and the gate length ranges from L = 50 nm to 1 μm. The relatively high p-type doping ($\sim 10^{18}$ cm^{-3}) of the channel wire is chosen to ensure a depletion length shorter than half the channel length in order to have a fully developed potential barrier in this n-p-n structure and so to keep the conductance threshold at a large enough positive gate voltage. The characteristics at room temperature of these nanoscale FinFETs look therefore similar to

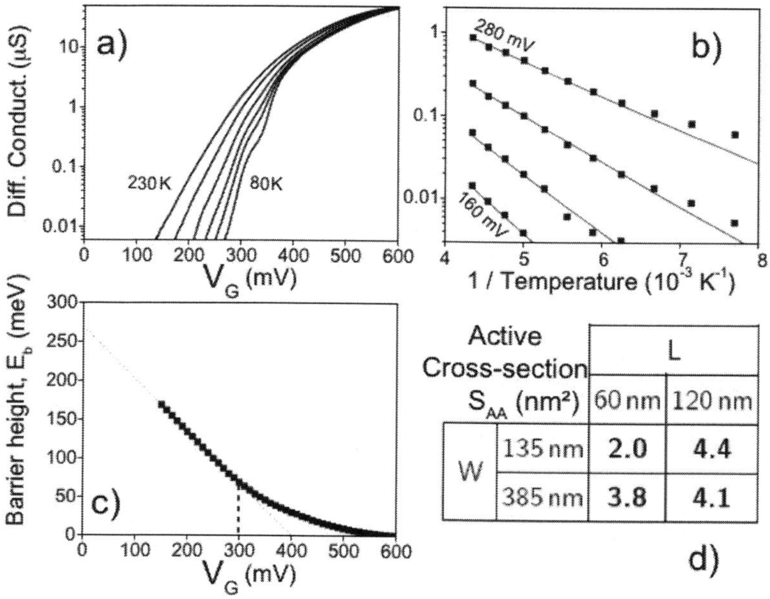

Figure 10.2. (a) Differential conductance vs gate voltage for a short and wide fin ($L = 60$ nm, $W = 385$ nm). (b) Differential conductance plotted vs the inverse of the temperature for the same sample. The conductance is thermally activated above 150 K. (c) Barrier height vs V_G changing behavior at 300 mV (same sample). (d) Measured cross section S_{AA} for the activated current of 4 samples with different lengths L and widths W.

those of their larger planar counterparts (see Fig. 10.1b at 300 K). For sub-threshold voltages, a thermionic barrier (E_b) (Sze, 1981) exists between the source and drain electron reservoirs and the transport is thermally activated at high enough temperature, as shown in Fig. 10.2a,b. For very short devices, G is simply given by the thermionic emission above the barrier according to the formula (Sze, 1981):

$$G_{3D} = S_{AA} A^* T \frac{e}{k_B} exp\left(-\frac{E_b(V_G)}{k_B T}\right) \qquad (10.1)$$

where the effective Richardson constant A^* for Si is $2.1\times$ 120 A cm^2 K^2, T is the temperature, k_B the Boltzmann constant, e the elementary charge and S_{AA} represents the active cross section, which can be interpreted as a good estimation of the portion of the physical cross section area through which the transport preferentially occurs (Sze, 1981).

10.2.2 *Analysis of the Thermionic Regime (High Temperatures)*

Several samples have been measured in this thermionic regime (80 K $\leqslant T \leqslant$ 250 K) and their conductance has been fitted using Eq. (10.1) to obtain E_b and S_{AA} (see Fig. 10.2c,d). The two 385 nm wide samples have the same cross section $S_{AA} \approx 4$ nm^2 although their length differ by a factor of 2. It is therefore possible to conclude that, in the sub-threshold regime transport is dominated by thermionic emission in these devices. The two 135 nm-wide samples, however, have different S_{AA} values, but this cannot imply a diffusive transport since the longest sample has the largest conductance. Another result is that the cross section $S_{AA} \approx 4$ nm^2 is much smaller than the channel width W (135 or 385 nm) multiplied by the channel interface thickness (about 1 nm). This result is consistent with the corner effect that produces a lower conduction band (stronger electric field) along the two edges of the wire, where the current will flow preferentially (Fig. 10.3b). The barrier height E_b versus gate voltage is plotted in Fig. 10.2c. The data extrapolated to zero gate voltage are consistent with a 220 meV barrier height calculated for a p-type channel in contact with a n++ gate through a 1.4 nm SiO_2 dielectric (Sze, 1981). The linear dependence of the barrier height shows a good channel/gate coupling ratio, $\alpha = dE_b/(dV_G) = 0.68$, due to the triple-gate geometry with a thin gate oxide. At higher gate voltage (above 300 mV), the coupling ratio decreases and a finite barrier survives up to large voltages.

10.2.3 *Analysis of the Coulomb Blockade Regime (Low Temperatures)*

Analysis of the low-temperature transport (4 K $\leqslant T \leqslant$ 60 K, see below) shows that the gate action remains constant inside the channel where localised states are formed. Two confining barriers are formed in the access regions (between channel and contacts), where the concentration of implanted arsenic atoms is

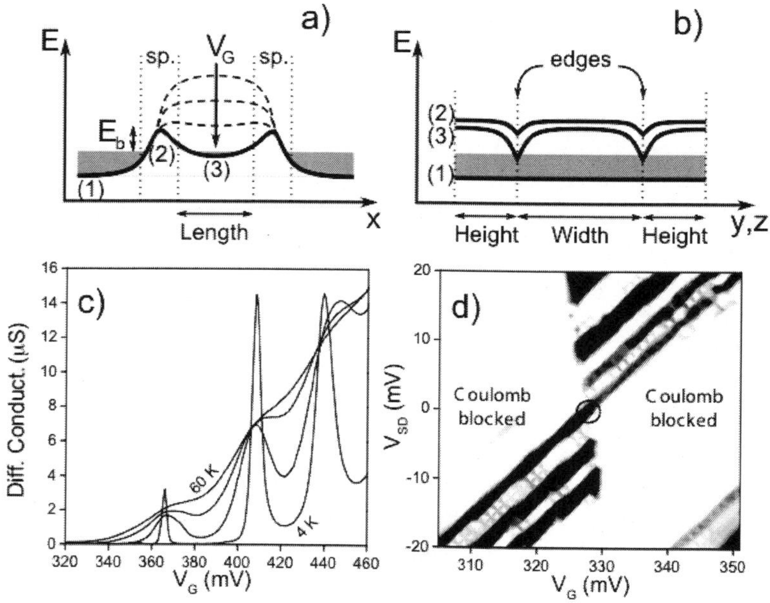

Figure 10.3. (a) Conduction band edge profile with the highest barrier in the channel or in the access regions below the spacers (sp.) depending on the gate voltage. (b) Band edge along the gate oxide interface (1) in the contacts, (2) in the barriers, and (3) in the channel. The corner effect produces two channels with low barriers at the wire edges. (c) Differential conductance vs gate voltage for a short and wide channel ($L = 60$ nm, $W = 385$ nm) showing Coulomb blockade peaks up to high temperatures (20 K steps). (d) Stability diagram, i.e., conductance vs gate and bias voltages at 4.2 K. The circle indicates a zero bias conductance peak, which develops into a triangular sector at finite bias.

reduced by the masking silicon nitride spacers placed next to the gate (see Fig. 10.3a). For long channels and at low temperatures the conductance develops fluctuations versus gate voltage (see Fig. 10.1b) with a pattern that reproduces after thermal cycling (at least for the main features). These fluctuations are caused by quantum interferences in the channel. For gate voltages close to the threshold, charge localization occurs, especially for short fins. In fact, when short channel devices are cooled down to 4.2 K, conductance pattern develops a series of peaks, as can be seen in Fig. 10.3c, that can be attributed to Coulomb blockade of electrons in the potential

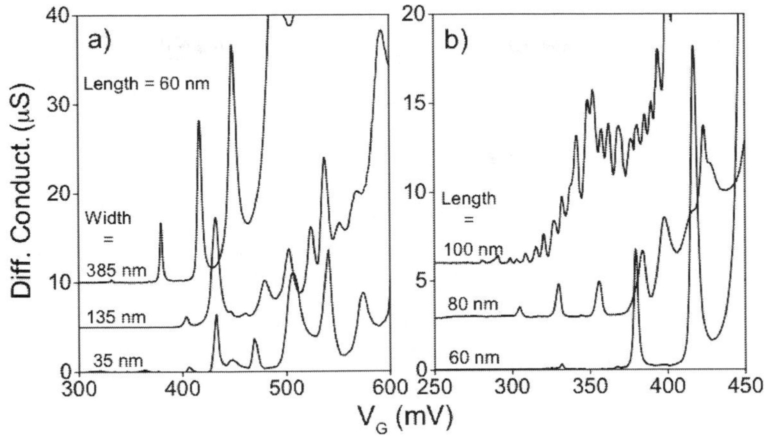

Figure 10.4. Differential conductance vs V_G at 4.2 K for several devices. (a) Short fins ($L = 60$ nm) of different widths ($W = 35, 135, 385$ nm) have a similar peak spacing. (b) Devices with longer fins ($L = 60, 80, 100$ nm) have a smaller peak spacing (the widths are different). The curves have been shifted for clarity.

well created in the channel by the two tunnel barriers of the low-doped access regions (Sellier *et al.*, 2007). This interpretation is supported by the channel-length dependence of the peak spacing discussed later. An explanation in terms of a quantum well formed by an impurity can be ruled out. An impurity or defect could not accept many electrons, i.e., more than 20 for the 100 nm sample in Fig. 10.4b, since they represent a single charge or empty state.

10.2.4 *Interpretation of the Results*

These results can be interpreted as follows: Devices with shorter channel act as quantum dots where the conduction electrons are spatially localised and are Coulomb blockade for the transport by a finite charging energy bias. In the stability diagram of a quantum dot (see Fig. 10.3d), the slopes of a triangular conducting sector give the ratios of the capacitances C_G, C_S, and C_D between the dot and, respectively, the gate, source, and drain electrodes. In this way the dot/gate coupling $\alpha = C_G/(C_G + C_S + C_D) = 0.78$ (0.65) for the first (second) resonance is found. These values are close to the channel/gate coupling of 0.68 obtained independently in the same sample from the gate voltage dependence of the barrier height in the middle of the channel at higher temperatures. This result indicates that the gate coupling in the centre of the device remains constant and supports the idea of a minimum in the conduction band, as sketched in (Fig. 10.3b). The peak spacing, ΔV_G, is the change in gate voltage that increases by 1 the number of electrons in the dot located at the silicon/oxide interface. This quantity provides the dot/gate capacitance $C_G = e/\Delta V_G$, and then the dot area $S = C_G/C_{ox}$ using the gate capacitance per unit area $C_{ox} = \epsilon_{ox}/t_{ox} = 0.025$ F/m^2. The peak spacings for the same gate length ($L = 60$ nm) but three different channel widths ($W = 35$, 135, and 385 nm) can be compared in Fig. 10.4a. Although the patterns are not very regular, an average peak spacing of about 30 mV is obtained for all of them, indicating similar dot areas whereas the effective width is varied by more than one order of magnitude.

10.2.5 *The Corner Effect*

The conductance patterns for three different lengths ($L = 60$, 80, and 100 nm) shown in (Fig. 10.4b) have decreasing average peak spacings ($\Delta V_G = 39$, 24, and 6 mV, respectively) and therefore increasing dot areas ($S_{AA} = 160$, 270, and 1100 nm^2). However, these areas are not strictly proportional to the gate length, so that the actual width could be length dependent or the actual dot length could be smaller than the gate length for very short fins. If it is assumed that the dot length equals the gate length, we obtain 2.7, 3.4, and 11 nm for the dot width, i.e., a small fraction of the total Si/oxide interface width $W_{eff} = W + 2H = 150$–500 nm. The observation of similar dot widths of a few nanometers for different fin widths of hundreds of nanometers is consistent with the idea of a dot located at the edge of the fin and thus with the corner effect (Doyle *et al.*, 2003; Fossum *et al.*, 2003).

10.2.6 *Temperature Dependence of the Conductance Peaks*

In addition to a large charging energy $E_c = \alpha e \Delta V_G$, these dots also have a large quantum level spacing ΔE, as can be deduced from the temperature dependence of the conductance peaks in Fig. 10.3c. When the temperature is lowered below the level spacing, the tunneling process involves a single quantum level at a time and the peak height starts to increase above the high temperature value (Sellier *et al.*, 2007). The crossover from the classical to the quantum regime of Coulomb blockade being around 15 K, it is possible to estimate the level spacing to be about 1.3 meV. If the value $L = 60$ nm is used for the gate length, in the expression $\Delta E = 3\pi^2\hbar^2/2m^*L^2$ for the energy separation between the first and second states of a one-dimensional system, a level spacing $\Delta E = 1.6$ meV, similar to the experimental estimation, is found. This result supports the idea of a long dot extending over the whole gate length (assumed above to extract the dot width from the dot/gate capacitance).

10.2.7 *Conclusion*

In doped channel FinFETs, experiments show the existence of a few nanometers wide edge channel, which shows itself in the activated current amplitude, the Coulomb blockade peaks spacing, and the quantum levels spacing. These channels are formed along the edges the devices due to an enhanced band bending called corner effect. To utilize the full FinFET cross section for electron transport with a homogeneous current distribution, a lower sub-threshold current, and a larger on/off current ratio, this corner effect should be reduced. Better devices should have rounder corners on the scale of the depletion length and a lower doping concentration in the channel.

10.3 Transport in Undoped N-FinFETs

Section 10.2 showed that in doped FinFET the geometry and the mechanisms of sub-threshold transport are affected by the presence of screening. This screening may result in a reduction of active transistor area (i.e., corner effect) and in a sub-threshold swing (SS) degradation. Several models predicted that the introduction of an undoped channel FinFETs avoids the formation of the corner effect (Doyle *et al.*, 2003; Fossum *et al.*, 2003) in these devices. However, it has been found that even the undoped channel devices have a non-trivial, gate voltage (V_G) dependent current distribution; there is therefore the necessity to develop tools that could be used to investigate current distribution even in these intrinsic channel devices (Tettamanzi *et al.*, 2010). Design insights could be used to improve device characteristics towards their scaling to the nanometer size regime.

10.3.1 *Introduction to Transport in Undoped Devices*

For undoped FinFETs and for widths smaller than 5 nm, full volume inversion is expected to arise (Wong (2002) and references therein). Wider devices are expected to be in the regime of weak volume inversion (where the bands in the channel closely follow the potential of V_G) only for $V_G \ll V_{th}$ (Wong, 2002; Taur, 2000). Several groups have theoretically investigated the behavior of such weak volume inversion devices using both classical (Fossum *et al.*, 2003), and quantum (Ruiz *et al.*, 2007) computational models, but no experimental method that yields information on the location of the current-carrying regions of the channel exists prior to the work discussed in this section. Taur has studied this problem analytically for an undoped channel with double gate (DG) geometry, using a 1-D Poisson equation (Taur, 2000). The main conclusion emerging from this work is that when the gate voltage is increased, a crossover takes place between the behavior of the channel at $V_G \ll V_{th}$, and at $V_G \sim V_{th}$, caused by screening of induced carriers which subsequently increase the carrier density at the gate-channel interface. This section describes the first experimental observation of this prediction, furthermore the results of a 2D model are compared with experimental data, keeping in mind that the physical principles of this are fully analogues to the 1D case of Taur.

10.3.2 *Experimental Results*

Conductance versus temperature traces for a set of eight undoped FinFET devices with the same channel length, length ($L = 40$ nm) and channel height (H $= 65$ nm) but different channel widths,

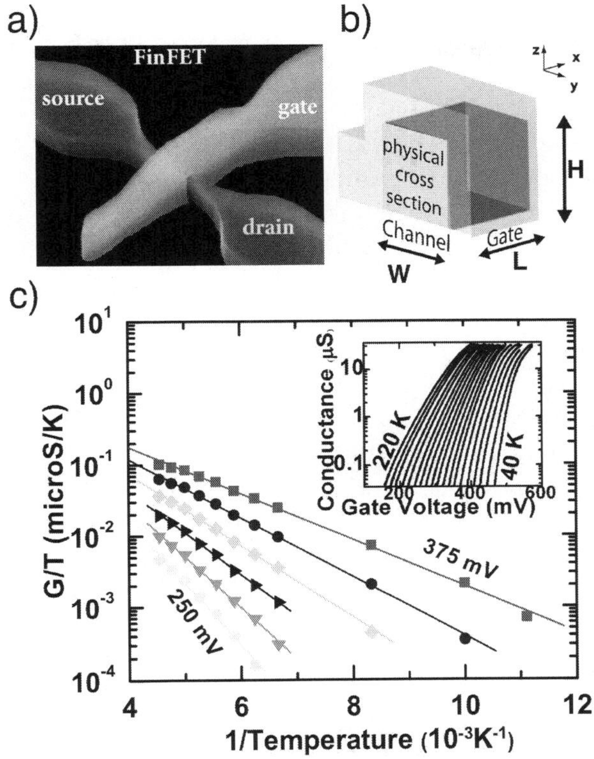

Figure 10.5. (a) Scanning electron microscope (SEM) image of typical FinFETs studied in this section. (b) Schematic view of the FinFETs as in Fig. 10.1 The gate (light yellow) covers three faces of the channel (dark grey). L, H and W represent the channel length, height and width respectively. The physical cross sectional area is shown in light grey. (c) Fits used to extrapolate E_b and S_{AA} in one of our $W = 55$ nm device. In the inset, differential conductance versus V_G data, for different temperatures, are shown.

($W = 25$, 55, 125, and 875 nm) are studied in this section. The discussion focuses on one device for each width since the same behavior for each of the devices of the same width is found consistently. The devices consist of a nanowire channel etched on a 65 nm Si intrinsic film with a wrap-around gate covering three faces of the channel (Fig. 10.5a,b) (Collaert *et al.*, 2005). They have a geometry identical to the ones discussed in Section 10.2 (Sellier *et al.*, 2007), but their channels are completely undoped. In the devices of this study, an HfSiO layer isolates a TiN layer from the intrinsic Si channel (Collaert *et al.*, 2005). Differential conductance data are taken at $V_{SD} = 0$ mV using a lock-in technique. Fig. 10.5c shows the $G\,/\,T$ versus $1000/T$ data obtained from the G versus V_G data taken at different temperatures (inset in Fig. 10.5c).

Using the data of Fig. 10.5c, results for the source (drain)-channel barrier height, E_b, versus V_G dependence and for the active cross-section area of the channel, S_{AA}, versus V_G dependence can be extrapolated using the thermionic fitting procedure as described in Section 10.2. The important fact is that S_{AA} can, also in the undoped case, be interpreted as a good estimation of the portion of the physical cross-section area through which the transport preferentially occurs. Note that Eq. (10.1) has only two parameters, S_{AA} and E_b, and the accuracy obtained in the fits made using this equation[1] demonstrates the validity of the use of this model for the study of sub-threshold transport also in these undoped channel FinFETs.

10.3.3 *Evolution of the Barrier Height with Gate Voltage*

Figure 10.6a examines the barrier height as a function of V_G. An expected decrease in E_b while increasing V_G is observed (as for doped devices, see Fig. 10.2c). The inset of Fig. 10.6a shows that, this effect is less pronounced for a wider device. The decrease is to be attributed to short-channel effects (SCEs) that influence the electronic characteristics even at low bias. This trend is also reflected by the data of Table 10.1, where the coupling factors obtained from our thermionic fits, $\alpha_1 = dE_b/dV_G$,[2] show a decrease for increasing width.

10.3.3.1 Capacitive coupling

In Table 10.1, the coupling between the potential of the channel interface and V_G, α_2, extracted from Coulomb blockade (CB)

[1] $R \sim 0.99$ for all fits of devices with width $\leqslant 125$ nm, as shown in Fig. 10.5c.

[2] See also Section 10.2, thus the electrostatic coupling between the gate and the bulk of the channel.

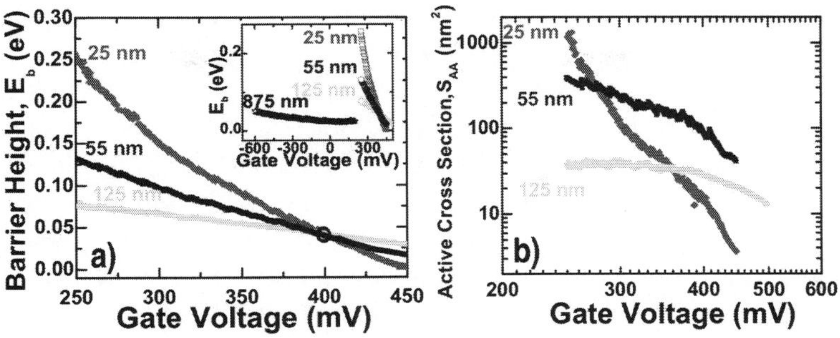

Figure 10.6. Data obtained using the model of Eq. 10.1: (a) E_b versus V_G for one device for each width from 25 nm to 125 nm. In the inset, calculated E_b versus V_G for all device widths are shown. (b) Results of the dependence of the active cross section, S_{AA}, versus V_G obtained for all devices with $W \leqslant$ 125 nm.

Table 10.1. Summary of the characteristics gate channel capacitive coupling of devices reported in this study, obtained from the results of Fit as in Fig. 10.2a (α_1) and from Coulomb Blockage (CB) measurements at 4.2 K (α_2)

Width (nm)	α_1	α_2
25	1	0.7
55	0.7	0.8
125	0.14	0.8
875	0.03	0.8

measurements (at 4.2 K) of confined states that are present at the Channel/Gate interface (Hinds *et al.*, 2000) is also shown. α_2, is found to be a constant independent of W. In CB theory, α_2 is the ratio between the electrochemical potential of the confined states and the change in V_G. This ratio can be estimated from the so-called stability diagram (Sellier *et al.*, 2007) as it is shown in Section 10.2. Overall, these results lead to the conclusion that the coupling to the channel interface remains constant for increasing W, whereas the coupling to the centre of the channel does not. In the 875 nm devices, SCEs are so strong (see inset Fig. 10.6a), that the thermionic theory loses accuracy; hence the results of these devices will not be discussed any further. All the E_b versus V_G curves, as depicted in Figure 10.6a, cross each other at around 0.4 V (outlined by the black circle), before complete inversion of the channel takes place at $V_{th} \sim 0.5$ V (Collaert *et al.*, 2005). This suggests that for these devices and at $V_G = 0.4$ V, the work function of the TiN is equal to the affinity of the Si channel in our devices (flat bands condition). The same value has also been verified in other measurements using capacitance-voltage ($C-V$) techniques (Singanamalla *et al.*, 2006), independently from the W of the channel. This fact confirm, that, also for these devices, similarly to the ones described in section 10.2, activated transport over the channel barrier is indeed observed. However, for these undoped devices, the barrier is formed by the Metal/Oxide/Semiconductor interface, which at $V_G = 0.4$ V will not dependent on W. The crossing point in Fig. 10.6 (a) is not located exactly at $E_b = 0$ meV, but is at 50 meV. This feature is attributed to the presence, at the Channel-Gate boundary, of interface states (already found in CB measurements) that can store charge, repel electrons and therefore raise-up the barrier by a small amount. In Si/SiO_2 systems that have been studied in the past, these states were estimated to give an energy shift quantifiable between 70 and 120 meV (Hinds *et al.*, 2000), in line with the data of this section.

10.3.4 *Evolution of the Active Cross Section with Gate Voltage*

The data of S_{AA} for these undoped FinFETs show a surprising different evolution with increasing V_G's if compared to what has been observed in the previous section 10.2 for doped channel devices. Fig. 10.6b shows S_{AA} as a function of V_G extrapolated using Eq. (10.1). These results are then compared to the analytical model (Taur, 2000) discussed before and to the self-consistent simulations performed as described in (Neophytou *et al.*, 2008; Paul *et al.*, 2009; Lee *et al.*, 2009; Klimeck *et al.*, 2009). At low V_G, devices with $W = 25$ nm show an active cross sectional area of around 1000 nm^2 (see Fig. 10.6b). This is almost equal to the physical cross sectional area of the channel at these widths. At higher V_G, the active cross sectional decreases to a few nm^2. The interpretation of this data is as follows: at low V_G, transport in these devices is uniformly distributed everywhere in the physical cross section of the channel (weak volume inversion). But with the increase of V_G, an increase of carrier density in the region near the interface, which leads to a reduction of S_{AA}, arises. This interpretation corresponds with the screening mechanism discussed in Taur (2000). Subsequently the action of the gate on the centre of the channel is suppressed. Devices that have 55 nm and 125 nm widths behave in a fashion similar to the ones with 25 nm, but show a less pronounced decreasing trend and counter intuitive small values for S_{AA}, as a progressive reduction of α_1 (i.e., of the gate-to-channel coupling) for increasing W is indeed observed. This is not a surprise as the barrier in these larger devices is lower and more carriers are allowed to migrate to the interface enhancing the screening effect. These results give, for the first time, an experimental insight into the mechanisms of conduction in undoped FinFETs.

10.3.5 *Comparison with Simulation*

State-of-the-art-simulations, done using an atomistic 10 band $sp^3d^5s^*$ Tight-binding (TB) model (Klimeck *et al.*, 2002; Lee *et al.*, 2009), have been used to perform electronic structure calculation, coupled self-consistently with a 2D Poisson solver (Neophytou *et al.*, 2008), and terminal characteristics using a ballistic top of the barrier (ToB) model (Paul *et al.*, 2009) have been obtained. Due to the extensively large cross-section of the device that combines up to 44,192 atoms in the simulation domain, a new NEMO 3D code (Lee *et al.*, 2009) has been integrated into the top of the barrier analysis (Paul *et al.*, 2009). This expanded modeling capability has made possible to compare experiment and simulations results. The effects of the variation of the potential in the source-drain direction are not expected to play a role in the simulated devices since V_{SD} is very small (Paul *et al.*, 2009; Tettamanzi *et al.*, 2010). Also, the gate length is long enough to suppress the tunneling current from source to drain (Paul *et al.*, 2009; Tettamanzi *et al.*, 2010). In fact, using a geometry identical to the one of the FinFETs used in the experiments discussed in this section, with $W = 25$ nm, $H = 65$ nm and under similar biases, the simulated current distribution shows a crossover from a situation of weak volume inversion at $V_G = 0$ mV (Fig. 10.7a)

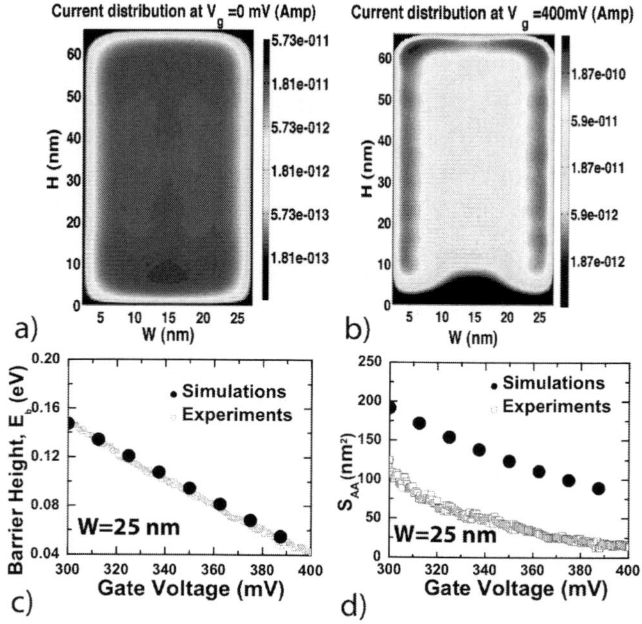

Figure 10.7. Current distributions, for (a) $V_G = 0$ mV, (b) $V_G = 400$ mV, obtained using TB simulations for a geometry having $L = 65$ nm and $W = 25$ nm. Comparison of the simulated (c) E_b and (d) S_{AA} with the experimental data for a $W = 25$ nm device.

to a situation of transport confined prevalently at the interface at $V_G = 400$ mV (Fig. 10.7b).

The simulated spatial current distribution (Fig. 10.7) gives a good indication of where the mobile charges predominately flow in the channel. From calculation too, a reduction of S_{AA} with increasing V_G is obtained (see Fig. 10.7d). However, this reduction is not as sharp as in the experimental data, as these simulations have been performed at $T = 300$ K and also due to the absence of interface states (expected to enhance the effect of screening in real devices as it will be discussed in section 10.4) (Hinds *et al.*, 2000; Sellier *et al.*, 2007). As a final benchmark to this experimental method, the results of the TB simulations have been used to calculate the current and the conductance at different temperatures and to extract, using again Eq. (10.1), simulated E_b and S_{AA} for a $W = 25$ nm device. In fact, in Fig. 10.7c,d, the simulated values are compared to the experiments and it is found that it is possible to predict experimental results with good accuracy, although the simulations overestimate the values of S_{AA} (probably for the same reasons discussed for Fig. 10.7b). In any case, the comparison between experimental and simulation give a demonstration of the reliability of the method developed in this section (Tettamanzi *et al.*, 2010). This opens the way of its systematic use to obtain information about the magnitude and the position of carriers in FET devices in general and not only in FinFET structures. In these investigations, possible modifications of A^* due to the constrained geometry (Ragi and Romero, 2006) of the devices have been neglected, as it is found to be negligible, and tunneling regimes of transport (Appenzeller *et al.*, 2004) have been excluded due to different temperatures dependences.

10.3.6 *Conclusion*

In conclusion, the results presented in section 10.3 are the first experimental study of the behavior of the active cross-section area as a function of V_G for undoped FinFETs. In particular, conductance traces for a set of undoped FinFETs having the same channel length and height but different width, together with TB simulations for the device of $W = 25$ nm have been presented. For all these small devices ($W \leqslant 125$ nm), a mechanism of inversion of the bands from flat band to band bending in the interface regions respectively, all as a function of V_G, has been proposed and demonstrated. Therefore this section discusses the first-ever direct observation of the theoretical results suggested by Taur. The validity of thermionic approach as a tool for the investigation of sub-threshold transport in undoped FET devices has been confirmed and some answers to the fundamental technological questions, such as how to localize and quantify areas of transport have been provided.

10.4 Interface Trap Density Metrology of Undoped N-FinFETs

10.4.1 *Introduction*

In sections 10.2 and 10.3, it has been demonstrated that, by using thermionic emission, it is possible to measure (1) the active channel

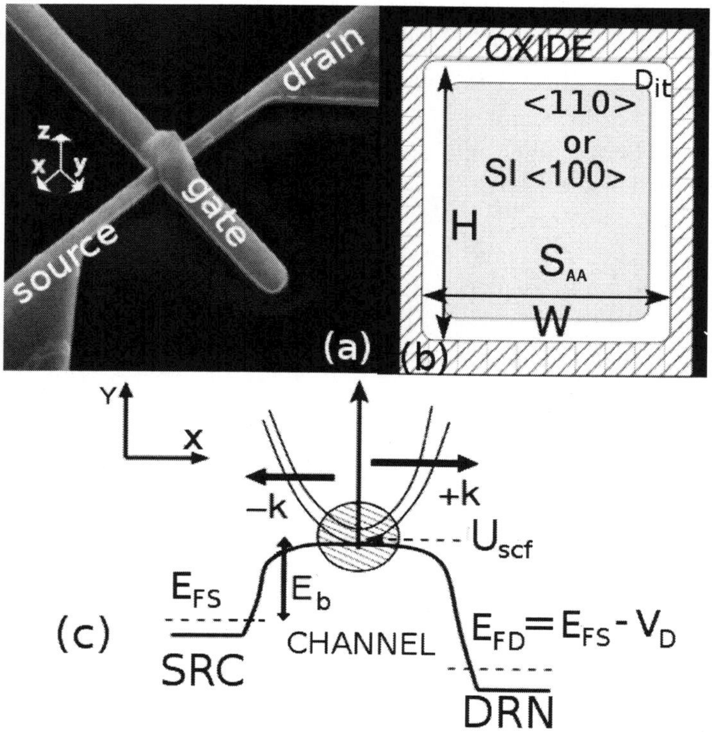

Figure 10.8. (a) Scanning-electron-microscope (SEM) image of a Si n-FinFET with [100] channel orientation and single fin. (b) The schematic of the cross sectional cut in the Y-Z plane of a typical tri-gated FinFET. The active cross-section (S_{AA}) is in gray, H and W are the physical height and width, respectively. (c) Ballistic top of the barrier model employed for calculating the thermionic current in the FinFETs.

cross-section area (S_{AA}) (see Fig. 10.8b), and (2) the source to channel barrier height (E_b), hence opening new ways to investigate FinFETs. Furthermore, in Section 10.3, it was found that for undoped FinFETs, although the trends of the S_{AA} values obtained by mean of experiments and of theoretical simulations were identical, differences in the absolute values were observed. These differences were found to be caused by the presence of interface states at the metal–oxide–semiconductor interface of the experimental devices (Tettamanzi *et al.*, 2010; Lee *et al.*, 2003). These states can trap electrons and enhance screening, therefore reducing the action of the gate on the channel, and as a final result, a decrease in the absolute value of S_{AA} in the experimental data is observed. Typical D_{it} frequency or time dependent measurements cannot be performed on ultimate devices but only on custom designed structures (Kapila *et al.*, 2007). Such custom structures may only be partially reflective towards the possibly surface orientation-dependent and geometry-dependent D_{it}.

10.4.2 *Aim*

In this section, a simple set of methods for the direct estimation of D_{it} in ultimate devices is provided. The comparison between the values of D_{it} obtained with these two methods and the values obtained using a method implemented in the past (Kapila *et al.*, 2007) show similar trends. A new approach to trap density metrology is of critical importance as CMOS scaling takes device dimensions into the nanometer regime. At these scales, quantities such as D_{it} can vary rapidly with device geometry, rendering old techniques inadequate as they cannot be applied directly in these ultra-scaled devices.

In this section it is shown that by using simple mathematical manipulations and the difference between experimental and simulated values of S_{AA} and of the capacitive coupling, α (see also previous sections), it is possible to infer the value of the interface trap density (D_{it}). Furthermore, to shed more light into the complicated transport phenomena that can arise in these undoped FinFETs, the work of previous sections is expanded and more careful investigations of the evolution of S_{AA} and of E_b are performed. For theoretically investigating these devices, the atomic representation is used. The band structure is obtained using a 10 band $sp^3d^5s^*$ TB model with spin orbit coupling (SO) (Klimeck *et al.*, 2002; Boykin *et al.*, 2004; Neophytou *et al.*, 2008), which is confirmed to be well suited for modeling the band-structure of these confined silicon channels, since TB can easily take into account the material, geometrical, strain and potential fluctuations at the atomic scale (Neophytou *et al.*, 2008). This model takes also into account the coupling of the conduction and the valence bands which is neglected in simple models like the effective mass approximation (EMA). As shown in Section 10.3, semi-classical "Top of the barrier" (ToB) model accurately captures the thermionic transport (Fig. 10.8c) (Neophytou *et al.*, 2008; Paul *et al.*, 2009; Tettamanzi *et al.*, 2010), the same model can also shed more light on the inner details of the transport, which is discussed next.

10.4.3 *New Implementation of Interface Trap Metrology*

In the undoped devices studied here, qualitatively similar theoretical and experimental trends for the active cross section area versus V_G and barrier height versus V_G are found (Tettamanzi *et al.*, 2010). However, the theoretically obtained values quantitatively over-estimated the experimental values. The reduced experimental values can be attributed to the presence of interface traps in these FinFETs (Tettamanzi *et al.*, 2011; Lee *et al.*, 2003; Kapila *et al.*, 2007). The effect of interface traps on the channel property are even more dominant in the extremely thin FinFETs (Tettamanzi *et al.*, 2011). In this section it is shown how this difference in S_{AA} and E_b can be utilized for the direct estimation of the interface trap density (D_{it}) in FinFETs, thereby eliminating the need to implement special FinFETs geometries to determine D_{it} (Kapila *et al.*, 2007) and providing a new tool for performing interface trap metrology.

This paragraph has been divided into the following sections. Section 10.4.4 provides the details about the FinFETs for which interface trap density metrology has been implemented and the fundamentals of the experimental procedures that are in line with Sections 10.2 and 10.3. The details about the self-consistent calculations are provided in Section 10.4.5 and more insight on the theoretical extraction of E_b and S_{AA} is outlined in Section 10.4.6. Section 10.4.7 provides the details of the two procedures for obtaining the interface trap density. The theoretical and experimental results and the discussion on them are given in Section 10.4.8, while Section 10.4.9 discussed current distributions. The conclusions are summarized in Section 10.4.10.

10.4.4 *Device and Experimental Details*

The undoped n-FinFETs used in this work (A–G, see Table 10.2) consist of nanowire channels etched on a Si intrinsic film with a

Table 10.2. Si n-FinFETs used in the trap metrology study along with their labels. The surface hydrogen annealing detail is also shown. The channel is intrinsic Si, while the source and the drain are n-type doped for all the FinFETs

Label	H (nm)	W (nm)	L (nm)	Channel orientation (X)	H_2 anneal
A	65	25	40	[100]	Yes
B	65	25	40	[100]	No
C	65	~5	40	[100]	No
D	40	18	40	[110]	Yes
E	40	18	40	[110]	Yes
F	40	~3–5	40	[110]	Yes
G	65	~7	40	[100]	Yes

wrap-around gate covering the three faces of the channels (Fig. 10.8a) (Collaert *et al.*, 2005) identical to the ones discussed in Section 10.3. FinFETs with two different channel orientations of [100] ((FinFETs A–C and G)) and [110] ((FinFETs D–F)) have been used (see Table 10.2). All the FinFETs have the same channel length ($L = 40$ nm). The channel height (H) is either 40 nm or 65 nm (Table 10.2). The channel width (W) varies between 3 and 25 nm. An HfSiO (high-κ) layer isolates a TiN layer from the intrinsic Si channel (Collaert *et al.*, 2005). These FinFETs have either one channel (FinFETs A-C and G) or ten channels (FinFETs D-F). These devices have two different surface treatments (with or without H_2 annealing) as shown in Table 10.2.

Measurement procedure: The experimental value of E_b and S_{AA} are obtained using the differential conductance method introduced in sections 10.2 and 10.3. The conductance data are taken at $V_{SD} = 0$ V using a lock-in technique. The full experimental method and the required ambient conditions have been outlined in detail in (Tettamanzi *et al.*, 2010). In the next section we discuss the theoretical approach to calculate the values of E_b and S_{AA} in tri-gated n-FinFETs.

10.4.5 *Modeling Approach*

To obtain the self-consistent charge and potential and transport characteristics in the n-FinFETs, the electronic structure is calculated using an atomistic 10 band $sp^3d^5s^*$ semi-empirical TB (Klimeck *et al.*, 2002) as discussed in Section 10.3. Using thermionic fitting procedure (Tettamanzi *et al.*, 2010), E_b, α and S_{AA} can be extracted using the experimental and theoretical conductance (G) using Eq. (10.1) for a 3D system (Sze, 1981). This equation will hold only when the cross-section size of the FinFET is large enough (i.e., W, $H > 20$ nm) to be considered a 3D bulk system. In this study, S_{AA} is extracted for FinFETs with W(H) $\approx$ 25 nm (65 nm). When the $3D$ approximation is not true anymore (i.e., W or $H \lesssim 20$ nm), only E_b and α can be correctly extrapolated (Tettamanzi *et al.*, 2010). Since the FinFETs studied here show (i) negligible source-to-drain tunneling current and (ii) reduced SCEs (Tettamanzi *et al.*, 2010), the ToB model is applicable to such devices (Paul *et al.*, 2009). For the simulations, all the FinFETs are n-type doped in the source and drain to a value of 5×10^{19} cm^{-3}. A 1.5 nm SiO_2 cover is assumed. Next the procedure used to calculate E_b and S_{AA} are discussed more in detail.

10.4.6 *Extraction of Barrier Height and the Active Cross Area Section*

For pure thermionic emission any carrier energetic enough to surmount the barrier from the source to the channel (C) (Fig. 10.8c) will reach the drain provided the transport in the channel is close to ballistic. The source/drain in FETs are typically close to thermal and electrical equilibrium (since heavy scattering in the contacts is assumed which leads to instantaneous carrier relaxation). This allows the use of the realistic assumption that most of the carriers in the Source/Drain are thermalized at their respective Fermi-levels (E_{fs}, E_{fd} in Fig. 10.8c). Also the channel potential (U_{scf}) can be determined under the application of V_G using the self-consistent scheme (Paul *et al.*, 2009; Lee *et al.*, 2009). Hence, for the source-to-channel homo-junction inside a FET, the barrier height (E_b) can be determined as a function of V_G,

$$E_b(V_G) = U_{scf}(V_G) - E_{fs}. \tag{10.2}$$

This definition of E_b implicitly contains the temperature dependence since the simulations are performed at different temperatures

(T) which feature in the Fermi distribution of the Source/Drain, but, as it will be shown in Section 10.4.8, the temperature dependence of E_b in the sub-threshold region is very weak. Therefore, all the theoretical E_b results shown in this chapter are at $T \approx 300$ K.

The study of thermionic emission model is applicable when the barrier height is much larger than the thermal broadening ($E_b \gg k_B T$ (Sze, 1981)). For this reason, Eq. (10.2) works only in the sub-threshold region where E_b is well defined (Paul *et al.*, 2009) and once the FinFET is above the threshold, E_b ($\leq K_B T$) is not a well-defined quantity anymore (Paul *et al.*, 2009). Furthermore, when the cross-section size of the FinFET is not large enough (i.e., W, $H \leqslant 20$ nm) to be considered in a 3D bulk limit, S_{AA} cannot be extracted using Eq. (10.1) since the system is close to 1D. For a 1D system the G, under a small drain bias (V_{SD}) at a temperature T, is given by the following (for a single energy band),

$$G_{1D} = \frac{2e^2}{h} \cdot \left[1 + exp(\frac{E_b(V_G)}{k_B T})\right]^{-1} \tag{10.3}$$

where h is the Planck's constant. Since Eq. (10.3) lacks any area description, G for 1D systems is no more a good method to extract S_{AA}. Below we will present an approach to solve this problem and to distinguish a 1D system from a 3D system. A part of all these limitations and as described in Sections 10.2 and 10.3, S_{AA} can be extracted using Eq. (10.1).

10.4.7 *Trap Extraction Methods*

In Tettamanzi *et al.* (2010) (see also Section 10.3), it was observed that the active cross-section area ($S_{AA,sim}$) obtained theoretically is over-estimating the experimental value ($S_{AA,exp}$). In Section 10.4.8 it will be further shown that also the theoretical E_b value can over estimate the experimental E_b value. These mismatches can be attributed to the presence of traps at the oxide–channel interface of multi-gate FETs where these traps can enhance the electro-static screening and suppress the action of the gate on the channel (Kapila *et al.*, 2007; Lee *et al.*, 2003; Tettamanzi *et al.*, 2010). This simple idea is a powerful tool used for the estimation of interface trap density (D_{it}) in these undoped Si n-FinFETs.

10.4.7.1 Method I: D_{it} from active area

Based on the difference between the simulated and the experimental active area (S_{AA}) values, a method to calculate the density of interface trap charges, σ_{it}, in the FinFETs is outlined. The method is based on the assumption that the total charge in the channel at a given V_G must be the same in the experiments and in the simulations. This requirement leads to the following:

$$S_{AA,sim} \cdot L_{ch} \cdot \rho_{sim} = S_{AA,expt} \cdot L_{ch} \cdot \rho_{expt} + e \cdot \sigma_{it} \cdot L_{ch} \cdot P \quad (10.4)$$

where $S_{AA,sim}$ ($S_{AA,expt}$) is the simulated (experimental) active area, P is the perimeter of the channel under the gate ($P = W + 2H$) and ρ_{sim} (ρ_{expt}) is the simulated (experimental) charge density. Close to the oxide channel interface it is possible to locally assume that ρ_{expt} is obtained from ρ_{sim} and σ_{it} as,

$$\rho_{expt} = \rho_{sim} - \rho_{it} = \rho_{sim} - (e \cdot \sigma_{it} \cdot P)/(W \cdot H) \quad (10.5)$$

Using Eqs. (10.4) and (10.5) the final expression for σ_{it} is obtained as,

$$\sigma_{it}(V_G) = \frac{\rho_{sim}(V_G) S_{AA,sim}(V_G)}{e \cdot P} \times \left[\frac{\left[1 - \frac{S_{AA,expt}(V_G)}{S_{AA,sim}(V_G)}\right]}{\left[1 - \frac{S_{AA,expt}(V_{gs})}{W \cdot H}\right]} \right] \quad [\#/\mathrm{cm}^2] \quad (10.6)$$

This method is useful for wider devices for which Eq. (10.1) is valid. For very thin FinFETs (close to a 1D system) this method cannot be utilized.

Assumptions in Method I: In the calculation of σ_{it} several assumptions were made. The extra charge contribution completely stems from the interface trap density (D_{it}) and any contribution from the bulk trap states has been neglected. Also all the interface traps are assumed to be completely filled which implies $\sigma_{it} \cong D_{it}$. This method of extraction works best for undoped channel since any filling of the impurity/dopant states is neglected in the calculation. Also the interface trap density is assumed to constant for the top and the side walls of the FinFET which is generally not the case (Kapila *et al.*, 2007; Lee *et al.*, 2003). Orientation-dependent D_{it} for different surfaces could be included as a further refinement.

10.4.7.2 Method II: D_{it} from barrier control

The second method does not utilize the E_b value directly but its derivative w.r.t. V_G. The term $\alpha = |dE_b/dV_G|$ represents the channel to gate coupling (Sellier *et al.*, 2007; Tettamanzi *et al.*, 2010). The presence of interface traps weakens this coupling due to the electrostatic screening. This method of trap extraction is based on the difference in the experimental and the simulated α value. The α value can be represented in terms of the channel and the oxide capacitance. The equivalent capacitance model for a MOSFET with and without interface traps (D_{it}) is shown in Fig. 10.9. The α value can be associated with the oxide, interface, and semiconductor capacitance, which is given in Eq. (38) on page 383 in Sze (1981). This relation leads to the following:

$$\left|\frac{dE_b}{dV_G}\right| = 1 - \frac{C_{tot}}{C_{ox}}, \tag{10.7}$$

where C_{tot} is the total capacitance. For the two cases, as shown in Fig. 10.9, the total capacitance is given by

$$C_{tot}^{exp} = \frac{C_{ox} \cdot (C_d + C_{it})}{C_d + C_{ox} + C_{it}}, \tag{10.8}$$

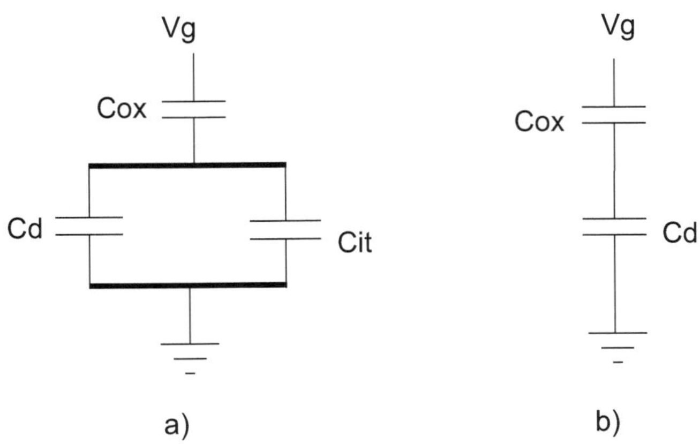

Figure 10.9. Equivalent circuits (a) with interface-trap capacitance (C_{it}) and (b) without interface capacitance. C_d and C_{ox} are the depletion and the oxide capacitance, respectively. The idea for this equivalent circuit is obtained from page 381 in Sze (1981).

$$C_{tot}^{sim} = \frac{C_d \cdot C_{ox}}{C_d + C_{ox}}, \tag{10.9}$$

where C_{it}, C_{ox}, and C_d are the interface trap capacitance, the oxide capacitance and the semi-conductor capacitance, respectively. Eq. (10.8) represents the capacitance in the experimental device and Eq. (10.9) represents the capacitance in the simulated device under ideal conditions without any interface traps. Combining Eqs. (10.7), (10.8), and (10.9) and after some mathematical manipulations, it is possible to obtain,

$$\frac{1}{\alpha_{exp}} = \frac{1}{\alpha_{sim}} + \frac{C_{it}}{C_{ox}}, \tag{10.10}$$

Manipulating Eq. (10.10) gives the following relation for C_{it}

$$C_{it} = C_{ox} \cdot \left(\frac{1}{\alpha_{sim}}\right) \cdot \left[\frac{\alpha_{sim}}{\alpha_{exp}} - 1\right] \tag{10.11}$$

Also C_{it} can be related to the interface charge density (σ_{it}) as (Sze, 1981),

$$C_{it} = e \cdot \frac{\partial \sigma_{it}}{\partial V_G} \tag{10.12}$$

where e is the electronic charge. In Eq. (10.11) all the values are dependent on V_G except C_{ox}. Combining Eqs. 10.11 and 10.12 and integrating w.r.t. V_G yields the final expression for the integrated interface charge density in these FinFETs as

$$\sigma_{it} = \frac{C_{ox}}{e} \cdot \int_{V1}^{V2=V_{th}} \left(\frac{1}{\alpha_{sim}(V_G)}\right) \times \left[\frac{\alpha_{sim}(V_G)}{\alpha_{exp}(V_G)} - 1\right] dV_G \quad [\#/\mathrm{cm}^2], \tag{10.13}$$

where V_{th} is the threshold voltage of the FinFET and V1 is the minimum V_G for which $\alpha_{exp/sim}$ is $\approx$ 1. Of course, the integration range for Eq. (10.13) is in the sub-threshold region. This method has the advantage that it is independent of the dimensionality of the FinFET. Hence, Eq. (10.13) can be used for wide as well as for thin FinFETs.

Assumptions in Method II: The most important assumption is that the rate of change of the surface potential ($\Psi(V_G)$) is the same as E_b w.r.t. V_G. The extra charge contribution completely originates from the density of interface trap charges (σ_{it}) and any contribution from the bulk trap states have been neglected. Also all the interface traps are assumed to be completely filled which implies $\sigma_{it} = D_{it}$. This method works best when the change in the DC and the AC signal is low enough, such that the interface traps can follow the change in the bias sweep (Sze, 1981).

10.4.7.3 Limitations of the methods

To apply these trap metrology methods properly, is important to understand their limitations, which are presented in this section. One of the main limitation is how closely the simulated FinFET structure resembles the experimental device structure. This depends both on the SEM/TEM imaging as well the type of simulator used. In the present case a FinFET cross-section structure is created by using the TEM image making the simulated structure as close to the experimental device as possible. With the development of better TCAD tools, the proximity of the simulated structure to experimental structure has increased. This allows good confidence in the simulated conductance values then used for the interface trap calculations. Furthermore, the simulated G is calculated as close to ideal as possible and all the differences between the ideal and experimental G are attributed to the traps, which may not be true always. An important difference between the two methods is that they are calculated over different V_G ranges. This is important since the trap filling and their behavior changes within the V_G range which should be taken into account accurately. One must also be aware of the embedded assumption of complete interface trap filling and the neglect of the bulk traps.

10.4.8 *Results and Discussion*

In this section the theoretical results as well as their comparison with the experimental data are provided and discussed.

10.4.8.1 Temperature dependence of the barrier height

The source-to-channel barrier height has been assumed to be temperature independent in the sub-threshold region. Figure 10.10

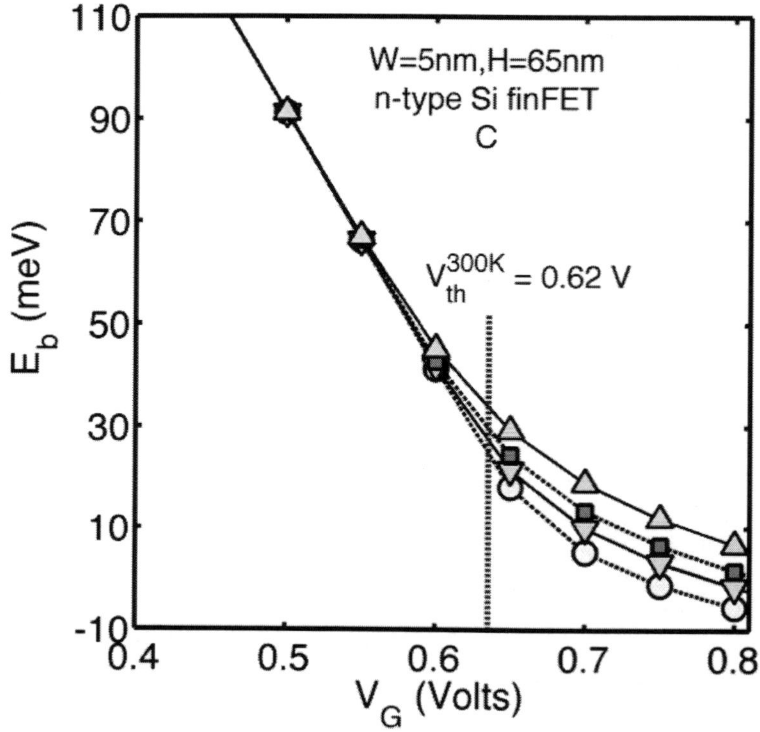

Figure 10.10. Temperature dependence of the simulated barrier height (E_b) in the n-FinFET C from 140 K to 300 K, (circle are for 140 K, down triangles for 200 K, squares for 240 K and up triangles for 300 K). At $T = 300$ K, V_{th} of the FinFET is 0.62 V. The overlap of the curves at different temperatures with V_G, below V_{th} at 300 K, shows a weak temperature dependence of E_b in the sub-threshold region. The impact of temperature becomes prominent after V_G goes above V_{th}.

shows the results of a temperature dependent ToB calculations and proves that the barrier height (E_b) is only weakly temperature dependent in the sub-threshold regime. In the subthreshold region, the E_b value for FinFET C, is same at four different temperatures ($T = 140$ K, 200 K, 240 K and 300 K). The variation with temperature becomes more prominent when the FinFET transitions into the on-state. Since, E_b has a weak temperature dependence in the sub-threshold region it is then possible to evaluate E_b from the 300 K simulations only.

10.4.8.2 Evolution of the barrier height and of the active cross-section area with V_G

Experimentally, it has been shown that for undoped silicon n-FinFETs (Tettamanzi *et al.*, 2010), E_b reduces as V_G increases. Theoretically, the E_b value is determined using Eq. (10.2), which depends on the self-consistent channel potential (U_{scf}). As the gate bias increases, the channel can support more charge. This is obtained by pushing the channel conduction band lower in energy to be populated more by the source and drain Fermi level (Neophytou *et al.*, 2008). Figures 10.11 and 10.12 show the experimental and theoretical evolution of E_b in FinFETs G, C and D, E, respectively. Theory provides correct quantitative trend for E_b with V_G. *Few important observations here are, (i) theoretical* E_b *value is always higher than experimental value and (ii) [110] Si devices (D and E) show larger mismatch to the experimental values.* The reason for the first point is suggested to be the presence of interface traps in the FinFETs which screen the gate from the channel (Tettamanzi

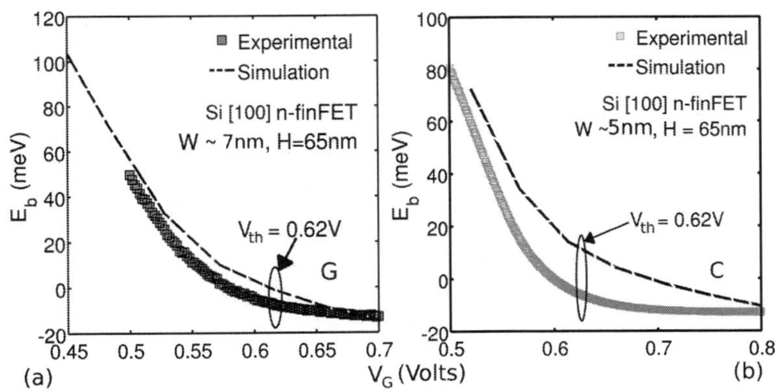

Figure 10.11. Experimental and simulated barrier height (E_b) in n-FinFET (a) G and (b) C. Both the devices have same V_{th}. Both experiment and simulation show a decreasing value of E_b with V_G, but the absolute values are different.

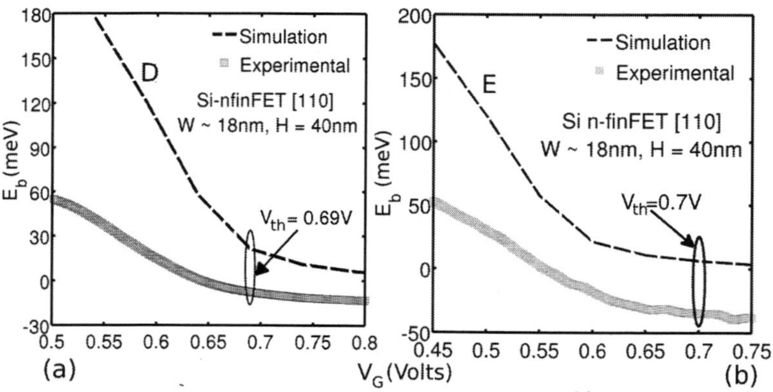

Figure 10.12. Experimental and simulated barrier height (E_b) in n-FinFETs (a) D and (b) E. Both the devices have similar V_{th}. Both experiment and simulation show a decreasing value of E_b with V_G, but the absolute values are different.

et al., 2010). The second observation can be understood by the fact that [110] channels with (110) sidewalls have more interface trap density due to the higher surface bond density (Sze, 1981) and bad etching on the (110) sidewalls (Kapila *et al.*, 2007).

The active cross section area (S_{AA}) represents the part of the channel where the charge flows (Tettamanzi *et al.*, 2010). Experimentally S_{AA} is shown to be decreasing with gate bias since the inversion charge moves closer to the interface that electrostatically screens the inner part of the channel from the gate (Tettamanzi *et al.*, 2010, 2011). This gives a good indication of how much channel area is used for transporting the charge. Figure 10.13a,b show the experimental evolution of S_{AA} in FinFET B and E, respectively. The theoretical value of S_{AA} decreases with V_G which is in qualitative agreement to the experimental observation (Tettamanzi *et al.*, 2010). However, the absolute values do not match. In fact theory over-estimates the experimental S_{AA} value (Fig. 10.13), which is attributed to the interface traps.

10.4.8.3 Trap density evaluation

In this section the results on D_{it} in the undoped Si n-FinFETs are presented:

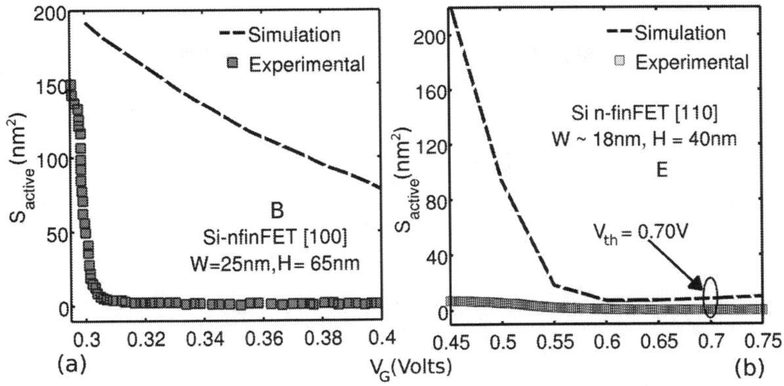

Figure 10.13. Experimental and simulated channel active cross-section (S_{AA}) in n-FinFETs (a) B and (b) E. Both experiment and simulation show a decreasing value of S_{AA} with V_G, but the absolute values are different.

D_{it} using S_{AA}: method I

This approach is based on method I (see section 10.4.7 for details). The calculated D_{it} values for FinFET B and E are 1.06e12 cm^{-2} and 1.81e12 cm^{-2} (Fig. 10.14 (a) and (b), respectively). The D_{it} values compare quite well with the experimental D_{it} values presented in (Kapila *et al.*, 2007) and also shown in Table 10.3. As expected the D_{it} value for FinFET E (with [110] channel and (110) sidewalls) is

Table 10.3. Values of D_{it} obtained from all the n-FinFETs

Device	Method	D_{it} (10^{11} cm^{-2})	FET type	Obs.
L = 140 nm*	Charge Pumping	1.725	Special body tied FET	—
L = 240 nm*		2.072		—
A	I	5.560	Std. FET	H_2 anneal, reduces D_{it}
B	I	10.60	Std. FET	
	II	8.860	Std. FET	
C	II	9.26	Std. FET	Thin fin, more D_{it}
D	II	18.31	Std. FET	(110) side-wall, thin fin, more etching, more D_{it}
E	I	18.1	Std. FET	
	II	15.3	Std. FET	
F	II	36.3	Std. FET	
G	II	4.33	Std. FET	H_2 anneal, less D_{it}

Source: From Kapila *et al.* (2007).

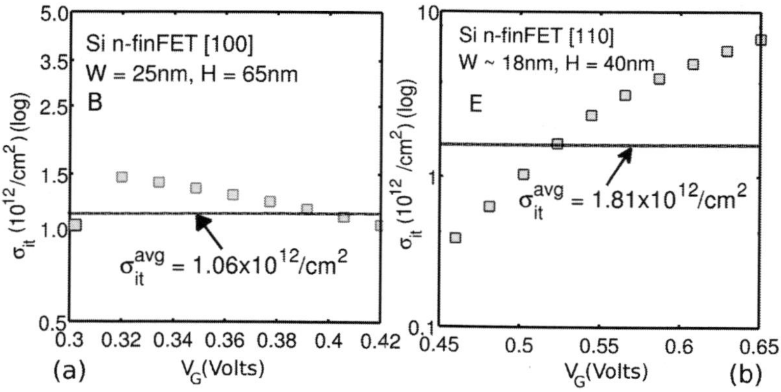

Figure 10.14. Extracted trap density using the difference in active device area (method I) for n-FinFETs (a) B and (b) E.

higher than FinFET B ([100] channel with (100) sidewalls). This is attributed to the higher D_{it} ($\sim 2\times$) on the (110) surfaces (Kapila *et al.*, 2007). The results presented in this section show $\sim 1.8\times$ more D_{it} for (110) sidewalls, in close agreement to previous experiments (Kapila *et al.*, 2007). This method allows to calculate the D_{it} in the actual FinFETs rather than custom made FETs.

D_{it} using $-dE_b/dV_G$ |: Method II

This approach is based on method II (see section 10.4.7 for details). The C_{ox} value, needed in this method, is taken as ~0.0173 F/m^2, which is assumed to be the same for all the devices since these FinFETs have similar oxide thickness. The calculated D_{it} values for FinFET C and E are 9.26e11 cm^{-2} and 1.563e12 cm^{-2} (Fig.10.15 (a) and (b), respectively). These calculations also show that [110] channel device (FinFET E) shows higher D_{it} compared to the [100] channel device (FinFET C), again consistent with the observations made in (Kapila *et al.*, 2007). The advantage of this method is that it can be used to obtain D_{it} in extremely thin FinFETs (close to 1D system) unlike method I which is applicable only to wider FinFETs (due to the reasons discussed in section 10.4.6).

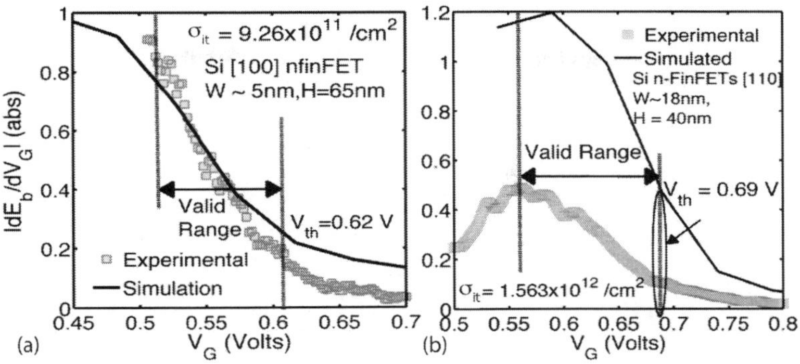

Figure 10.15. Experimental and simulated value of α in n-FinFETs (a) C and (b) E.

10.4.8.4 Discussion of the two methods and D_{it} trends

The D_{it} values for all the FinFETs used in this study are shown in Table 10.3. The important outcomes about the two methods are outlined below:

- The D_{it} values obtained by the two methods compare very well with the experimental measurement in (Kapila *et al.*, 2007) for similar sized FinFETs (A and B). This shows the validity of these new methods.
- The D_{it} values calculated using method I and II (for B and E) compare very well with each other which shows that the two methods are complimentary (Tettamanzi *et al.*, 2011).
- The D_{it} values calculated for the two similar FinFETs (E and F) compare very well showing the reproducibility of the methods.

The calculated D_{it} values also reflect some important trends about the FinFET width scaling and surfaces (Table 10.3). The central points are

- Hydrogen passivation considerably reduces D_{it} (Lee *et al.*, 2003). This is observed for FinFETs A and B where H_2 passivation results in $\sim 2\times$ less D_{it} in FinFET A.

- Width scaling requires more etching which also increases D_{it} (Kapila *et al.*, 2007). The same trend is observed in devices A to C and D to F (decreasing W).
- (110) sidewalls show higher D_{it} compared to (100) sidewalls (Kapila *et al.*, 2007). The same trend is also observed for FinFETs A, B, C, G ((100) sidewall) compared to FinFETs D, E, and F ((110) sidewall).

10.4.9 *Current Distribution*

The charge flow in n-FinFETs shows a very strong dependence on the geometrical confinement. For very small width FinFET the entire body gets inverted and shows a very little change in S_{AA} with V_G. For wider FinFETs the current flow starts from a weak volume inversion and moves to surface inversion as V_G increases (Tettamanzi *et al.*, 2010). The theoretical spatial current calculation reveals similar trend which is shown in Fig. 10.16 For extremely thin

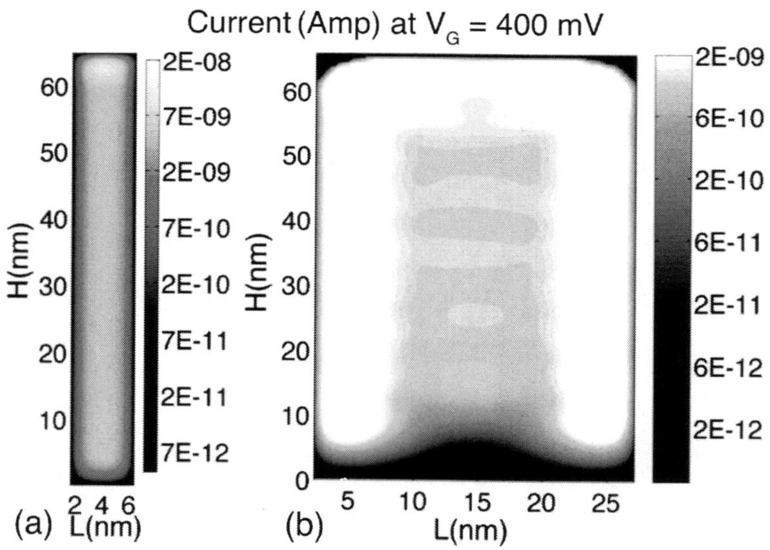

Figure 10.16. Simulated spatial current distribution in the [100] undoped Si n-FinFET intrinsic with H = 65 nm and (a) W = 5 nm and (b) W = 25 nm. $V_G = 0.4$ V and $V_{SD} = 30$ mV at 300 K. 5 nm device shows a complete volume inversion. In the 25 nm device the current mainly flows at the edges.

n-FinFETs ($W = 5$ nm, $H = 65$ nm) the charge flow is prevalently through the entire body (volume inversion) compared to the wider n-FinFETs ($W = 25$ nm, $H = 65$ nm) where the charge flows at the edges. This reflects the fact that thinner FinFETs show better channel area utilisation for the charge flow. However, an important practical limitation comes from the fact that extremely thin FinFETs also require more etching, which increases D_{it} and hence can limit the action of thin FinFETs. The advancement of fabrication methods and strain technology may improve the performance of thin FinFETs as shown by some experimental works (Wong, 2002).

10.4.10 *Conclusion*

A new D_{it} determination methodology for state-of-the-art n-FinFETs is presented. Two complementary approaches provide (a) the gate bias (V_G) dependence of D_{it} (Method I) and, (b) the total D_{it} (Method II).

The following trends are observed:

(i) The hydrogen annealing step in the fabrication process substantially reduces D_{it} in good agreement with Ref. (Lee *et al.*, 2003)
(ii) The scaling of the W of the devices (i.e., from A to C or from D (E) to F) increases the density of interface states
(iii) The change in the orientation of the channel (and therefore the sidewall surface where the interface traps are formed) from [100] (device A or C) to [110] (device D (E) or F) remarkably increases the density of interface states
(iv) By comparison of the value of D_{it} obtained for device B in the two approaches (i.e., see Fig. 10.13 and Table 10.3) and the value of D_{it} obtained for two identical devices (D and E) using the same approach (Method II), compatibility and reproducibility of the methods are demonstrated.

The reported trends are similar to the one suggested in the literature (Lee *et al.*, 2003; Xiong *et al.*, 2004). The simple Top-of-the-barrier model, combined with Tight-binding calculations, explains very well the thermally activated sub-threshold transport in state-of-the-art Si FinFETs. The qualitative evolution of E_b and S_{AA} with V_G are well explained by the theory. Furthermore, the mismatch in the quantitative values of E_b and S_{AA} led to the development of two new interface trap density calculation methods. The advantage of these methods is that they do not require any special structure as needed by the present experimental methods. Hence the interface quality of the ultimate channel can be obtained. These methods are shown to provide consistent and reproducible results which compare very well with the independent experimental trap measurement results. The calculated trends of interface trap density with channel width scaling, channel orientation and hydrogen passivation of the surfaces compare well with the experimental observations. The volume inversion observed in thin width FinFETs is more efficient, in term of volume utilization. However, it could lead to a better utilization of FETs channel only if surfaces roughness and the density of interface traps, created during the extreme etching necessary for these device to be fabricated, can be reduced.

10.5 Final Conclusions

This chapter discusses how, by making use of a classical tool such as the thermionic emission theory in combination with state-of-the-art tight binding simulations, it is possible to provide precious information on the transport characteristics of ultra-scaled Si n-FinFETs. In fact, it is demonstrated here that the amplitude of the energy barrier, of the region of transport in the channel and of the interface trap density, are all quantities that can be directly estimated in state-of-the-art FinFETs. Due to the rapid scaling of CMOS-FET technology, the techniques introduced in this chapter could become routine tools for device improvement and optimization.

References

Appenzeller, J., Radosavljević, Knoc, J., and Avouris, P. (2004). *Phys. Rev. Lett.* **92**, p. 048301.

Boykin, T. B., Klimeck, G., and Oyafuso, F. (2004). *Phys. Rev. B* **69**, 115201.

Collaert, N., Demand, M., Ferain, I., Lisoni, J., Singanamalla, Zimmerman, P., Yim, Y.-S., Schram, T., Mannaert, G., Goodwin, M., Hooker, J. C., Neuilly, F., Kim, M. C., Meyer, K. D., Gent, S. D., Boullart, W., Jurczak, M. and Biesemans, S. (2005). *Symp VLSI Tech.*, p. 108.

Doyle, B., Datta, S., amd S. Hareland, M. D., Jin, B., Kavalieros, J., Linton, T., Murthy, A., Rios, R. and Chau, R. (2003). *Electron Device Lett., IEEE* **24**, p. 263.

Fossum, J., Yang, J.-W. and Trivedi, V. P. (2003). *Electron Device Lett., IEEE* **24**, p. 745.

Hinds, B. J., Nishiguchi, K., Dutta, A., Yamanaka, T., Hatanani, S. and Oda, S. (2000). *Jpn. J. Appl. Phys.* **39**, p. 4637.

Hisamo, D., Lee, W.-C., Kedzierski, J., Takeuchi, H., Asano, K., Kuo, C., Anderson, E., King, T.-J., Bokor, J. and Hu, C. (2000). *IEEE, Trans. Electron. Devices* **47**, p. 2320.

Kapila, G., Kaczer, B., Nackaerts, A., Collaert, N. and Groeseneken, G. (2007). *Electron Device Lett., IEEE* **28**, 3, pp. 232–234, DOI:10.1109/LED.2007.891263.

Klimeck, G., Ahmed, S., Kharche, N., Korkusinski, M., Usman, M., Prada, M. and Boykin, T. B. (2009). *(INVITED) Special Issue on Nanoelectronic Device Modeling in IEEE, Trans. on Elec. Dev.* **54**, pp. 2090–2099.

Klimeck, G., Oyafuso, F., Boykin, T. B., Bowen, R. C. and von Allmen, P. (2002). *Comput. Model. Eng. Sci.* **3**, 5, pp. 601–642.

Lee, J.-S., Choi, Y.-K., Ha, D., Balasubramanian, S., King, T.-J. and Bokor, J. (2003). *Electron Device Lett., IEEE* **24**, 3, pp. 186–188, DOI:10.1109/LED.2003.809526.

Lee, S., Ryu, H., Jiang, Z. and Klimeck, G. (2009). *13th International Workshop on Computational Electronics (IWCE)* DOI:10.1109/IWCE.2009.5091117.

Neophytou, N., Paul, A., Lundstrom, M. and Klimeck, G. (2008). *IEEE, Trans. on Elec. Dev.* **55**, pp. 1286–1297.

Paul, A., Mehrotra, S., Luisier, M. and Klimeck, G. (2009). *13th International Workshop on Computational Electronics (IWCE)* DOI: 10.1103/WCE.2009.5091134.

Ragi, R. and Romero, M. A. (2006). *Microelectron. J.* **37**, p. 1261.

Ruiz, F. J. G., Godoy, A., Gámiz, F., Sampedro, C. and Donetti, L. (2007). *IEEE, Trans. on Elec. Dev.* **54**, p. 3369.

Sellier, H., Lansbergen, G. P., Caro, J., Rogge, S., Collaert, N., Ferain, I., Jurczak, M. and Biesemans, S. (2007). *Appl. Phys. Lett.* **90**, p. 073502.

Singanamalla, R., Yu, H. Y., Pourtois, G., Ferain, I., Anil, K. G., Kubicek, S., Hoffmann, T. Y., Jurczak, M., Biesemans, S. and Meyer, K. D. (2006). *Electron Device Lett., IEEE* **27**, p. 332.

Sze, S. M. (1981). *Physics of Semiconductor Devices*, Wiley, New York.

Taur, Y. (2000). *Electron Device Lett., IEEE* **21**, p. 245.

Tettamanzi, G., Paul, A., Lansbergen, G., Verduijn, J., Lee, S., Collaert, N., Biesemans, S., Klimeck, G. and Rogge, S. (2010). *Electron Device Lett., IEEE* **31**, 2, pp. 150–152, DOI: 10.1109/LED.2009.2036134.

Tettamanzi, G., Paul, A., Lee, S., Mehrotra, S., Collaert, N., Biesemans, S., Klimeck, G. and Rogge, S. (2011). *Electron Device Lett., IEEE* **32**, 4, pp. 440–442, DOI: 10.1109/LED.2011.2106150.

Wong, H.-S. P. (2002). *IBM J. Res. Dev.* **46**, p. 133.

Xiong, W., Gebara, G., Zaman, J., Gostkowski, M., Nguyen, B., Smith, G., Lewis, D., Cleavelin, C. R., Wise, R., Yu, S., Pas, M., King, T.-J. and Colinge, J. P. (2004). *Electron Device Lett., IEEE* **25**, p. 541.

Chapter 11

Dopant Metrology in Advanced FinFETs

G. Lansbergen,[a] R. Rahman,[b] G. C. Tettamanzi,[a,c] J. Verduijn,[a,c] L. C. L. Hollenberg,[d] G. Klimeck,[e,f] and S. Rogge[a,c]

[a]*Kavli Institute of Nanoscience, Delft University of Technology, Lorentzweg 1, 2628 CJ Delft, The Netherlands*
[b]*Sandia National Laboratories, Albuquerque, NM 87185, USA*
[c]*CQC2T, University of New South Wales, Sydney, NSW 2052, Australia*
[d]*CQC2T, School of Physics, University of Melbourne, VIC 3010, Australia*
[e]*Network for Computational Nanotechnology, Purdue University, West Lafayette, Indiana 47907, USA*
[f]*Jet Propulsion Laboratory, California Institute of Technology, Pasadena, California 91109, USA*
g.tettamanzi@unsw.edu.au

11.1 Introduction

Ultra-scaled FinFET transistors bear unique fingerprint-like device-to-device differences attributed to random single impurities. This chapter describes how, through correlation of experimental data with multimillion atom tight-binding simulations using the NEMO 3-D code, it is possible to identify the impurity's chemical species and determine their concentration, local electric field and depth below the Si/SiO_2 interface. The ability to model the excited states rather than just the ground state is the critical component of

CMOS Nanoelectronics: Innovative Devices, Architectures, and Applications
Edited by Nadine Collaert

ISBN 978-981-4364-02-7 (Hardcover), 978-981-4364-03-4 (eBook)
www.panstanford.com

the analysis and allows the demonstration of a new approach to atomistic impurity metrology.

11.2 Recent Progress in Donor Spectroscopy

Modern transistors are getting so small that it is increasingly difficult to use traditional techniques for their study and their characterisation (Sze, 1981). This is particularly true for the identification of the impurity chemical species present in the channel and for the quantification of their concentration. Different groups have recently investigated the effects of ultra-scaling in silicon field effect transistor (FET) geometries and interesting results have emerged:

- Bjork *et al.* (2008) have shown that screening due to interface traps in ultra-scaled silicon nanowires can cause substantial increase on the ionization energy of the dopant. This result has profound implications for the design of future FET devices.
- Pierre *et al.* (2010) and Wacquez *et al.* (2010) have shown that the presence of a single dopant in the channel of a trigate FET can dramatically alter its electrical signature, even at room temperature.
- Fuechsle *et al.* (2010) have studied the band structure effects on single-crystal silicon geometries for which the source, the drain and the gates are fabricated using an atomically sharp doping procedure (Schofield *et al.*, 2003). Therefore they have investigated on the consequences of scaling a device up to the single atom limit.
- Tabe *et al.* (2010) have demonstrated that, in ultra scaled silicon FET devices, even in the presence of a dopant-rich environment, it is possible to observe the signature of a single dopant.

Overall, all these studies have allowed a better understanding of the effects that arise due to the ultra-scaled environment, however, they have also indicated that, for the successful design of future Complementary-Metal-Oxide-Semiconductor (CMOS) devices, a substantial amount of knowledge is still missing. As an example it is not yet clear how CMOS technology will be able to overcome critical challenges such as scaling-induced variability of device characteristics (Wacquez *et al.*, 2010; Asenov, 1999).

As a consequence, it is of interest to discuss in detail a method that can be used to demonstrate atomic impurity metrology (Lansbergen *et al.*, 2008a,b). In fact, through correlation of experimental data with multimillion atom simulations in NEMO 3-D, the impurity's chemical species can be identified and their concentration, local electric field and depth below the Si/SiO_2 interface can be determined (Lansbergen *et al.*, 2008a,b). Furthermore, the extension of the dopants in the source/drain (S/D) regions can be measured by spectroscopy of confined states in the channel (Lansbergen *et al.*, 2008a,b). Lastly, the effective current distribution in the channel can be determined by means of thermionic emission theory (Sellier *et al.*, 2007). Following these lines, the goal of this chapter is to introduce a new dopant metrology technique to be used for ultra-scaled CMOS devices.

11.3 Transport-Based Dopant Metrology in Advanced FinFETS

Direct or impurity-mediated tunnelling between source and drain competes with the thermally activated current and thereby affects the sub-threshold swing. Advanced Si MOSFET devices have shrunk to dimensions where the magnitude of the sub-threshold swing is dominated by the nature of individual impurities in the channel region. Due to the random nature of the impurity distribution, parameters such as excited band levels (Fuechsle *et al.*, 2010), ionization energy, threshold voltage and leakage current show device-to-device fluctuations (Asenov, 1999; Ono *et al.*, 2007; Khalafalla *et al.*, 2007, 2009; Tabe *et al.*, 2010; Pierre *et al.*, 2010; Wacquez *et al.*, 2010; Bjork *et al.*, 2008). An atomistic point of view is imperative to understand and determine the underlying donor characteristics in the channel. Several recent experiments have showed that the fingerprint of a single dopant can be identified in low-temperature transport through such devices (Calvet *et al.*, 2007; Hofheinz *et al.*, 2006; Tabe *et al.*, 2010; Pierre *et al.*, 2010; Wacquez *et al.*, 2010; Lansbergen *et al.*, 2008b; Sellier *et al.*, 2006), suggesting a new method to characterize devices down to the level of a single impurity. In the context of quantum state control in quantum computing, it was shown that it is possible to model the orbital levels of a single donor in the channel of scaled FinFETs by means of multi-million atom modeling (Lansbergen *et al.*, 2008b; Rahman *et al.*, 2009). In this chapter it is shown that the aforementioned technique can be used to perform single donor mapping in advanced Si FinFETs. By carefully examining the fingerprints of isolated donors in an ensemble of devices, the chemical species, concentration, and local field of donors in the channel region can be determined in a non-intrusive fashion.

11.4 Devices

The FinFET devices used in this study consist of crystalline silicon wires (fins) with large contacts patterned by 193 nm optical-lithography and dry etching from silicon-on-insulator (see Fig. 11.1a). After a boron channel implantation, a 100 nm polycrystalline silicon layer was deposited on top of a nitrided oxide (1.4 nm equivalent SiO_2 oxide thickness). A phosphorus (P) implant was used for pre-doping and the structure was subsequently patterned using an oxide hard mask to form a narrow gate. Next, high-angle arsenic (As) implantations were used for source or drain extensions, while the channel was protected by the gate and 50 nm wide nitride spacers and remained p type. Finally, As and P implants and a NiSi metallic silicide were used to complete the source or drain electrodes. The samples described in this chapter all have a gate length of 60 nm.

Transport measurements are performed on an ensemble of devices at a temperature of 4 K and a search for the fingerprints of isolated donors is performed (see previous chapter). These single donors are located in or near the active cross section of the channel, i.e., the cross section of the FET body where the potential is lowest and the electrical transport thus takes place. Large electric fields

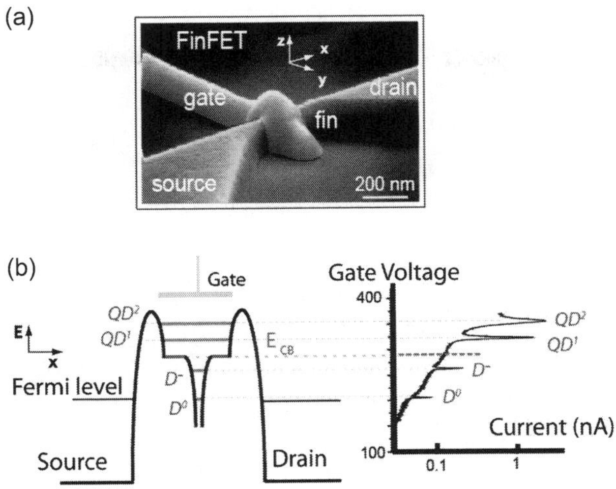

Figure 11.1. Geometry and electrical characteristics of a single donor located in the channel of a FinFET device. (a) Scanning Electron Micrograph of a typical FinFET device. (b) Band diagram along the x-direction with the D^0-state in resonance combined with the measured source/drain current versus gate voltage for a typical sample. QD^1 and QD^2 indicate resonances of a quantum dot, formed by the confinement provided by the corner effect and residual barriers in the access regions between source/drain and channel. The gate voltage where the band edge in the channel is aligned with the Fermi energy E_F in source/drain, indicated by E_{CB}, is estimated by subtracting one unit of addition energy from QD^1. Below the band edge, there are resonances ascribed to the D^0 and D^- charge states of a single donor. © 2008 IEEE. Reprinted, with permission, from Lansbergen, G. P., Rahman, R., Wellard, C. J., Caro, J., Collaert, N., Biesemans, S., Klimeck, G., Hollenberg, L. C. L., and Rogge, S. (2008). Transport-based dopant metrology in advanced finFETS, pp. 1–4, doi:10.1109/IEDM.2008.4796794.

induced by the gate or even corner effects can reduce the active cross section to dimensions much smaller than the FET body (Sellier *et al.*, 2007). Furthermore, as described in the previous chapter, corner effects play a major role in these devices, as indicated by an active cross section of only 4 nm^2, determined by thermionic transport measurements (Sellier *et al.*, 2007).

A single donor's fingerprint is characterized by a pair of resonances in the source–drain current, I_{SD}, versus gate voltage, V_G, characteristics at low V_{SD} (Fig. 11.1b). The positions of a pair of resonances in V_G are an indication of the energy of the one-electron

(D^0) and two electron charge states (D^-). A large quantum dot present in the channel (with charge states indicated by QD^1 and QD^2) is also observed, which allows a rough determination of the position of the band edge in the active area. While the quantum dot in the channel is almost always found, only about one out of seven devices shows the fingerprint of a donors. The identification of the resonances of the donor is based on the determined binding energy, charging energy and the odd-even spin filling (Sellier *et al.*, 2006). Next, the excited energy levels of the one-electron (D^0)-state are determined by sweeping both the V_G and V_{SD} biases and measuring the differential conductance (dI_{SD}/dV_{SD}) in the appropriate bias space see Fig. 11.2. In this so-called stability diagram the typical diamond-shaped region associated with Coulomb-blocked transport between the D^0 and D^- states is observed. The total electronic transport in the conducting regions increases as an excited level of the D^0-state enters the bias window defined by source/drain, giving the stability diagram its characteristic pattern (Sellier *et al.*, 2006, 2007) indicated by the dashed black lines. The red dots indicate the combinations of V_{SD} and V_G where the ground state is at the Fermi energy of the drain and an excited state is at the Fermi energy of the source. It is the bias voltage V_{SD} in this combination that is a direct measure for the energy of the excited state ($eV_{SD,N} = E_N$), where E_N is the energy relative to the ground state and N is the level index). The excited states as determined in this fashion are depicted in Table 11.1. These levels are not bulk-like but heavily influenced by the local electric field and the nearby interface (Smit *et al.*, 2003; Calderón *et al.*, 2006; Rahman *et al.*, 2009).

Finally, the measured level spectrum is compared to a multi-million atom tight-binding NEMO 3-D calculation (Klimeck *et al.*, 2009) of the system taking two possible chemical species, As and P, into account. NEMO 3-D solves for the eigenvalues of the single electron Schrödinger all band equation in a tight-binding approach (Klimeck *et al.*, 2002). The NEMO simulation package is based on about 14 years of development at Texas Instruments, NASA Jet Propulsion Laboratory, and Purdue University (Klimeck *et al.*, 2002, 2009). Each atom is explicitly represented and the electronic structure of the valence electrons is represented by ten $sp^3d^5s^*$ orbitals. Spin can be included explicitly into the basis by doubling the

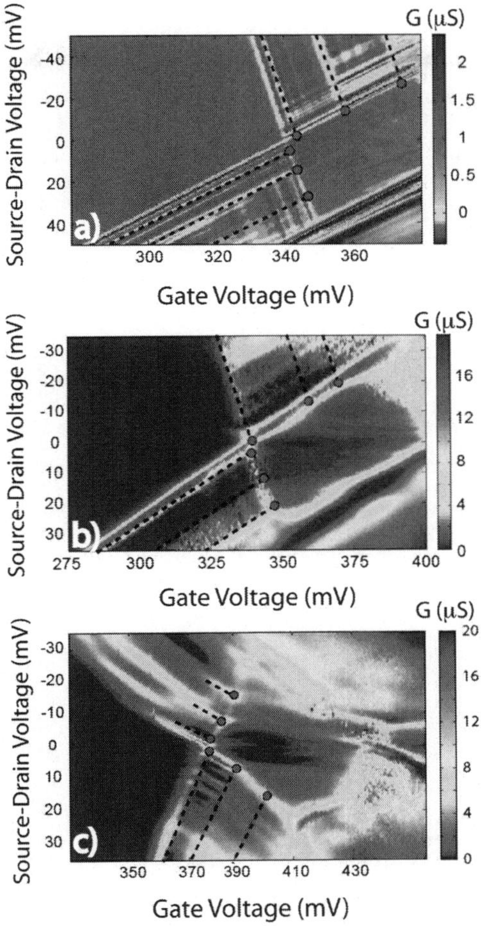

Figure 11.2. Source/drain differential conductance of the D^0 charge state as a function of bias voltage and gate voltage of typical single donor FinFET devices. The excited states, indicated by the black dashed lines, form the fingerprint by which the donor properties can be identified. The dots are a direct indication for the energy of these states ($E_i = eV_{SD}$, with E_i the i-th excited state and e the unit charge.) (a) Sample 13G14: Excited states are observed at 3.5, 15.5 and 26.4 meV (b) Sample 10G16: Excited states are observed at 2, 15, and 23 meV. (c) Sample GLJ17: Excited states are observed at 2, 7.7, and 15.5 meV. © 2008 IEEE. Reprinted, with permission, from Lansbergen, G. P., Rahman, R., Wellard, C. J., Caro, J., Collaert, N., Biesemans, S., Klimeck, G., Hollenberg, L. C. L., and Rogge, S. (2008). Transport-based dopant metrology in advanced finFETS, pp. 1–4, doi:10.1109/IEDM.2008.4796794.

Table 11.1. First three measured excited states of each sample (see for example Fig. 11.2) versus the best fit to the NEMO 3-D model (as depicted in Fig. 11.3). The fit yields a unique combination of (F, d) for each single donor device. The measurement error for each level is estimated to be around 0.5 meV

Device		E1 (meV)	E2 (meV)	E3 (meV)	d (nm)	F (MV/m)	s (meV)
10G16	Exp	2	15	23			
	TB	2.2	15.6	23.0	3.3	37.3	0.59
11G14	Exp	4.5	13.5	25			
	TB	4.5	13.5	25.0	3.5	31.6	0.04
13G14	Exp	3.5	15.5	26.4			
	TB	3.6	15.7	26.3	3.2	35.4	0.17
HSJ18	Exp	5	10	21.5			
	TB	4.5	9.9	21.8	4.1	26.1	0.63
GLG14	Exp	1.3	10	13.2			
	TB	1.3	10	12.4	5.2	23.1	0.28
GLJ17	Exp	2	7.7	15.5			
	TB	1.3	7.7	15.8	4.9	21.9	0.77

Source: © 2008 IEEE. Reprinted, with permission, from Lansbergen, G. P., Rahman, R., Wellard, C. J., Caro, J., Collaert, N., Biesemans, S., Klimeck, G., Hollenberg, L. C. L., and Rogge, S. (2008). Transport-based dopant metrology in advanced finFETS, pp. 1–4, doi:10.1109/IEDM.2008.4796794.

number of orbitals. Spins are coupled through spin-orbit coupling resulting in accurate valence band states. The five d orbitals help shape the curvature of the conduction bands to achieve appropriate masses and symmetries at X and L. The tight-binding parameters are tuned to reproduce the bulk silicon properties under various strain conditions faithfully. For systems where the primary interest is in the conduction band properties and if no magnetic fields need to be considered, spin can safely be ignored without any significant loss of accuracy. Effects due to crystal symmetry, strain, local disorder, and interfaces can be explicitly included in the model through direct atomic representation.

The single impurity states are modeled with a simple Coulomb potential away from the impurity site and a central on-site core correction to match experimentally observed bulk-like impurity energies. The simulation domain for a bulk-like single impurity must be large enough such that the hard wall boundary conditions imposed by the finite simulation domain are not felt by the central impurity. With a simulation domain of $30.4 \times 30.4 \times 30.4$ nm^3

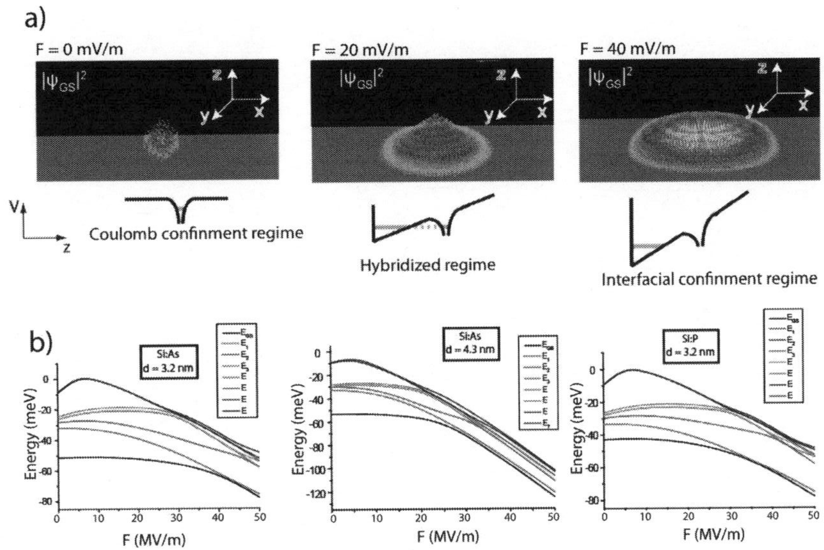

Figure 11.3. (a) Calculated wave-function density of an As donor with $d = 4.3$ nm for three different fields. The gray plane indicates the SiO_2-interface. From low-fields (where the donor has a bulk-like spectrum) to high fields, the donor electron makes a transition from being localized on the donor to being localized at the silicon interface. (b) First eight eigen-levels of an As donor 3.2 and 4.3 nm below the interface and a P donor 3.2 nm below the SiO_2 interface as a function of electric field (F) calculated in a tight-binding model (NEMO 3-D). Note that we measure excited states relative to ground state (lower black line in this graph.) © 2008 IEEE. Reprinted, with permission, from Lansbergen, G. P., Rahman, R., Wellard, C. J., Caro, J., Collaert, N., Biesemans, S., Klimeck, G., Hollenberg, L. C. L., and Rogge, S. (2008). Transport-based dopant metrology in advanced finFETS, pp. 1–4, doi:10.1109/IEDM.2008.4796794. See also Color Insert.

corresponding to about 1.4 million silicon atoms the impurity eigenstates move less than 1 μeV with further domain size increases. A critical modeling capability here is the need to be able to compute reliably the ground states as well as the excited states of the impurity system, as that is a significant component of the impurity fingerprint. Figure 11.3b shows typical eigenstate spectra for an As donor (two donor depths) and a P donor as a function of electric field. Three electric field regimes can be distinguished (Fig. 11.3a). At the low field limit ($F \sim 0$ mV/m) the spectrum of a bulk As donor is obtained. In the high field limit ($F \sim 40$ MV/m) the electron is pulled into a triangular well formed at the interface and the donor is ionized (Smit *et al.*, 2003; Calderón *et al.*, 2006; Lansbergen *et al.*, 2008b). In the cross-over regime ($F \sim 20$ MV/m) the electron is de-localized over the donor- and triangular well potential and the level spectrum consists of levels associated with the donors, levels associated with the triangular well at the gate interface (formed by the local field) and hybridized combinations of the two (Calderón *et al.*, 2006; Lansbergen *et al.*, 2008b; Rahman *et al.*, 2009).

The measured level spectra are least-square fitted to a calculation over a sufficiently sized region of F–d (field and donor depth parameter space). At least three excited levels per donor are taken into account to make the fit over-determined. The fitting procedure is performed for two different species of donor atoms, As and P, which were both used in the fabrication process. The concentration of donors in or near the active area of the FET channel can be estimated by comparing how many times a single donor is identified with the relevant volume where donors can be found.

11.5 Results

Of the 42 devices that have been examined, six have been found to exhibit the fingerprint of a single donor in the transport characteristics. These devices were subsequently measured carefully and the D^0 level spectrum was fitted. The quality of the fits, indicated by $\chi 2$, across the six samples is 0.92 ($\chi 2 < 1$ means a good fit) assuming As donors. For P donors, we find a $\chi 2$ of 10.22 (although two of the six are comparable in quality.) Based on the fits, the donors active in the devices are assumed to be As. The (over-determined) fit furthermore yields a unique combination of (F, d) for each single donor device, as shown in Table 11.1, together with the measured level spectra, and their fits.

Finally, it is also possible to obtain the donor concentration. As mentioned before, the active cross section of the devices are heavily reduced by a corner effect (Sellier *et al.*, 2007). The identified donors are either in or near these corners, and from the least-square fit we actually know the donor depths range from $\sim$3 to 6 nm below the Si/SiO_2 interface, see Table 11.1. The part of the FinFET channel where donors are found is a volume spanned by the donor depths and the gate length (60 nm), and a single donor device is found in average only in one out of seven devices that are measured. This means that for each $\sim$1000 nm^3 of measured material it is possible to found one As dopant, and, as a consequence, a local As concentration of about 10^{18} cm^{-3} can be extrapolated.

11.6 Conclusions

In this chapter a novel method for dopant metrology is introduced. The excellent quantitative agreement between the measured and modeled level spectra gives an indication of the high level of confidence of this method to determine the chemical species and local field of single impurities in silicon FinFET transistors. Furthermore, the local concentration of donors near the active cross section of the FinFET can be estimated. The present method offers opportunities for non-invasive characterisation down to the level of a single donor and could be a future tool in the guidance of device processing. This is especially true for such CMOS devices for which variability problems are increasing dramatically with ultra-scaling and this justifies the importance of the method described here.

Acknowledgments

G.P.L., G.C.T., J.V., and S.R. acknowledge financial support from the EC FP7 FET-proactive NanoICT projects MOLOC (215750) and AFSiD (214989) and the Dutch Fundamenteel Onderzoek der Materie FOM.

G.C.T., J.V., L.C.L.H., and S.R. acknowledge financial support from the ARC-CQC2T (project number CE110001027). L.C.L.H. acknowledges the US National Security Agency and the US Army Research Office under contract number W911NF-08-1-0527. R.R. and G. K. acknowledge financial support from U.S. National Security Agency (NSA) and the Army Research Office (ARO) under Contract No. W911NF-04-1-0290. The work at Purdue and JPL is supported by grants from the Army Research Office. The work at the Jet Propulsion Laboratory, California Institute of Technology, is supported by grants from the National Aeronautics and Space Administration. R.R. acknowledges the financial support from Sandia, which is a multiprogram laboratory operated by SandiaCorporation, a Lockheed Martin Company, for the United States Department of Energys National Nuclear Security Administration under Contract No. DE-AC04-94AL85000. GCT is supported by an ARC-DECRA Fellowship, project ID DE120100702.

References

Asenov, A. (1999). Random dopant induced threshold voltage lowering and fluctuations in sub 50 nm mosfets: a statistical 3d 'atomistic' simulation study, *Nanotechnology* **10**, 2, p. 153, URL http://stacks.iop.org/0957-4484/10/i=2/a=309.

Bjork, M. T., Schmid, H., Knoch, J., Riel, H., and Riess, W. (2008). Donor deactivation in silicon nano-structures, *Nat. Nano* **4**, pp. 103–107, doi: 10.1038/nnano.2008.400.

Calderón, M. J., Koiller, B., Hu, X., and Das Sarma, S. (2006). Quantum control of donor electrons at the Si-SiO_2 interface, *Phys. Rev. Lett.* **96**, p. 096802, doi:10.1103/PhysRevLett.96.096802, URL http://link.aps.org/doi/10.1103/PhysRevLett.96.096802.

Calvet, L. E., Wheeler, R. G., and Reed, M. A. (2007). Observation of the linear stark effect in a single acceptor in Si, *Phys. Rev. Lett.* **98**, p. 096805, doi:10.1103/PhysRevLett.98.096805, URL http://link.aps.org/doi/10.1103/PhysRevLett.98.096805.

Fuechsle, M., Mahapatra, S., Zwanenburg, F. A., Friesen, M., Eriksson, M. A., and Simmons, M. Y. (2010). Spectroscopy of few-electron single-crystal silicon quantum dots, *Nat. Nano* **5**, pp. 502–505, doi:10.1038/nnano.2010.95.

Hofheinz, M., Jehl, X., Sanquer, M., Molas, G., Vinet, M., and Deleonibus, S. (2006). *Eur. Phys. J. B.* **54**, p. 299.

Khalafalla, M. A. H., Ono, Y., Nishiguchi, K., and Fujiwara, A. (2007). *Appl. Phys. Lett.* **91**, p. 263513.

Khalafalla, M. A. H., Ono, Y., Nishiguchi, K., and Fujiwara, A. (2009). *Appl. Phys. Lett.* **94**, p. 223501.

Klimeck, G., Ahmed, S., Kharche, N., Korkusinski, M., Usman, M., Prada, M., and Boykin, T. B. (2009). Atomistic simulation of realistically sized nano-devices using nemo 3-D: Part II — Applications", *(INVITED) Special Issue on Nanoelectronic Device Modeling in IEEE, Trans. Elecron Devices* **54**, pp. 2090–2099.

Klimeck, G., Oyafuso, F., Boykin, T. B., Bowen, R. C., and von Allmen, P. (2002). Development of a nanoelectronic 3-D (NEMO 3-D) simulator for multimillion atom simulations and its application to alloyed quantum dots, *Comput. Model. Eng. Sci.* **3**, 5, pp. 601–642.

Lansbergen, G. P., Rahman, R., Wellard, C. J., Caro, J., Collaert, N., Biesemans, S., Klimeck, G., Hollenberg, L. C. L., and Rogge, S. (2008a). Transport-based dopant metrology in advanced finFETS, pp. 1–4, doi:10.1109/IEDM.2008.4796794.

Lansbergen, G. P., Rahman, R., Wellard, C. J., Woo, I., Caro, J., Collaert, N., Biesemans, S., Klimeck, G., Hollenberg, L. C. L., and Rogge, S. (2008b). Quantum confinement and symmetry transition of a single gated donor electron in silicon *Nat. Phys.* **4**, p. 656.

Ono, Y., Fujiwara, A., Nishiguchi, K., Yamaguchi, H., Inokawa, H., and Takahashi, Y. (2007). Conductance modulation by individual acceptors in Si nanoscale field-effect transistors, *Appl. Phys. Lett.* **90**, p. 102106.

Pierre, M., Wacquez, R., Jehl, X., Sanquer, M., Vinet, M., and Cueto, O. (2010). Single-donor ionization energies in a nanoscale CMOS channel, *Nat. Nano* **5**, pp. 133–137, doi:10.1038/nnano.2009.373.

Rahman, R., Lansbergen, G. P., Park, S. H., Verduijn, J., Klimeck, G., Rogge, S., and Hollenberg, L. C. L. (2009). Orbital stark effect and quantum confinement transition of donors in silicon, *Phys. Rev. B* **80**, p. 165314, doi:10.1103/Phys.Rev.B.80.165314, URL http://link.aps.org/doi/10.1103/PhysRevB.80.165314.

Schofield, S. R., Curson, N. J., Simmons, M. Y., Rueß, F. J., Hallam, T., Oberbeck, L., and Clark, R. G. (2003). Atomically precise placement of single dopants in Si, *Phys. Rev. Lett.* **91**, 13, p. 136104, doi:10.1103/PhysRevLett.91.136104.

Sellier, H., Lansbergen, G. P., Caro, J., Rogge, S., Collaert, N., Ferain, I., Jurczak, M., and Biesemans, S. (2006). Transport spectroscopy of a single dopant in a gated silicon nanowire, *Phys. Rev. Lett.* **97**, p. 206805, 10.1103/PhysRevLett.97.206805, URL http://link.aps.org/doi/10.1103/PhysRevLett.97.206805.

Sellier, H., Lansbergen, G. P., Caro, J., Rogge, S., Collaert, N., Ferain, I., Jurczak, M., and Biesemans, S. (2007). Subthreshold channels at the edges of nanoscale triple-gate silicon transistors, *Appl. Phys. Lett.* **90**, p. 073502.

Smit, G. D. J., Rogge, S., Caro, J., and Klapwijk, T. M. (2003). Gate-induced ionization of single dopant atoms, *Phys. Rev. B* **68**, p. 193302, doi:10.1103/PhysRevB.68.193302, URL http://link.aps.org/doi/10.1103/PhysRevB.68.193302.

Sze, S. M. (1981). *Physics of Semiconductor Devices*, Wiley, New York.

Tabe, M., Moraru, D., Ligowski, M., Anwar, M., Jablonski, R., Ono, Y., and Mizuno, T. (2010). Single-electron transport through single dopants in a dopant-rich environment, *Phys. Rev. Lett.* **105**, 1, p. 016803, doi: 10.1103/PhysRevLett.105.016803.

Wacquez, R., Vinet, M., Pierre, M., Roche, B., Jehl, X., Cueto, O., Verduijn, J., Tettamanzi, G., Rogge, S., Deshpande, V., Previtali, B., Vizioz, C., Pauliac-Vaujour, S., Comboroure, C., Bove, N., Faynot, O., and Sanquer, M. (2010). Single Dopant Impact on Electrical Characteristics of SOI NMOSFETs with Effective Length Down to 10 nm, *Symp. VLSI Tech.*, p. 193.

Index

Color Insert

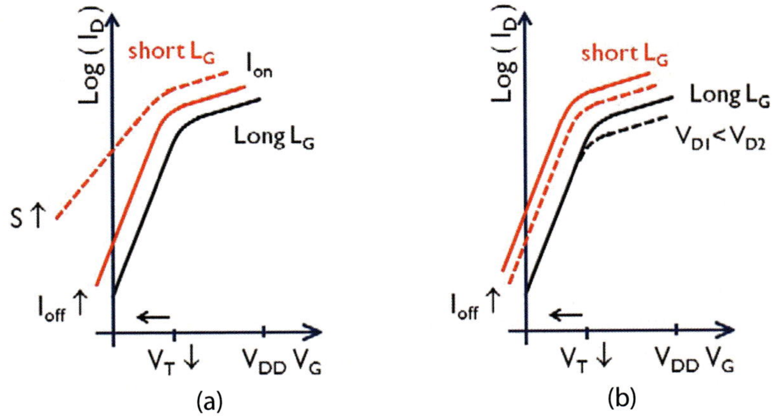

Figure 1.3

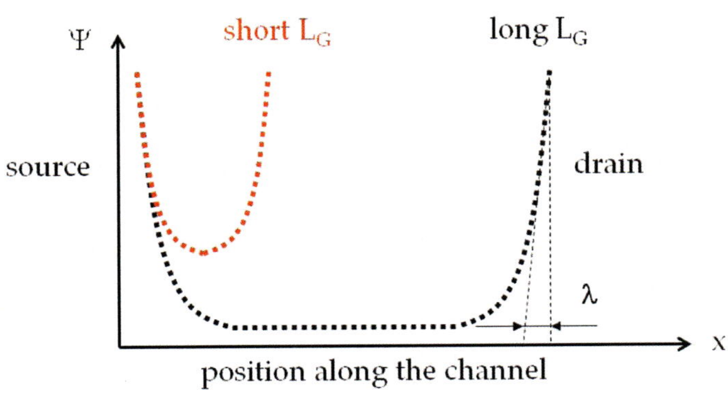

Figure 1.4

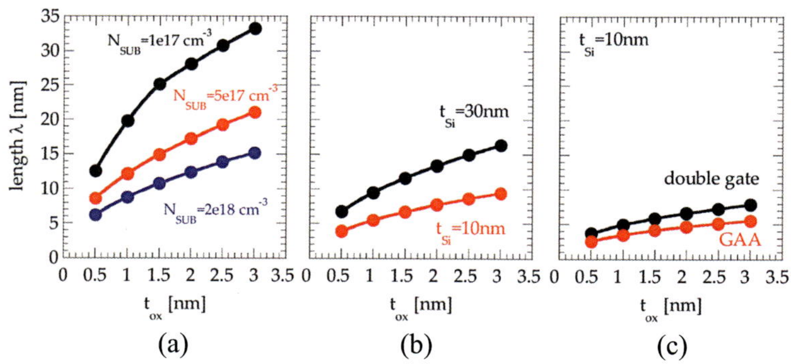

Figure 1.5

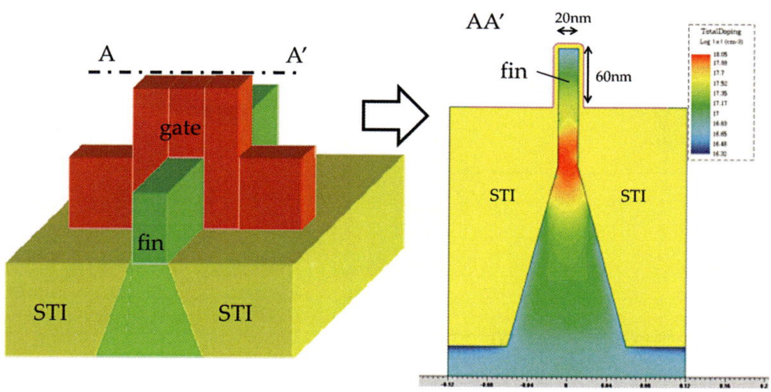

Figure 1.8

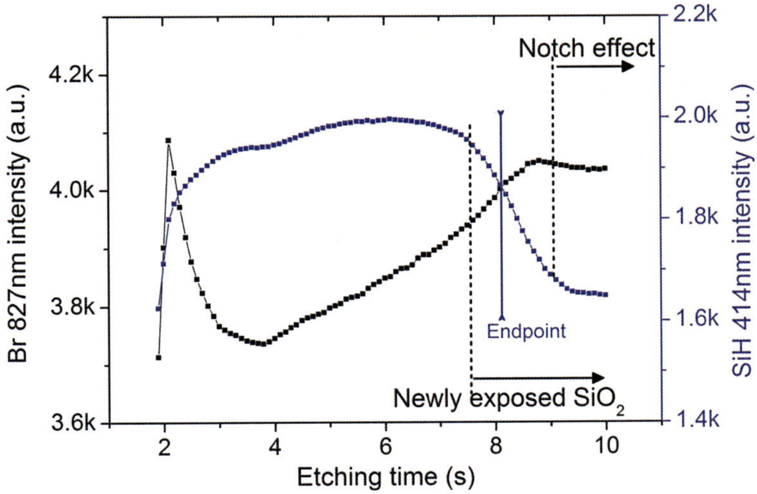

Figure 2.6

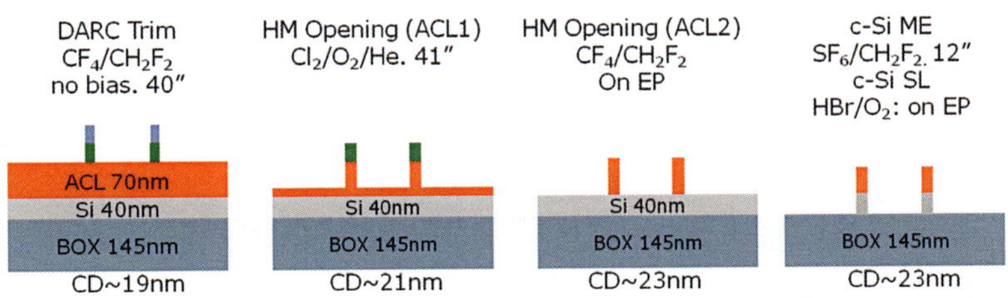

Figure 2.8

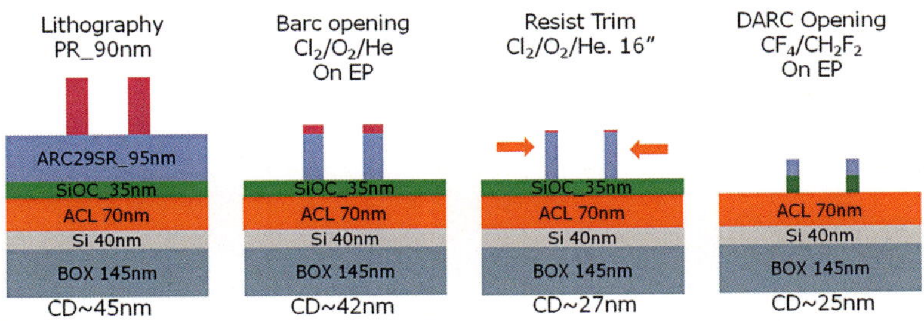

Figure 2.9

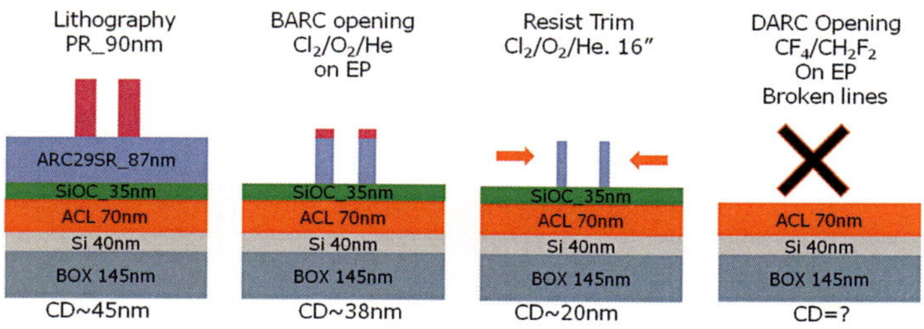

Figure 2.10

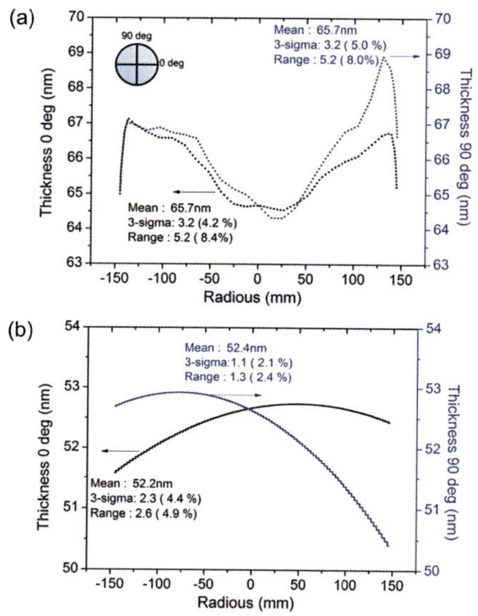

Figure 2.13

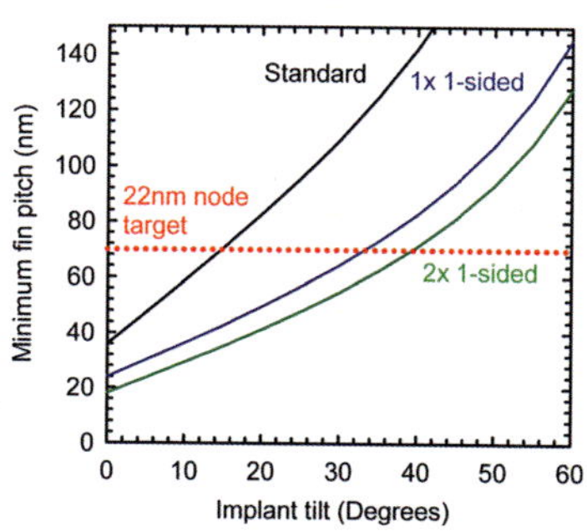

Figure 4.8

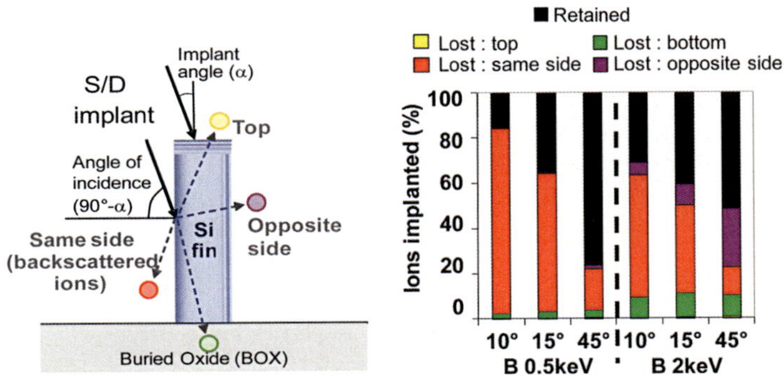

Figure 4.9

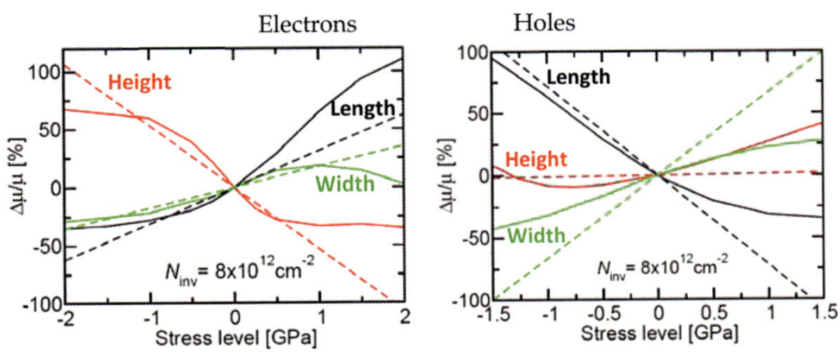

Figure 4.21

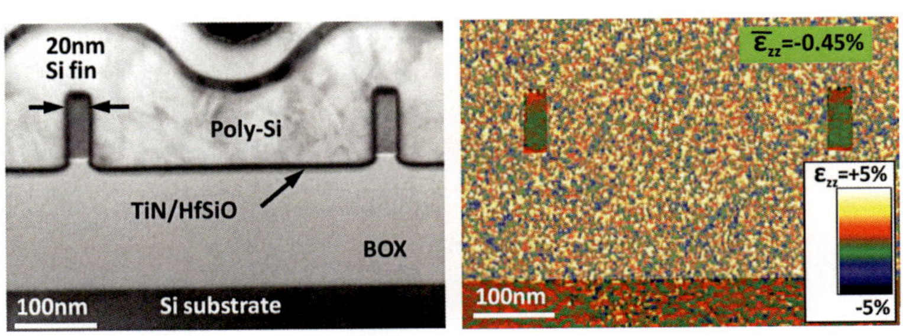

Figure 4.22

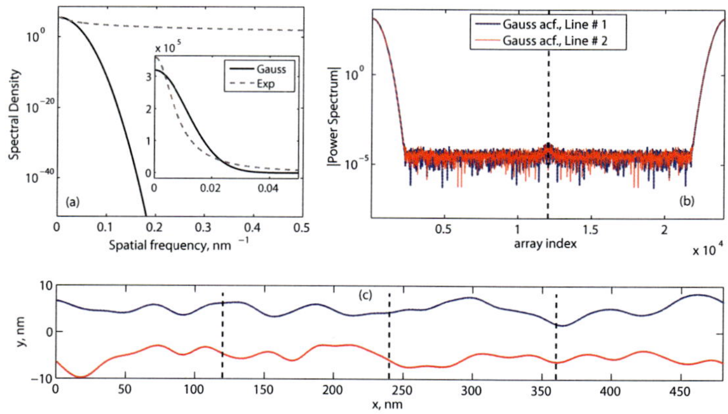

Figure 5.3

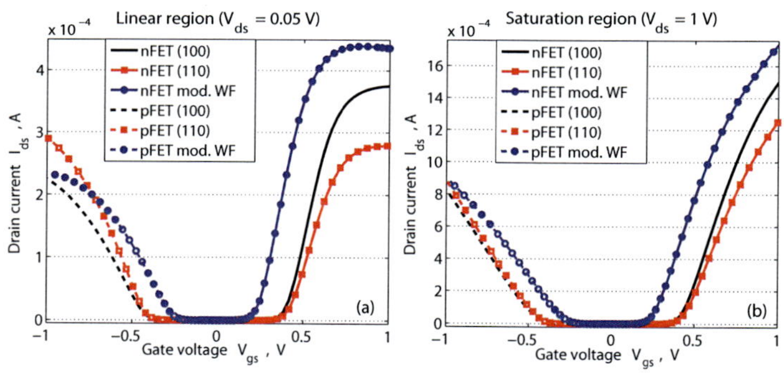

Figure 5.4

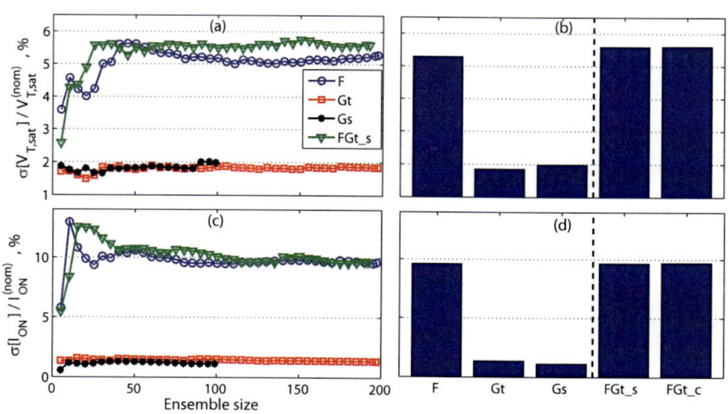

Figure 5.6

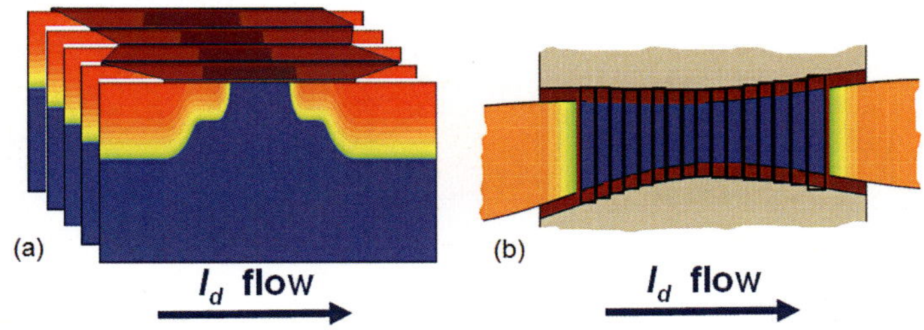

Figure 5.9

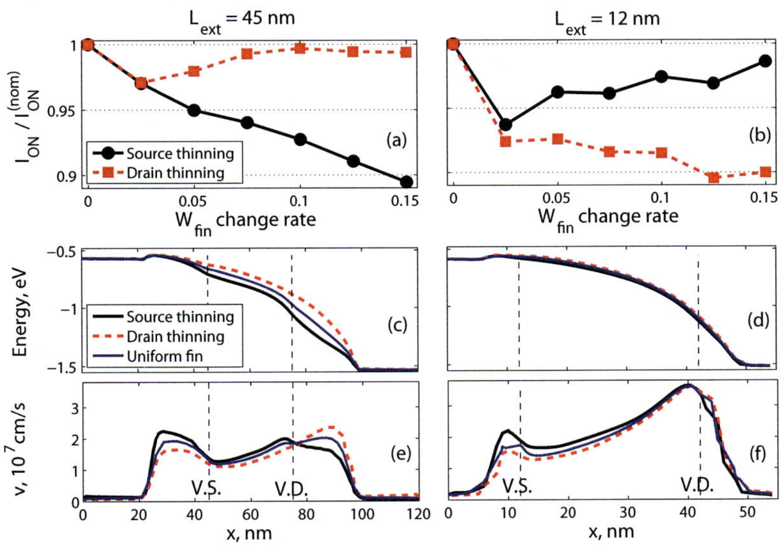

Figure 5.19

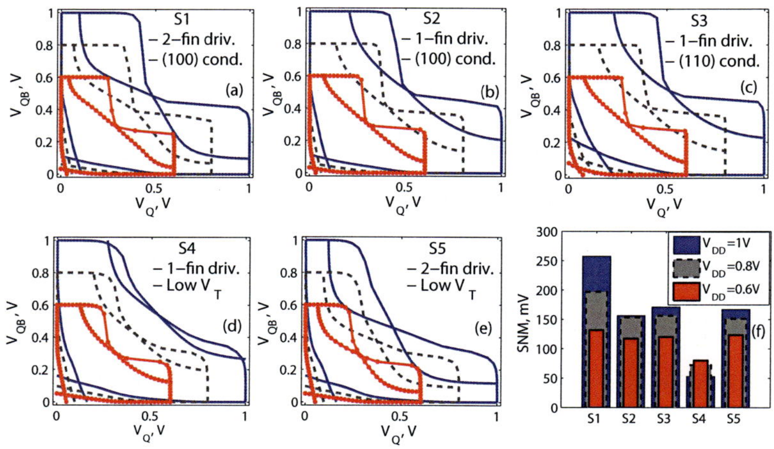

Figure 5.21

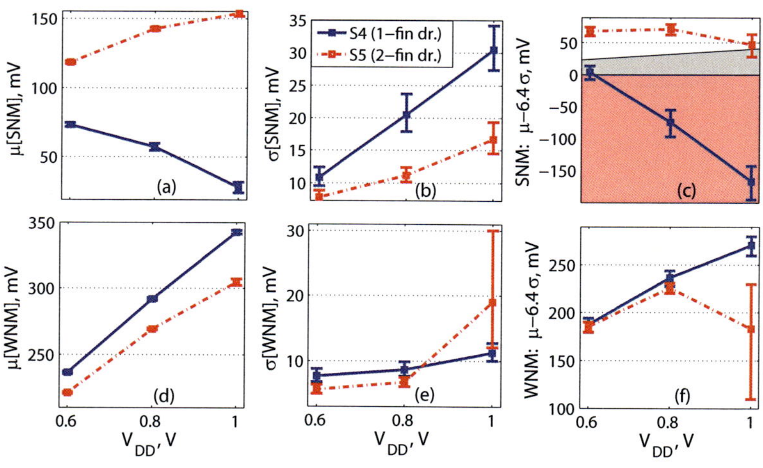

Figure 5.27

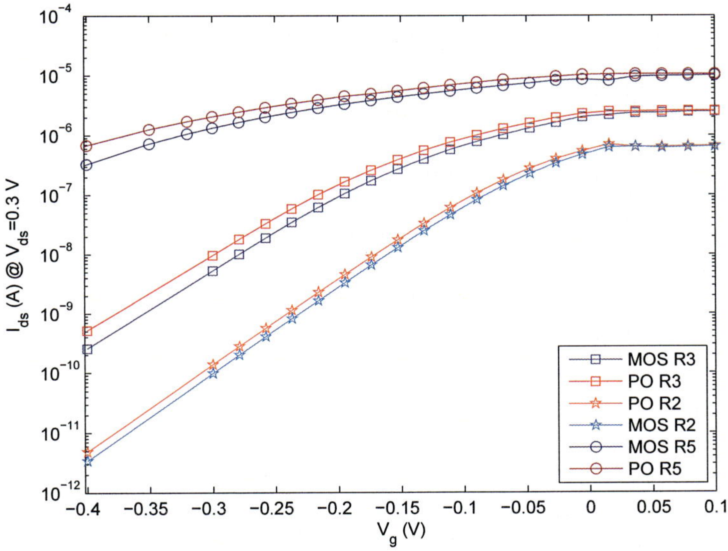

Figure 8.12

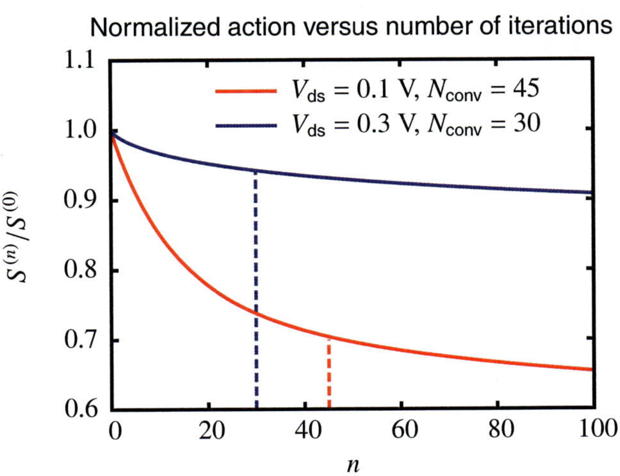

Figure 9.3

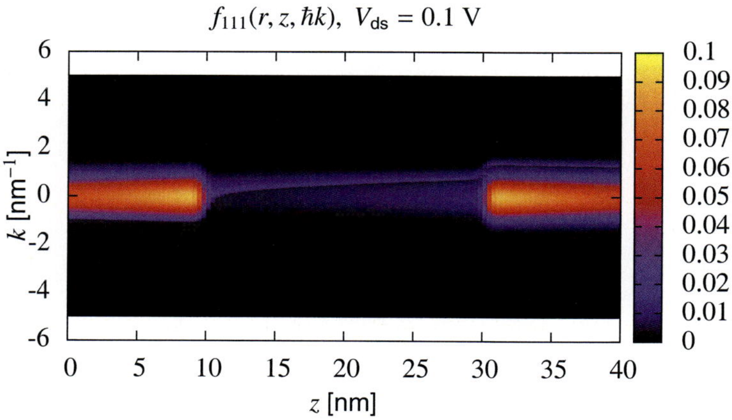
$f_{111}(r, z, \hbar k)$, V_{ds} = 0.1 V
k [nm^{-1}]
z [nm]
6
4
2
0
-2
-4
-6
0
5
10
15
20
25
30
35
40
0.1
0.09
0.08
0.07
0.06
0.05
0.04
0.03
0.02
0.01
0

(a)

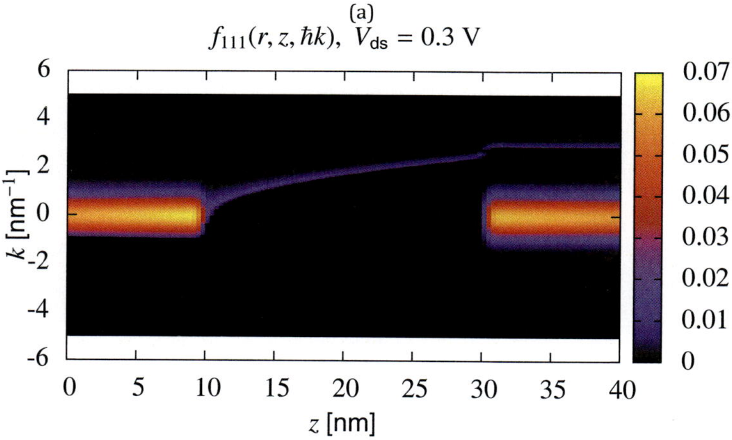
$f_{111}(r, z, \hbar k)$, V_{ds} = 0.3 V
k [nm^{-1}]
z [nm]
6
4
2
0
-2
-4
-6
0
5
10
15
20
25
30
35
40
0.07
0.06
0.05
0.04
0.03
0.02
0.01
0

(b)

Figure 9.4

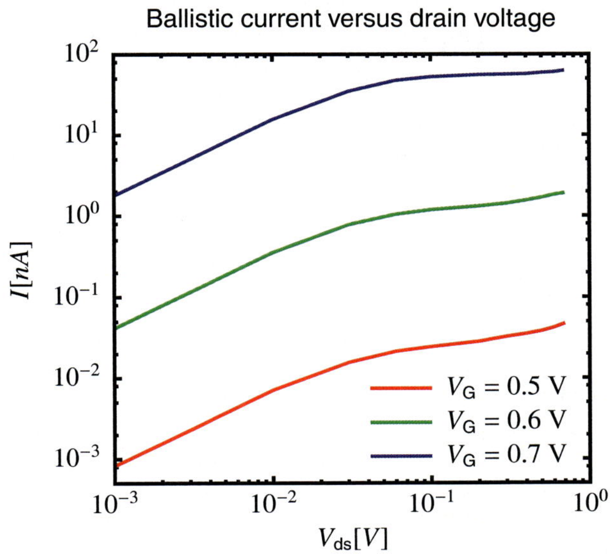
Ballistic current versus drain voltage
10^2
10^1
10^0
10^{-1}
10^{-2}
10^{-3}
$I[nA]$
$V_G = 0.5$ V
$V_G = 0.6$ V
$V_G = 0.7$ V
10^{-3}
10^{-2}
10^{-1}
10^0
$V_{ds}[V]$

Figure 9.5

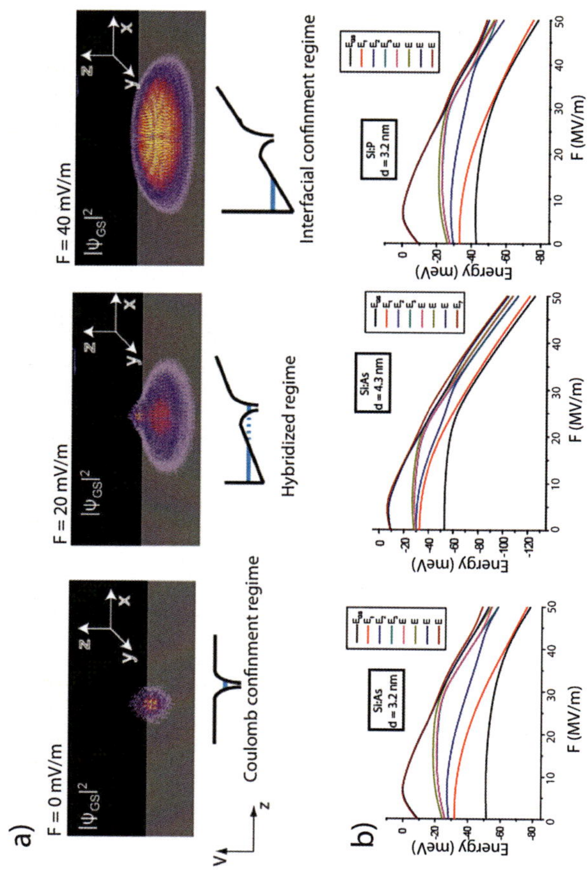
a)
F = 0 mV/m
F = 20 mV/m
F = 40 mV/m
|ψ_GS|^2
Coulomb confinement regime
Hybridized regime
Interfacial confinement regime
b)
Energy (meV)
F (MV/m)
Si:As d = 3.2 nm
Si:As d = 4.3 nm
Si:P d = 3.2 nm

Figure 11.3